Impulse Control Disorders

In the last decade, much needed attention and research have been focused on the group of psychiatric conditions termed "impulse control disorders," or ICDs. Pathological gambling, compulsive shopping, kleptomania, hypersexuality, and Internet "addiction," among other disorders, are characterized by a recurrent urge to perform a repetitive behavior that is gratifying at the moment but causes significant long-term distress and disability. Despite the high rate of comorbidity with obsessive-compulsive disorder, ICDs are now clearly distinguished from this disorder by a unique clinical approach for diagnosis and treatment. A wide array of psychopharmacologic and psychotherapeutic options are now available for treating these disorders. Drs. Elias Aboujaoude and Lorrin M. Koran have compiled the world's foremost experts in ICD research and treatment to create a comprehensive book on the frequency, evolution, treatment, and related public policy, public health, forensic, and medical issues of these disorders. This is the first book to bring together medical and social knowledge bases related to impulse control disorders.

ELIAS ABOUJAOUDE, MD, is Director of the Impulse Disorders Clinic at the Stanford University School of Medicine, Stanford, California.

LORRIN M. KORAN, MD, is Professor of Psychiatry, Emeritus, and Director of the Obsessive-Compulsive Disorder Clinic at Stanford University School of Medicine, Stanford, California.

Impulse Control Disorders

Edited by

ELIAS ABOUJAOUDE
Stanford University School of Medicine, Stanford, California

LORRIN M. KORAN
Stanford University School of Medicine, Stanford, California

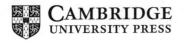
CAMBRIDGE
UNIVERSITY PRESS

CAMBRIDGE UNIVERSITY PRESS
Cambridge, New York, Melbourne, Madrid, Cape Town, Singapore,
São Paulo, Delhi, Dubai, Tokyo

Cambridge University Press
32 Avenue of the Americas, New York, NY 10013-2473, USA

www.cambridge.org
Information on this title: www.cambridge.org/9780521898706

First published 2010

Printed in the United States of America

A catalog record for this publication is available from the British Library.

Library of Congress Cataloging in Publication data

Impulse control disorders / edited by Elias Aboujaoude, Lorrin M. Koran.
   p.; cm.
Includes bibliographical references and index.
ISBN 978-0-521-89870-6 (hardback)
1. Impulse control disorders.   I. Aboujaoude, Elias –   II. Koran, Lorrin M.
[DNLM: 1. Impulse Control Disorders – therapy.   2. Impulse Control Disorders – etiology.
3. Socioeconomic Factors. WM 190 I343 2009]
RC569.5.I46I467   2009
616.85′84 – dc22   2009013485

ISBN   978-0-521-89870-6 Hardback

Every effort has been made in preparing this book to provide accurate and
up-to-date information that is in accord with accepted standards and practice at the time
of publication. Although case histories are drawn from actual cases, every effort
has been made to disguise the identities of the individuals involved. Nevertheless, the
authors, editors, and publishers can make no warranties that the information
contained herein is totally free from error, not least because clinical standards are
constantly changing through research and regulation. The authors, editors, and
publishers therefore disclaim all liability for direct or consequential damages resulting
from the use of material contained in this book. Readers are strongly advised to pay
careful attention to information provided by the manufacturer of any drugs or
equipment that they plan to use.

to my mother
Elias Aboujaoude

to Alexander and Jason Koran, explorers and
shapers of the future
Lorrin M. Koran

Contents

Color plates follow page 2.

Contributors

Elias Aboujaoude, MD
Impulse Control Disorders Clinic
Stanford University School of Medicine
Stanford, California
E-mail: eaboujaoude@stanford.edu

Tina S. Alster, MD
Washington Institute of Dermatologic
    Laser Surgery
Washington, DC
E-mail: talster@skinlaser.com

April Lane Benson, PhD
Stopping Overshopping, LLC
Institute for Contemporary
    Psychotherapy
New York, New York
E-mail: aprilbensonphd@gmail.com

Wolfgang Berner, MD
Institute of Sex Research and Forensic
    Psychiatry
University Medical Center
    Hamburg-Eppendorf
Hamburg, Germany
E-mail: bemer@uke.uni-hamburg.de

Donald W. Black, MD
Department of Psychiatry
University of Iowa Carver College of
    Medicine
Iowa City, Iowa
E-mail: donald-black@uiowa.edu

Dana Bodnik, MD
Ness Zionah and Beer Ya'acov Mental
    Health Center
Tel Aviv University
Tel Aviv, Israel

Peer Briken, MD
Institute of Sex Research and Forensic
    Psychiatry
University Medical Center
    Hamburg-Eppendorf

Hamburg, Germany
E-mail: briken@uke.uni-hamburg.de

Raul Caetano, MD, MPH, PhD
School of Public Health
University of Texas
Houston, Texas
E-mail: raul.caetano@utsouthwestern.edu

Celal Çalıkuşu, MD
Bakirkoy Research Hospital for Psychiatry
    and Neurology
Istanbul, Turkey
E-mail: celalcalikusu@gmail.com

Joan C. Chrisler, PhD
Department of Psychology
Connecticut College
New London, Connecticut
E-mail: jcchr@conncoll.edu

Emil F. Coccaro, MD
Department of Psychiatry and Behavioral
    Neuroscience
University of Chicago Pritzker School of
    Medicine
Chicago, Illinois
E-mail: ecoccaro@yoda.bsd.uchicago.edu

Pinhas N. Dannon, MD
Ness Zionah and Beer Ya'acov Mental
    Health Center
Tel Aviv University
Tel Aviv, Israel
E-mail: pinhasd@post.tau.ac.il

Helga Dittmar, PhD
Department of Psychology
University of Sussex
Sussex, United Kingdom
E-mail: H.E.Dittmar@sussex.ac.uk

Sheila Ferguson, MD
Department of Psychology
Connecticut College
New London, Connecticut

Candice Germain, MD
Department of Psychiatry
Bichat-Claude Bernard Hospital
Paris, France
E-mail: candicepatrick@aol.com

Jon E. Grant, MD, JD, MPH
Department of Psychiatry
University of Minnesota
Minneapolis, Minnesota
E-mail: grant045@umn.edu

John H. Greist, MD
Department of Psychiatry
University of Wisconsin School of
   Medicine and Public Health
Madison, Wisconsin
E-mail: jgreist@healthtechsys.com

Andreas Hill, MD
Institute of Sex Research and Forensic
   Psychiatry
University Medical Center
   Hamburg-Eppendorf
Hamburg, Germany
E-mail: hill@uke.uni-hamburg.de

Lorrin M. Koran, MD
Obsessive-Compulsive Disorder Clinic
Department of Psychiatry and Behavioral
   Sciences
Stanford University School of Medicine
Stanford, California
E-mail: lkoran@stanford.edu

Michel Lejoyeux, MD, PhD
Department of Psychiatry
Bichat-Claude Bernard Hospital
Paris, France
E-mail: michel.lejoyeux@bch.aphp.fr

Laura M. Letson, MPA
President, Integrity 1st
P.O. Box 5754
Endicott, New York 13763
E-mail: letson101@aol.com

Timothy Liu, MD
Department of Psychiatry
Yale University School of Medicine
New Haven, Connecticut
E-mail: tcl25@email.med.yale.edu

Eileen M. Luna-Firebaugh, PhD
Department of American Indian Studies
University of Arizona

Tucson, Arizona
E-mail: eluna@u.arizona.edu

Michael S. McCloskey, PhD
Department of Psychiatry and Behavioral
   Neuroscience
University of Chicago Pritzker School of
   Medicine
Chicago, Illinois

Duane C. McKay, DDS
Dentistry (Private Practice)
Los Angeles, California

Christy M. McKinney, PhD, MPH
Department of Epidemiology
School of Public Health
University of Texas
Houston, Texas
E-mail:
   christy.mckinney@utsouthwestern.edu

Amy McMichael, MD
Department of Dermatology
Wake Forest University School of Medicine
Winston-Salem, North Carolina
E-mail: amcmicha@wfubmc.edu

Drew Miller, MD
Department of Dermatology
Wake Forest University School of Medicine
Winston-Salem, North Carolina

Brad Novak, MD
Department of Psychiatry
University of California, San Francisco
   School of Medicine
San Francisco, California
and
Department of Psychiatry
Stanford University School of Medicine
Stanford, California
and
Human Services Agency
City and County of San Francisco
San Francisco, California
E-mail: Bradley_novak@yahoo.com

Brian L. Odlaug, BA
Department of Psychiatry
University of Minnesota Medical Center
Fairview, Minnesota

Christina S. Pearson
Trichtillomania Learning Center
Santa Cruz, California
E-mail: trichster@aol.com

Guy Porter, BA, MBBS (Hons)
Faculty of Medicine
University of Sydney
Sydney, New South Wales, Australia

Marc N. Potenza, MD, PhD
Department of Psychiatry
Yale University School of Medicine
New Haven, Connecticut
E-mail: marc.potenza@yale.edu

Paul Schwartzman, MS, DAPA, LMHC
Fairport Counseling Services
Fairport, New York
E-mail: fairportcs@frontiernet.net

William M. Spice, MRCP
Sexual Health and HIV Medicine
Worcestershire Primary Care Trust
Worcester, United Kingdom
E-mail: william.spice@worcspct.nhs.uk

Vladan Starcevic, MD, PhD, FRANZCP
Discipline of Psychological Medicine
University of Sydney
Sydney, New South Wales, Australia
and
Department of Psychological Medicine
Nepean Hospital
Sydney/Penrith, New South Wales,
    Australia
E-mail: starcev@wahs.nsw.gov.au

Özlem Tecer, MD
Cerrahpasa Medical Faculty
Istanbul University
Istanbul, Turkey
E-mail: ozlemtecer@gmail.com

Benjamin T. P. Tucker, BA
Department of Psychology

University of Wisconsin
Milwaukee, Wisconsin

Michael R. Walther, BS
Department of Psychology
University of Wisconsin
Milwaukee, Wisconsin

Rungsima Wanitphakdeedecha, MD
Department of Dermatology
Faculty of Medicine
Sirraj Hospital
Mahidol University
Bangkok, Thailand
E-mail: sirwn@mahidol.ac.th

Sven E. Widmalm, DDS, Dr Odont
School of Dentistry
University of Michigan
Ann Arbor, Michigan
E-mail: sew@umich.edu

Timothy Ivor Williams, MD
School of Psychology
Berkshire Healthcare NHS Foundation
    Trust
Bracknell, United Kingdom
and
University of Reading
Reading, Berkshire, United Kingdom
E-mail: sxswiams@reading.ac.uk

Reeta Wolfsohn, CMSW
Center for Financial Social Work
Asheville, North Carolina

Douglas W. Woods, PhD
Department of Psychology
University of Wisconsin
Milwaukee, Wisconsin
E-mail: dwoods@uwm.edu

Acknowledgments

We wish to express our deep appreciation to Nona Gamel, MSW, who devoted many hours to transcribing our editorial jottings into readable text and carefully reviewed the entire manuscript for those errors that can escape an editor's eye. We also wish to thank Marc Strauss of Cambridge University Press, who first suggested that we create a textbook bringing together the new information available regarding impulse control disorders. We are deeply grateful to our authors, who took the time to codify their knowledge for the benefit of patients, their families, the public, and policymakers.

Introduction

The last decade has brought the impulse control disorders (ICDs) much-needed attention and has seen the accumulation of a modest body of clinical research results. Yet, clinicians wanting to provide cutting-edge pharmacological and psychotherapeutic care for these disorders have no up-to-date, comprehensive resource to consult. Given this unmet need, we have attempted to create a practical, authoritative clinical guide to the ICDs that summarizes the current state of knowledge.

An individual's disorder often both reflects and affects society. Thus, we wished not only to present the information and guidance needed to offer excellent clinical care but also to provide clinicians, policymakers, patients and families, and advocacy groups with information regarding societal aspects of ICDs. We therefore include companion chapters for each clinical disorder to discuss social factors affecting the onset or course of the disorder, legal system considerations, social costs (including familial and financial costs), and public health issues. We hope that these chapters will stimulate discussion regarding programs, laws, and public policies that can help prevent or treat various impulse control disorders or that can mitigate their widespread unfortunate social effects.

Each clinical chapter is organized into sections discussing:

- History of psychiatric attention to the disorder
- Diagnosis, both in DSM-IV and ICD-10
- Differential diagnosis
- Clinical picture, including the effects of symptoms on functioning
- Assessment instruments
- Prevalence
- Age at onset
- Natural history
- Effects of the disorder on quality of life
- Biological data that have treatment implications
- Comorbid conditions
- Treatments, both psychotherapeutic and psychopharmacological
- Self-help materials, when available

For many impulse control disorders, information on these topics is sparse or absent. To the extent possible, we present clinically useful information in detail, including resources for patients and families. In addition, Appendix I contains a treatment-planning guide for each disorder to help the clinician conduct the necessary evaluations and create a comprehensive treatment plan. Appendix II includes rating instruments that may be useful in defining each disorder's severity when the patient is first seen and in monitoring response to treatments.

The societal aspect chapters vary widely. The discussion of the social aspects of pathological gambling, for instance, explores financial and workplace impacts; relationship to crime; how federal and state governments, the gambling industry, the media and film industries, retailers, and even schools and community-based organizations encourage gambling; gambling's contributions to homelessness, domestic violence, and divorce; and, how these unfortunate consequences could be mitigated by social interventions. A separate chapter discusses the intricate politics and economics of Indian gaming in the United States.

The chapter on the social aspects of kleptomania describes the legal system complexities surrounding the disorder. The companion chapter to compulsive buying disorder describes how advertising agencies, credit card issuers, the media, and retailers strive to "associate products we don't need with feelings we deeply desire" and so contribute to the problem of compulsive buying. This chapter lays out how a cultural focus on materialism promotes pernicious debt and degrades both interpersonal relationships and participation in civic life. The companion chapter regarding hypersexuality discusses the commercial sex industry and the health – including mental health – risks it entails for sex workers, as well as the substance abuse and legal problems they face.

Although not all behavior symptomatic of intermittent explosive disorder is physically violent, the disorder does account for a portion of the emotional and physical abuse suffered by many individuals. As a result, we have included a chapter that describes the epidemiology and health-related consequences of intimate partner violence and reviews the means to identify, educate, and treat the estimated 4.8 million women and 2.9 million men who are victimized in the United States each year. A second companion chapter describes the physical health and mental health consequences of violence against women, along with economic consequences and impact on the next generation. This chapter concludes with an exploration of primary, secondary, and tertiary prevention efforts that exist or could be created to diminish this evil.

Problematic Internet use may be the disorder of our time. To complement the clinical chapter on this topic, we included a chapter on the social effects of the virtual violence contained in video games and in so many venues on the World Wide Web. "Are we in danger of becoming desensitized to violence because our virtual lives are suffused with it?" is the important question that this chapter's authors explore.

Although pyromania accounts for only a small proportion of fire setting and arson, we have included a companion chapter reviewing the magnitude and costs of arson and the legal and community responses to it. The chapter also discusses how the legal and mental health systems interface and can collaborate to contain this sometimes lethal calamity.

For trichotillomania, skin-picking disorder, and nail biting – ICDs that can be associated with significant medical consequences – we include contributions from nonpsychiatric medical experts to complement the clinical chapters and to provide more thorough reviews. Hence, dermatological perspectives are discussed in two chapters that complement the trichotillomania and skin-picking–disorder chapters, and a dentist's clinical perspective is presented to complement the chapter on nail biting.

Finally, because nonprofit resource, support, and advocacy groups frequently provide patient and public education, and because they can attract public attention and research funding to a given disorder, we include a chapter describing a successful effort to create a nonprofit organization, the Trichotillomania Learning Center. This narrative contains many rarely discussed and extremely helpful points for anyone who chooses to follow the author's courageous example.

Our book contains the distilled knowledge of a distinguished group of international experts from the fields of psychiatry, medicine, public policy, and the law, in addition to other disciplines pertinent to understanding and managing impulse control disorders. We are deeply grateful to our contributing authors. They have helped us create a book that we think readers will find is a comprehensive resource regarding disorders that are costly and painful for the afflicted individual and for society at large but that too often are underestimated, underdiagnosed, and undertreated.

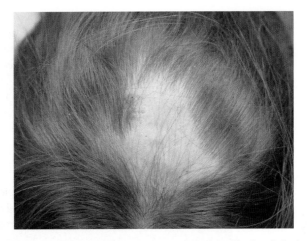

Figure 9.1   Irregular bordered TTM scalp patch with scarring, excoriation, and broken hairs in a teenager.

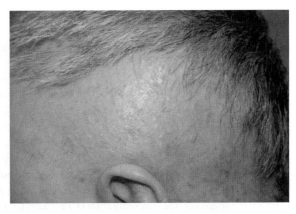

Figure 9.2   Side view. TTM broken hairs in an elderly woman with several other psychiatric diagnoses.

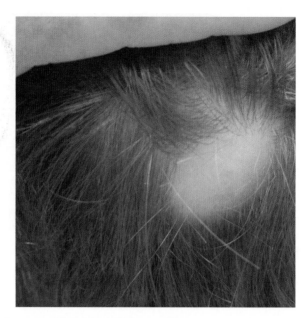

Figure 9.3   Patch of alopecia areata with fine blond hair regrowing.

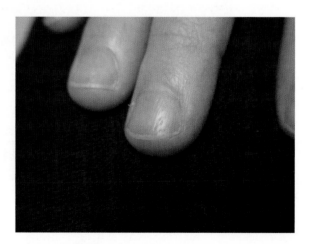

Figure 9.4   Nail pitting that can be seen with alopecia areata.

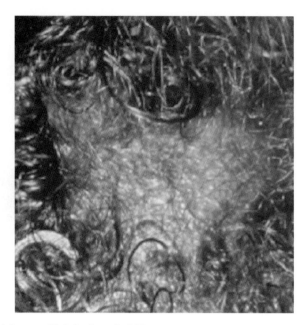

Figure 9.5   Broken hairs of tinea capitis infection mimicking TTM.

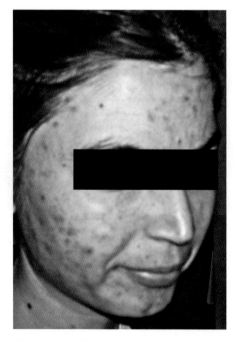

Figure 11.1   Excoriations on the face of a woman with skin picking disorder (Çalıkuşu, 2008).

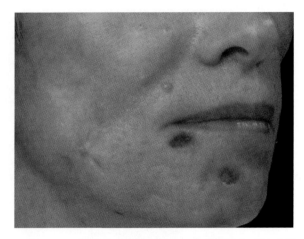

Figure 12.1   Disfiguring ulcers and scars on the face resulting from uncontrollable skin picking.

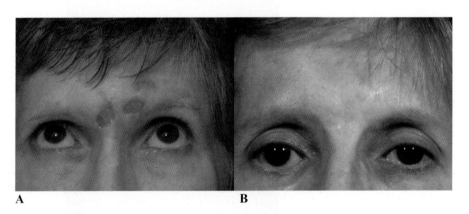

A   B

Figure 12.2   Facial ulcerations and scars before (A) and after (B) 585-nm pulsed dye laser irradiation.

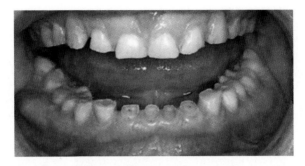

Figure 14.1   Bruxism. Severe wear of all teeth, especially those in the lower jaw.

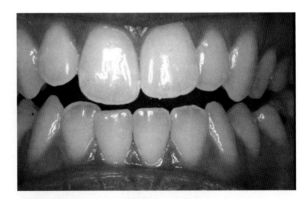

Figure 14.2   Anterior open bite in a teenage girl. Such opening can be caused by thumb or finger sucking, but can also develop because of pathological changes in the TMJs caused by rheumatoid arthritis.

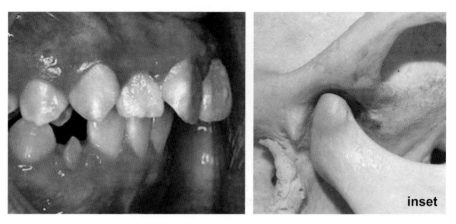

inset

Figure 14.3   The figure shows how upper and lower teeth come together when a young nail-biting patient with a large horizontal overbite achieves maximal intercuspation/centric occlusion (CO). Intercuspation is the fitting together of the cusps of opposing teeth, creating an occlusion (bite) between the upper and lower dentitions. The inset in the lower right corner illustrates normal skeletal relationships between condyle and fossa when biting in CO.

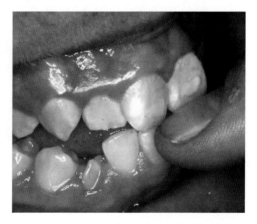

Figure 14.4   The patient in Figure 14.1 now protrudes the lower jaw to bite her fingernail. The upper left corner inset shows the effect on the nail. The lower right corner inset illustrates how the condyle is moved forward during lower jaw protrusion into an unphysiological position where clenching may harm the internal TMJ structures.

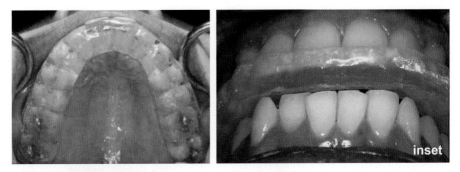

Figure 14.5   A typical occlusal splint made of plastic for covering the upper teeth. The inset shows an anterior view of the splint and the teeth.

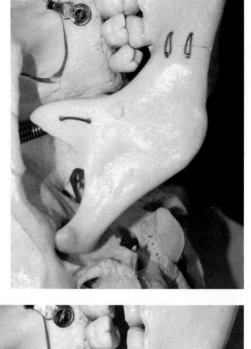

(b)

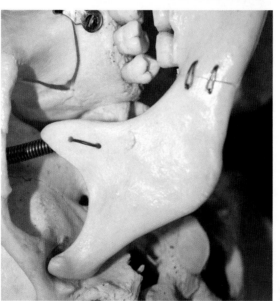

(a)

Figure 14.6   The figure illustrates how, on the left (a), the extruded third upper right molar interferes by preventing the jaw from closing, with the condyle remaining in an optimal position by rotating around the hinge axis without translation. On the right (b), the teeth are in maximal intercuspation and the condyle has been forced into a position anterior to the one on the left.

Section I

Acquisitive Impulses

Compulsive Buying: Clinical Aspects

Donald W. Black, MD

History

Shopping is a major leisure activity for most people in the United States and other developed countries (Farrell 2003). Kowinski (1985) has pointed out that the enclosed shopping mall is a central element in U.S. society, where more time is spent than anywhere else outside of home or work. Shopping experiences provide pleasure and relaxation; yet, for some, excessive shopping is an irresistible and costly way of life (Elliott 1994). These are the compulsive buyers whose lives are organized around a variety of shopping experiences and whose behavior has prompted concerns that it can lead to a clinical disorder.

Examples of profligate spending have been described for centuries, although these reports mainly involve the wealthy and powerful. Marie Antoinette, queen of France during the turbulent time before the revolution, was known for her extravagance (Castelot 1957; Erickson 1991). Mary Todd Lincoln, wife of President Abraham Lincoln, had spending binges that greatly distressed her husband (Baker 1987). Publisher and magnate William Randolph Hearst had an insatiable appetite for art and antiques that nearly drove him to bankruptcy during the Great Depression of the 1930s (Swanberg 1961). Jacqueline Kennedy Onassis, known for her personal charm and great fashion sense, was an obsessive shopper whose uncontrolled behavior dismayed both of her husbands (Heymann 1989). Even the late Princess Diana, a clotheshorse and media star, was widely reported to have an intense interest in shopping and spending (Davies 1996). Whether these individuals had a compulsive buying disorder (CBD) is a matter of debate, yet all were observed to have episodes of excessive and sometimes senseless spending that contributed to their financial downfall or personal problems and, in the case of Marie Antoinette, may well have cost her her life.

Apart from these accounts, the first clinical description of compulsive buying dates to 1915, when German psychiatrist Emil Kraepelin (1915) wrote about "buying maniacs," or "oniomanics," otherwise ordinary persons with uncontrolled shopping and spending behavior. He was later quoted by Swiss psychiatrist Eugen Bleuler (1930) in his *Lehrbuch der Psychiatrie* (*Textbook of Psychiatry*):

As a last category, Kraepelin mentions the buying maniacs (oniomaniacs) in whom even buying is compulsive and leads to senseless contraction of debts with continuous delay of payment until a catastrophe clears the situation a little – a little bit never altogether because they never admit all their debts. According to Kraepelin, here, too, it always involves women. The usually frivolous debt makers and who in this way wish to get the means for pleasure naturally do not belong here. The particular element is impulsiveness; they cannot help it, which sometimes even expresses itself in the fact that not withstanding a good school intelligence, the patients are absolutely incapable to think differently and to conceive the senseless consequences of their act, and the possibilities of not doing it. They do not even feel the impulse, but they act out their nature like the caterpillar which devours the leaf. (p. 540)

Both Kraepelin and Bleuler considered "oniomania" an example of a *reactive impulse*, or *impulsive insanity*, and placed it alongside kleptomania and pyromania. They appear to have been influenced by French psychiatrist Jean Esquirol's (1838) earlier concept of *monomania*, a term he used to describe persons with a pathological preoccupation who otherwise functioned well.

Despite this early work, CBD attracted little attention except for rare clinical case presentations in the psychoanalytic literature (Krueger 1988; Lawrence 1990; Stekel 1924; Winestine 1985). Interest was rekindled in the late 1980s and early 1990s through a convergence of events. Consumer behavior researchers showed the disorder to be widespread (Elliott 1994; Magee 1994; O'Guinn and Faber 1989), and a report appeared in the psychiatric literature describing three women and their response to antidepressant medication (McElroy et al. 1991). Three independent clinical case series followed on the heels of this report, involving a total of 90 subjects (Christenson et al. 1994; McElroy et al. 1994; Schlosser et al. 1994); the results were remarkably similar, even though the methods differed. These reports painted a picture of a definable, persistent clinical disorder that mainly affected women in early to mid-adulthood, many of whom had substantial psychiatric comorbidity.

Diagnosis and Classification

Compulsive buying disorder is not included in contemporary diagnostic systems, such as the *Diagnostic and Statistical Manual of Mental Disorders–Text Revision* (DSM-IV-TR) (American Psychiatric Association 2000) or the *International Classification of Diseases,* 10th edition (World Health Organization 1992), yet several definitions have been proposed. Following in the tradition of criteria-based diagnoses, McElroy et al. (1994) developed an operational definition that emphasizes cognitive and behavioral aspects of the disorder as well as associated impairment from marked subjective distress, interference in social or occupational functioning, or financial/legal problems; in addition, mania and hypomania have to be ruled out. These criteria have become standard in CBD research, although neither their reliability nor validity has been established. Although there is ample evidence of serious harm caused by compulsive buying and significant evidence of comorbidity, some writers have decried attempts to categorize CBD as an illness, attempts they see as part of an unfortunate trend toward "medicalizing" behavioral problems. This stance ignores the reality of CBD and trivializes and stigmatizes attempts to understand or treat it (Lee and Mysyk 2004).

Although DSM-IV-TR does not mention CBD, the disorder can be placed in the category "impulse control disorder not otherwise specified (Code 312.30)." The impulse control disorders share an inability to resist an "impulse, drive, or temptation to perform an act that is harmful to the person or to others" (American Psychiatric Association 2000, p. 663), symptoms that appear to describe CBD. The degree of harm caused by compulsive buying can vary widely. Most obvious is financial harm and distress; however, occupational, interpersonal, marital, social, and spiritual distress have all been reported (Christenson et al. 1994; Lejoyeux et al. 1997; Schlosser et al. 1994).

Other definitions have come from consumer behavior researchers or social psychologists. Faber and O'Guinn (1992) defined the disorder as "chronic buying episodes of a somewhat stereotyped fashion in which the consumer feels unable to stop or significantly moderate his behavior" (p. 738). Edwards (1993), another consumer behaviorist, suggests that compulsive buying is an "abnormal form of shopping and spending in which the afflicted consumer has an overpowering uncontrollable, chronic and repetitive urge to shop and spend (that functions) . . . as a means of alleviating negative feelings of stress and anxiety" (p. 67). Dittmar (2004) describes three cardinal features: irresistible impulse, loss of control, and carrying on despite adverse consequences. Some consumer behavior researchers consider CBD part of a spectrum of aberrant consumer behavior that includes pathological gambling, shoplifting, and credit abuse (Budden and Griffin 1996).

The appropriate classification of CBD remains elusive, a fact reflected by the many terms used to describe the condition: compulsive shopping, addictive shopping, shopaholism, compulsive buying, and even mall mania. McElroy et al. (1991) had suggested that compulsive shopping behavior might be related to "mood, obsessive-compulsive or impulse control disorders." Hollander (1993) later described a spectrum of disorders that he has related to obsessive-compulsive disorder, including CBD, while Lejoyeux et al. (1996) linked it to the mood disorders. Others (Glatt and Cook 1987; Goldman 2000; Krych 1989) have linked CBD to the addictive disorders, grouping it with alcohol and drug dependence. Other investigators have followed in the tradition pioneered by Kraepelin and Bleuler, classifying CBD as a disorder of impulse control. The relationship of CBD to other impulse control disorders was also recognized by Wilhelm Stekel (1924), an early follower of Freud, who proposed that inordinate buying was an incomplete or atypical form of kleptomania (Maier 1997).

Hollander and Allen (2006) have suggested that CBD be included in a new diagnostic category that combines behavioral and substance addictions. In this model, "behavioral addictions" include pathological gambling, kleptomania, pyromania, CBD, Internet addiction, and compulsive sexual behavior. The National Institute on Drug Abuse considers behavioral addictions to be relatively pure models of addiction because they are not contaminated by the presence of an exogenous substance (Holden 2001).

Differential Diagnosis

Ruling out bipolar disorder as the cause of excessive shopping and spending is essential. A manic patient's unrestrained spending typically corresponds to manic episodes and is accompanied by euphoric mood, grandiosity, unrealistic plans, and often a giddy, overly bright affect. The pattern of shopping and spending in the person with CBD lacks the periodicity seen in bipolar patients and points to an ongoing preoccupation (Kuzma and Black 2006). Although unlikely, clinicians should also rule out medical causes (e.g., neurological disorders, brain tumors).

Compulsive buying disorder must be distinguished from normal buying behavior, although the distinction is sometimes arbitrary. Frequent shopping does not by itself constitute evidence of the presence of CBD. For the person with CBD, the frequent shopping and spending has a compulsive and difficult-to-resist quality and leads to deleterious consequences. Although normal buying can also sometimes exhibit a compulsive quality, particularly around special holidays or birthdays, the pattern neither persists nor leads to distress or impairment. Persons who receive an inheritance or win a lottery may experience shopping sprees as well. The clinician needs to exercise judgment in applying the diagnostic criteria of McElroy et al. (1994) and be mindful of the need for evidence of resultant distress or impairment.

Clinical Picture

A distinct clinical picture of the compulsive shopper has emerged. Four distinct phases of CBD have been described, including: (1) anticipation; (2) preparation; (3) shopping; and (4) spending (Black 2007). In the first phase, the person with CBD experiences a thought or preoccupation either with having a specific item or with the act of shopping itself. This leads the individual to prepare for shopping and spending, e.g., deciding on when and where to go, how to dress, and even which credit cards to take. This phase is followed by the actual shopping experience, which many individuals with CBD describe as intensely exciting; some even describe experiencing a sexual feeling (Schlosser et al. 1994). The act is completed with the purchase, often followed by a sense of letdown or disappointment with oneself (Koran et al. 2006).

Perhaps the most important symptom is preoccupation with shopping and spending. This typically leads to spending many hours each week engaged in these behaviors (Christenson et al. 1994; Schlosser et al. 1994). Although it could be argued that a person could be a compulsive shopper and not spend, confining the interest to window shopping, this pattern is very uncommon in the author's experience. Persons with CBD often describe increasing anxiety that is relieved only when a purchase is made.

Compulsive buying disorder behaviors occur all year but can be more problematic during the Christmas holidays and others, as well as around the birthdays of family members and friends. Schlosser et al. (1994) reported that subjects showed a range of behaviors after a purchase: returning the item, failing to remove the item from the package, selling the item, or even giving it away. Compulsive shopping tends to be a private pleasure, and individuals with CBD typically shop alone (Schlosser et al. 1994). Compulsive shopping can occur in any venue: high-fashion department stores and boutiques, consignment shops, garage sales, or catalogs (Christenson et al. 1994). Dittmar (2007) has documented how CBD has gained a strong foothold in online buying.

Compulsive buyers are mainly interested in consumer goods such as clothing, shoes, crafts, jewelry, gifts, makeup, and compact discs/DVDs (Christenson et al. 1994; Mitchell et al. 2006; Schlosser et al. 1994). Research has not identified gender-specific buying patterns, but in the author's experience men with CBD tend to have a greater interest than women in electronic, automotive, and hardware goods. Compulsive shoppers often display a great fashion sense and have an intense interest in new clothing styles and products. They may report buying a product based on its attractiveness or because it was a "bargain" (Frost et al. 1998). Individually, items purchased tend not to be large or expensive, but many compulsive shoppers will buy in quantity, so that spending rapidly escalates. During a typical episode, compulsive shoppers have reported spending an average of $110 (Christenson et al. 1994), $92 (Schlosser et al. 1994), or $89 (Miltenberger et al. 2003). Compulsive buying disorder has little to do with intellect or educational level and has been observed to occur in mentally retarded persons (Otter and Black 2007).

Several writers have emphasized the emotional significance of the types of objects purchased, which may address personal and social identity needs (Dittmar 2007; Richards 1996). Richards (1996) stressed the role of clothing in developing a feminine identity and noted that voids in one's identity have their roots in failed parent–child interactions. Krueger (1988) observed that emotionally deprived persons unconsciously replace what is missing with objects in an attempt to "fill the emptiness of depression and the absence of self-regulation" (p. 582). These explanations for compulsive buying behaviors may apply to some, but certainly not all, persons with CBD. One study found that self-image concerns were more closely linked to the motivations underlying CBD in women than in men (Dittmar and Drury 2000).

Miltenberger et al. (2003) reported that negative emotions, such as anger, anxiety, boredom, and self-critical thoughts, were the most common antecedents to shopping binges; euphoria or relief of negative emotions has been the most common immediate emotional reaction (Elliott, Eccles, and Gournay 1996). Lejoyeux et al. (1996) concluded that for some persons "uncontrolled buying, like bulimia, can be used as a compensatory mechanism for depressive feelings" (p. 1528). Faber and Christenson (1996) commented on the close relationships among shopping, self-esteem, and negative emotions. Faber and O'Guinn (1992) concluded that shopping behavior is likely to become problematic when it provides a sense of recognition and acceptance for people with low self-esteem, allowing them to act out anger or aggression while providing an escape from day-to-day drudgery.

Natarajan and Goff (1991) have identified two independent factors in CBD: (1) buying urge or desire and (2) degree of control over buying. In their model, compulsive shoppers combine high urge with low control. This view is consistent with clinical reports that compulsive buyers are preoccupied with shopping and spending and despite trying to resist their urges, often have little success (Black 1996; Christenson et al. 1994; Marks 1990). For example, in the study of Christenson et al. (1994), 92% of persons with the disorder described often unsuccessful attempts to resist buying. Subjects indicated that the urge to buy resulted in a purchase 74% of the time. Typically, one to five hours passed between initially experiencing the urge to buy and the eventual purchase.

Income has relatively little to do with CBD because persons with a low income can be as preoccupied with shopping and spending as wealthier individuals (Black 2001; Dittmar 2007); level of income may lead one person to shop at a consignment shop, while the other shops at a high-end boutique. Koran et al. (2006) found that, compared with other respondents, individuals with CBD were more likely to report an income under $50,000; less likely to pay off credit card balances in full; and gave maladaptive responses regarding their consumer behavior. In this study, compulsive buyers engaged in "problem shopping" more frequently and for longer periods, and were more likely than other respondents to feel depressed after shopping, to make senseless and impulsive purchases, and to experience uncontrollable buying binges. These data are partially compatible with the findings of Black et al. (2001), who divided a sample of individuals with CBD into quartiles from most to least severe based on their Compulsive Buying Scale score (Faber and O'Guinn 1992). Greater severity was associated with lower gross income, a lower likelihood of having an income above the median, and spending a lower percentage of income on sale items. Subjects with more severe CBD were also more likely to have comorbid Axis I or Axis II disorders. These results suggest that more severe buying disorders occur in psychologically distressed persons with low incomes who have an impaired ability to control or to delay their urges to make inappropriate purchases.

Wealth does not protect against CBD either because the presence of CBD may cause or contribute to interpersonal, occupational, marital, or spiritual problems, even when it does not create financial problems. Many compulsive buyers who seek treatment have incomes well in excess of $100,000 (A. Benson, personal communication, 2008).

Identification and Assessment

In clinical practice, few patients refer themselves for treatment for a compulsive buying disorder. When CBD is a presenting problem, the patient has typically been referred by a financial counselor, lawyer, law enforcement officer, family member, or spouse (Black 2000). More frequently, compulsive buying reveals itself in the course of ongoing treatment. Some patients will begin to talk openly about the problem; with others, it emerges in the context of financial independence and responsibility issues, relationship problems, difficulties at work, or parenting problems. Compulsive buying may also present itself indirectly: a patient might wear something new or different to every session, arrive with shopping bags week after week, repeatedly give gifts to the therapist, or fall behind in paying the bill (Benson 2000).

Compulsive buyers are largely secretive about their disorder because it is a source of great shame, perhaps even more so than alcoholism or drug abuse. The latter are commonly thought of as diseases, or at least are recognized as serious problems requiring treatment. Compulsive buyers, on the other hand, worry that they will be considered materialistic and vacuous – judgments that likely reflect their self-perceptions (Benson 2000).

The diagnostic process begins with relatively nonintrusive inquiries, followed with more detailed inquiries regarding the person's shopping attitudes and behaviors (Black 2000). For general screening purposes, the clinician might ask:

- "Do you feel overly preoccupied with shopping and spending?"
- "Do you ever feel that your shopping behavior is excessive, inappropriate, or poorly controlled?"
- "Have your shopping desires, urges, fantasies, or behaviors ever been overly time consuming, caused you to feel upset or guilty, or led to serious problems in your life such as financial or legal problems or the loss of a relationship?"

Positive responses can be followed up with more detailed inquiries, such as how frequently the behavior occurs, what the individual prefers to buy, and how much money is spent. Attitudes and behaviors following purchases are also important to explore.

This exploration should be followed by a thorough assessment of the patient's psychiatric history, including medications, psychotherapy, and hospitalizations. This assessment is important because most compulsive buyers have a history of psychiatric comorbidity, and the presence of a disorder, such as major depression or panic disorder, may suggest a particular treatment strategy or approach or provide information that may be useful in counseling the patient. Taking a history of physical illnesses, surgical procedures, drug allergies, or medical treatment may help rule out medical causes of the compulsive buying, as noted earlier.

A family history should be obtained. Compulsive buying runs in some families (typically female relatives), and these families are often troubled by depression, alcoholism, or drug addiction (Black et al. 1998). Having grown up in a dysfunctional home in which one or more family members had a mental illness or an addictive disorder may have contributed to the patient's CBD. On the other hand, the patient may have learned inappropriate buying and spending behavior from his or her parent or other relatives.

The patient's social and personal history should be explored, including family life, history of childhood development, possible history of abuse, educational background, occupational history, intimate relationships and marriages, children, and finances or legal problems related to the disordered buying. This information will help in planning a comprehensive approach to the patient's problems.

Several instruments have been developed to either identify CBD or rate its severity. Canadian researchers developed the Compulsive Buying Measurement Scale (Valence, D'Astous, and Fortier 1988). These investigators selected 16 items thought to represent four basic dimensions of compulsive buying (tendency to spend, urge to buy or shop, post-purchase guilt, and family environment). A reliability analysis led to deleting three items representing family environment. A modified version of the scale, tested by German researchers (Scherhorn, Reisch, and Raab 1990) as the Addictive Buying Scale (ABS), had high reliability and construct validity. Like the Canadian instrument, the ABS discriminated normal from compulsive buying behavior.

The Compulsive Buying Scale (CBS) was developed by Faber and O'Guinn (1992) to distinguish normal from pathological buyers. They began with 29 items, each item reflecting important characteristics of compulsive buying derived from earlier work, and rated each item on a 5-point scale. Logistic regression analysis identified seven items representing specific behaviors, motivations, and feelings that together correctly classified 88% of the individuals tested. Many researchers consider the CBS a useful tool for identifying compulsive buyers and rating CBD severity.

Edwards (1993) developed a 13-item scale to assess important experiences and feelings about shopping and spending. The items were selected to measure dimensions of tendency to spend, frequency of shopping, spending feelings and experiences while shopping, impulsivity while shopping, unplanned purchasing, post-purchase guilt, and dysfunction resulting from spending. The scores can be used to classify consumers according to their level of compulsiveness in buying.

Other scales have not found wide use. Lejoyeux et al. (1997) developed a 19-item questionnaire to tap the basic features of CBD, but its psychometric properties have not been reported. Weun et al. (1998) developed the Impulse Buying Tendency Scale to assess the proclivity for impulse buying, which they distinguish from compulsive buying. Ridgeway et al. (2008) have developed the Compulsive-Impulsive Buying Scale, which measures compulsive buying as a construct incorporating elements of both an obsessive-compulsive and an impulse control disorder. The scale appears to be reliable and valid, and it performs

Table 1.1 Prevalence surveys of compulsive buying disorder

Study	Location	Diagnostic Method	Sample Size	Setting	Findings
Faber and O'Guinn 1992[1]	Illinois	CBS	292	General population	1.8%–8.1%
Dittmar 2005	England	CBS	194	General population	13.5%
Neuner et al. 2005[2]	Germany	ABS	1527/1017	General population	6.5%–8%
Koran et al. 2006[1]	United States	CBS	2513	General population	1.4%–5.8%
Magee 1994	Arizona	CBS	94	College students	16%
Hassay and Smith 1996	Manitoba, Canada	CBS	92	College students	12%
Roberts 1998	Texas	CBS	300	College students	6%
Dittmar 2005	England	CBS	195	Adolescents	44.1%
Grant et al. 2005	Minnesota	MIDI	204	Psychiatric outpatient clinic	9.5%

CBS = Compulsive Buying Scale; ABS = Addictive Buying Scale; MIDI = Minnesota Impulsive Disorders Interview.
[1] The study used conservative and liberal cut points with the CBS.
[2] The study involved interviews with East and West Germans from 1991 to 2001.

well in correlating with other theoretically related constructs. These instruments will be of interest mainly to researchers.

Monahan, Black, and Gabel (1995) modified the Yale Brown Obsessive-Compulsive Scale to create the YBOCS-Shopping Version (YBOCS-SV). The 10-item scale rates time involved, interference, distress, resistance, and degree of control for both cognitions and behaviors typical of CBD, yielding a score ranging from 0 to 40. The scale had adequate inter-rater reliability and was valid in measuring both severity and change during a clinical trial. Persons with CBD had a mean score of 21 (range 18–25) compared with a mean of 4 (range 1–7) for normal buyers.

Christenson et al. (1994) developed the Minnesota Impulsive Disorders Interview, a semistructured interview to assess the presence of CBD, kleptomania, trichotillomania, intermittent explosive disorder, compulsive sexual behavior, pathological gambling, and compulsive exercise. The instrument had a sensitivity of 100% and a specificity of 96.2% for CBD when compared with the diagnostic criteria of McElroy et al. (1994) (Grant et al. 2005).

Shopping logs or diaries may be helpful in understanding and treating persons with CBD. Patients can record their shopping experiences, accompanying mood, and the outcome (e.g., money spent, item purchased). This description of the patient's buying behavior may be helpful during treatment, for example, in a medication or behavior therapy trial (Benson 2006; Bernik et al. 1996; Black et al. 1997). The use of a daily log may be therapeutic as well by fostering the patient's awareness of the extent of the problem.

Prevalence

Prevalence surveys relevant to CBD have produced rates that range from 1.4% to 44%, the differences likely resulting from the populations examined and the research methods used (Table 1.1). In general, adolescents and college students had higher rates of CBD than general adult populations.

In perhaps the most widely cited study, Faber and O'Guinn (1992) estimated the prevalence of CBD at between 1.8% and 8.1% of the general population based on a mail survey in which the Compulsive Buying Scale (CBS) was returned by 292 individuals from a sample selected to approximate the demographic makeup of the general population of Illinois. The high and low prevalence estimates reflect different score thresholds set for CBD. The higher figure is based on a probability level of 0.70 (i.e., two standard deviations above the mean), while the lower figure is based on a more conservative probability level of 0.95 (i.e., three

Table 1.2 Studies involving individuals with compulsive buying disorder

Investigator(s)	Location	Subjects, n	Age, Years, Mean	% Female	Age at Onset, Years, Mean	Duration of Illness, Years, Mean
O'Guinn and Faber 1989	Los Angeles, CA	386	37	92	N/A	N/A
Scherhorn, Reisch, and Raab 1990	Germany	26	40	85	N/A	N/A
McElroy et al. 1994	Cincinnati, OH	20	39	80	30	9
Christenson et al. 1994	Minneapolis, MN	24	36	92	18	18
Schlosser et al. 1994	Iowa City, IA	46	31	80	19	12
Black et al. 1998	Iowa City, IA	33	40	94	N/A	N/A
Ninan et al. 2000	Cincinnati, OH; Boston, MA	42	41	81	N/A	N/A
Koran et al. 2002	Stanford, CA	24	44	92	22	22
Miltenberger et al. 2003	Fargo, ND	19	N/A	100*	18	N/A
Mitchell et al. 2006	Fargo, ND	39	45	100*	N/A	N/A

*Indicates that the sample recruited was female.

standard deviations above the mean). These authors recommend using the probability level of 0.70 with the CBS.

Dittmar (2005) conducted two studies that address prevalence. In the first, she queried 194 persons who responded to an unsolicited mail survey and were residentially matched to a group of persons with shopping problems. Using the CBS, she determined that 13.4% of the residentially matched comparison group met the cutoff for CBD. She also sampled 195 adolescents aged 16 to 18 years and found that 44.1% scored above the CBS scale cutoff, indicating the presence of a CBD.

More recently, Koran et al. (2006) used the CBS to identify compulsive buyers in a random telephone survey of 2,513 U.S. adults and estimated the point prevalence at 5.8% of respondents. The estimate was calculated by using CBS scores two standard deviations above the mean. A prevalence of 1.4% was calculated using the stricter criterion of three standard deviations above the mean.

Three small surveys of college students, all utilizing the CBS and a cutoff score of two standard deviations above the mean, produced modestly varying estimates. Magee (1994) reported that 16% of 94 undergraduates were compulsive buyers, while Hassay and Smith (1996) found that 12.2% of 92 undergraduates were compulsive buyers. Roberts (1998) reported that 6% of 300 college students met the cutoff for CBD. Lastly, Grant et al. (2005) utilized the Minnesota Impulsive Disorders Interview (MIDI) to assess CBD and reported a lifetime prevalence of 9.3% among 204 consecutively admitted psychiatric inpatients.

In an interesting study designed to address whether CBD is becoming more prevalent, Neuner, Raab, and Reisch (2005) reported that the frequency of compulsive buying in Germany increased between 1991 and 2001. Using the ABS, these investigators found that the frequency of CBD increased from 1% to 6.5% in East Germany and from 5% to 8% in West Germany. They attributed the rapid rise of CBD in the former East Germany in part to the acculturation process brought about by reunification.

Age at Onset and Gender

Compulsive buying disorder is reported to have an onset in the late teens or early 20s, which may correlate with emancipation from the nuclear family (Table 1.2) as well as with the age at which people can first establish credit (Black 2001). Roberts and Tanner (2000, 2002) showed that uncontrolled buying in adolescents is associated with a more generalized pattern of behavioral disinhibition that includes cigarette smoking, alcohol use, drug use, and early sex.

Community-based clinical studies and the survey results of Faber and O'Guinn suggest that from 80% to 94% of persons with CBD are women (Table 1.1) (Christenson et al. 1994; Faber and O'Guinn 1989; McElroy et al. 1994; Schlosser et al. 1994). In contrast, Koran et al. (2006) reported that the prevalence of CBD in their random telephone survey was nearly equal for men and women (5.5% and 6.0%, respectively). Their finding suggests that the reported gender difference may be artifactual and stem from women being more willing to acknowledge abnormal shopping behavior and participate in research. Men seem more likely to view their compulsive buying as "collecting." Dittmar (2004), considering the results of a general population survey in the United Kingdom, concluded that the gender difference is real and not an artifact of men being underrepresented in clinical samples. In her study, 92% of respondents labeled compulsive shoppers were women. That said, this survey's methods have not been published, making it difficult to assess the representativeness of the sample and the completeness of response.

Natural History and Course

Although there are no careful follow-up studies of CBD, cross-sectional studies suggest the disorder is chronic but fluctuating. Schlosser et al. (1994) reported that 59% of their subjects described their course as continuous and 41% as episodic. Of the 20 subjects in another study (McElroy et al. 1994), 60% reported a chronic course and 8% an episodic one. For the subjects in the studies listed in Table 1.2, CBD had been present from 9 to 18 years, although these clinical samples may be biased in favor of greater severity. The author has interviewed a woman in her mid-80s who had compulsively shopped for over 50 years. Recently, Aboujaoude, Gamel, and Koran (2003) suggested that persons who responded to treatment with citalopram were likely to remain in remission during a 1-year follow-up, suggesting that treatment can alter the natural history of the disorder.

Quality of Life

Formal quality of life data are limited, but research shows that CBD adversely impacts the lives of those with the disorder and their family members. First, most persons with CBD admit that the disorder is subjectively distressing and that they feel unable to control their behavior (Christenson et al. 1994; Schlosser et al. 1994). They report that the disorder has led to marital and family problems, including separation and divorce. Financial problems include substantial debt that can lead to bankruptcy. In some cases, individuals turn to crime to fuel their shopping or to repay their debts, for example, embezzling funds or shoplifting. The impact of CBD on emotional well-being and work functioning was noted earlier. Lejoyeux et al. (1997) report that CBD is associated with suicide attempts, although there are no reports of CBD leading to completed suicide.

Etiology and Pathophysiology

The cause of CBD is unknown, though speculation has settled on developmental, neurobiologic, and cultural influences.

Developmental

Psychoanalysts (Krueger 1988; Lawrence 1990; Stekel 1924; Winestine 1985) have suggested that early life events, including childhood sexual abuse, contribute to the development of CBD. Benson (2006) has observed several family constellations that she believes contribute: the physically abusive or neglectful parent; the emotionally neglectful parent who demands the child earn their love through "good" behavior; the absent parent who has little time or energy for the child; and families that have experienced financial reversals and fixate on lost luxury. In each scenario, possessions achieve importance as a means of easing suffering, boosting self-esteem, or restoring lost social status.

Genetic

There is some evidence that CBD runs in families and that within these families the rates of mood, anxiety, and substance use disorders exceed those of the general population. McElroy et al. (1994) reported that of 18 individuals with CBD, 17 had one or more first-degree relatives with major depression, 11 with alcohol or other substance abuse, and 3 with an anxiety disorder. Three had relatives with CBD as well. Black et al. (1998) used the family history method to assess 137 first-degree relatives of 31 persons with CBD. Relatives were significantly more likely than those in a comparison group to have depression, alcoholism, a drug use disorder, "any psychiatric disorder," and "more than one psychiatric disorder." Compulsive buying disorder was identified in 9.5% of the first-degree relatives but was not assessed in the comparison group. In two relevant molecular genetic studies, Devor et al. (1999) failed to find an association between two serotonin transporter gene polymorphisms and CBD, and Comings (1998) reported an association of CBD with the DRD1 receptor gene.

Pathophysiology

Neurobiologic theories have centered on disturbed neurotransmission, particularly involving the serotonergic, dopaminergic, or opioid systems. Selective serotonin reuptake inhibitors (SSRIs) have been used to treat CBD (Black, Monahan, and Gabel 1997, 2000; Koran et al. 2003, 2007; Ninan et al. 2000) in part because of hypothetical similarities between CBD and obsessive-compulsive disorder, a disorder known to respond to SSRIs (Hollander 1993). Dopamine has been theorized to play a role in "reward dependence," which has been claimed to foster behavioral addictions, such as CBD and pathological gambling (Holden 2001). Case reports suggesting benefit from the opiate antagonist naltrexone have led to speculation about the role of opiate receptors (Grant 2003; Kim 1998). There is no direct evidence, however, to support the role of these neurotransmitter systems in the etiology of CBD.

In a study with relevance to CBD, Knutson et al. (2007) used functional magnetic resonance imaging to explore neural circuits involved in purchasing decisions. The nucleus accumbens, a putative pleasure center, was activated when subjects were shown products they liked. When the item was priced lower than what the subject was willing to pay, the mesial prefrontal cortex (a brain region involved in decision making) became activated and the insula (a part of the brain that registers pain) showed less activity. The picture was reversed when the item was priced higher than the price the subject was willing to pay. Subjects then made the decision to buy, with high mesial prefrontal cortex activity indicating a decision to buy and high insula activity indicating a decision to refrain. This study supports the view that consumers balance immediate pleasure (purchasing) against immediate pain (price). Although the subjects were drawn from the general population, the study may help to explain compulsive shopping behavior; the pleasure of impulse buying is immediately registered, while the pain of delayed payment (i.e., from a credit card) is minimized.

Cultural Considerations

Because CBD occurs mainly in developed countries, cultural and social factors have been proposed as either causing or promoting the disorder (Black 2001; Dittmar 2007). The disorder has been described worldwide, with reports coming from the United States (Christenson et al. 1994; McElroy et al. 1994; Schlosser et al. 1994), Australia (Kyrios et al. 2002), Canada (Valence, D'Astous, and Fortier 1988), England (Dittmar 2004; Elliott 1994), Germany (Scherhorn et al. 1990), France (Lejoyeux et al. 1997), Holland (Otter and Black 2007), Mexico (Roberts and Sepulveda 1999), South Korea (Kwak, Zinkhan, and Crask 2003), Spain (Villarino, Otero-Lopez, and Casto 2001), and Brazil (Bernik et al. 1996). The presence of a market-based economy, the availability of a wide variety of goods, easily obtained credit, disposable income, and significant leisure time are elements considered

Table 1.3 Lifetime psychiatric comorbidity in persons with compulsive buying

Comorbid Disorder	Schlosser et al. 1994	Christenson et al. 1994	McElroy et al. 1994	Lejoyeux et al. 1997	Black et al. 1998	Ninan et al. 2000	Koran et al. 2002	Mitchell et al. 2006
Instrument used	DIS	SCID	SCID	MINI	SCID	SCID	MINI	SCID
Mood disorder, %	28	54	95	100	61	45	8	62
Anxiety disorder, %	41	50	80		42			26
Substance use disorder, %	30	46	40		21			33
Somatoform disorder, %	11		10					
Eating disorder, %	17	21	35	21	15		8	18
Impulse control disorder, %		21	40					

necessary for the development of CBD (Lee and Mysyk 2004). For these reasons, CBD is unlikely to occur in poorly developed (or developing) countries except among the wealthy elite or the growing middle classes (e.g., in India and China). Interestingly, a Web site specifically designed to offer resources to compulsive buyers and their families has attracted visitors from over 50 countries, suggesting that the disorder is nearly universal (A. Benson, personal communication, 2008).

Psychiatric Comorbidity

Psychiatric comorbidity is the rule in individuals with CBD. In the only studies in which comparison samples were used, Black et al. (1998) reported that major depression and "any" mood disorder were excessive, while Christenson et al. (1994) found that anxiety, substance use, eating, and impulse control disorder categories were all excessive. Data from the clinical studies summarized in Table 1.3 confirm high rates of major mental (Axis I) disorders, particularly the mood (21%–100%), anxiety (41%–80%), substance use (21%–46%), and eating (8%–35%) disorders. Disorders of impulse control are also relatively common (21%–40%).

The frequency of Axis II disorders in individuals with CBD was assessed by Schlosser et al. (1994) using both a self-report instrument and a structured interview. Nearly 60% of 46 subjects met criteria for at least one personality disorder through a consensus of both instruments. Although there was no special "shopping" personality, the most commonly identified personality disorders were the obsessive-compulsive (22%), avoidant (15%), and borderline (15%) types. Krueger (1988) observed that the four patients he treated using psychoanalysis each exhibited aspects of narcissistic character pathology.

Some investigators believe that CBD falls within an obsessive-compulsive spectrum. In clinical samples, from 3% (Black et al. 1998) to 35% (McElroy et al. 1994) of individuals with CBD have comorbid OCD. The presence of CBD may characterize a specific subset (10%) of OCD patients (du Toit et al. 2001; Hantouche et al. 1996, 1997), particularly those with hoarding, a special symptom that involves the acquisition of, and failure to discard, possessions that are of limited use or value (Frost et al. 1998). Yet, unlike the items retained by the typical hoarder, the items purchased by the compulsive shopper are not inherently valueless or useless.

With regard to impulse control disorders (ICDs), Black and Moyer (1998) and Grant and Kim (2003) each reported elevated rates of CBD among samples of pathological gamblers (23% and 8%, respectively). Likewise, other impulse control disorders are common among compulsive shoppers (Christenson et al. 1994; Koran et al. 2002; Lejoyeux et al. 1997; McElroy et al. 1994; Schlosser et al. 1994). Black, Belsare, and Schlosser (1999) reported that CBD was relatively frequent (19%) in a sample of individuals with compulsive computer use. A significant comorbidity with psychogenic excoriation, binge eating, and other impulsive behaviors has also been reported (Arnold, Auchenbach, and McElroy 2001; Carmin 1998; Faber et al. 1995).

Dimensional Traits

Lejoyeux et al. (1997) reported that depressed compulsive shoppers had higher scores than depressed normal buyers on the experience-seeking subscale of the Zuckerman Sensation Seeking Scale (Zuckerman 1994), as well as on cognitive impulsivity, motor impulsivity, nonplanning activity, and total scale scores for the Barratt Impulsiveness Scale (Barratt 1959). O'Guinn and Faber (1989) reported high levels of compulsivity, materialism, and fantasy but lower levels of self-esteem in compulsive buyers compared with normal buyers. Partially consistent with these results, Yurchisin and Johnson (2004) reported that compulsive buying behavior was negatively related to self-esteem and positively related to perceived social status associated with buying, materialism, and apparel-product acquisition. These findings suggest that many compulsive shoppers use possessions to raise their perceived social position, possibly in an attempt to boost low self-esteem.

Treatment

No treatment has been well established as effective for CBD, and both psychotherapies and medications have been recommended.

Psychotherapy

Several case studies report psychoanalytic treatment of CBD (Krueger 1988; Lawrence 1990; Schwartz 1992; Stekel 1924; Winestine 1985). Stekel described a woman whose compulsive buying was attributed to unconscious wishes for sexual adventure. Three months of psychoanalysis left her sexually responsive and free of her compulsive buying. Krueger described four cases to show that the CBD was motivated by a "dual attempt to regulate the affect and fragmented sense of self and to restore self-object equilibrium, symbolically or indirectly" (p. 583). None experienced clear-cut improvement from the therapy.

Winestine (1985) presented the case of a woman with a history of sexual abuse and fantasies of being the wife of a famous millionaire who had the power and funds to afford anything she wished. In identifying with this role, she was thought to be reversing her actual feelings of helplessness and inability to regulate her shopping and spending behavior: "The purchases offered some momentary fortification against her feelings of humiliation and worthlessness for being out of control" (p. 71). Lawrence (1990) wrote that compulsive shopping stems from an "intrapsychic need for nurturing from the external world" (p. 67); he may have been the first mental health professional to link compulsive buying with an attempt to deny death. More recently, Krueger (2000) described three additional cases and wrote that compulsive shoppers have a fragile sense of self and self-esteem that depends on the responses of others. Goldman (2000) surmised that compulsive buying often follows the disruption of an emotional bond, setting in motion a desperate need to appear attractive and desirable. Benson and Gengler (2004), in considering the different forms of individual therapy, suggest that many different psychodynamic explanations of compulsive buying have been proposed, usually related to the theoretical perspective of the therapist.

Cognitive-behavioral treatment (CBT) models for CBD have been developed over the past two decades. Lejoyeux et al. (1996) and Bernik et al. (1996) both suggested that cue exposure and response prevention may be helpful. Bernik et al. (1996) reported two patients with comorbid panic disorder and agoraphobia responsive to clomipramine whose uncontrolled buying did not respond to the drug. Both patients responded well to 3 to 4 weeks of daily cue exposure and response prevention, though no follow-up data were presented.

The first use of group therapy was described by Damon (1988). Later models were developed by Burgard and Mitchell (2000), Villarino, Otero-Lopez, and Casto (2001), and more recently by Benson and Gengler (2004). Mitchell et al. (2006) found that group CBT ($n = 28$ subjects) produced significant improvement compared with a wait list ($n = 11$ subjects) in a 12-week pilot study. Improvement attributed to CBT was maintained during a 6-month follow-up.

Benson (2006) has developed a comprehensive, guided self-help program that can be used by both individuals and groups. The program combines psychodynamic principles and exercises with self-monitoring, dialectical behavioral therapy, cognitive-behavioral therapy, and acceptance and commitment therapy. A detailed workbook with text and exercises, a shopping diary for self-monitoring during shopping, a CD-ROM with guided visualizations, and a reminder card to be carried at all times are included (www.Stoppingovershopping.com).

Medication

Treatment studies employing psychotropic medications have produced mixed results. In an early report, McElroy et al. (1991) described three women with comorbid mood or anxiety disorders who had a partial or full remission of compulsive buying behavior associated with fluoxetine, bupropion, or nortriptyline treatment. In a subsequent report, McElroy et al. (1994) described 20 additional patients, 9 of whom had partial or full remission during treatment with antidepressants, mainly serotonin reuptake inhibitors, usually in combination with a mood stabilizer. In most cases, the observation period was limited to a few weeks or months, and two of the patients who improved also received supportive or insight-oriented psychotherapy before receiving drug treatment.

Lejoyeux, Hourtane, and Ades (1995) reported that treatment of depression in two patients with comorbid CBD led to resolution of compulsive buying. In one case, clomipramine (150 mg/day) was used; in the other, no drug was specified.

Black, Monahan, and Gabel (1997), in a 9-week, open-label trial, reported that nine of ten nondepressed subjects with CBD who were given fluvoxamine showed benefit. Those who responded did so by week five. The fact that none were depressed appeared to refute the assertion by Lejoyeux, Hourtane, and Ades (1995) that the presence of comorbid depression explained the improvement in buying behavior during antidepressant treatment.

Two subsequent randomized controlled trials found fluvoxamine treatment was no better than placebo. Black et al. (2000) randomized 12 nondepressed patients with CBD to fluvoxamine and 11 to placebo. At the end of the 9-week trial, 50% of fluvoxamine recipients and 64% of placebo recipients had responded. Similarly, in a 12-week two-site trial in which 20 subjects received fluvoxamine and 17 a placebo, the intent-to-treat analysis failed to show a significant difference between the groups (Ninan et al. 2000).

In a 7-week open-label trial (Koran et al. 2002), 17 of 24 CBD patients (71%) responded to citalopram. In a subsequent study, 24 subjects received 7 weeks of open-label citalopram; 15 subjects (63%) were considered responders and entered into a double-blind phase in which they were randomly assigned to 9 weeks of treatment with citalopram or a placebo (Koran et al. 2003). Compulsive shopping symptoms returned in five of eight subjects (62.5%) assigned a placebo compared with none of the seven who continued taking citalopram. Surprisingly, in an identically designed discontinuation trial by the same investigators (Koran et al. 2007), escitalopram did not separate from the placebo. In this study, 19 of 26 women (73%) responded to open-label escitalopram, and 17 were then randomized to further treatment with the drug or placebo. At the end of the 9-week double-blind phase, five of eight (62.5%) escitalopram recipients had relapsed, compared with six of nine (66.7%) placebo recipients.

Grant (2003) and Kim (1998) have described cases in which individuals with CBD have improved with naltrexone treatment, suggesting that opiate antagonists may have a role in the treatment of CBD.

In conclusion, open-label medication trials have generally produced positive results, but controlled trials have not. Interpretation of these study results is complicated by placebo response rates as high as 64% (Black et al. 2000). Because the drug treatment study findings are mixed, no empirically well-supported treatment recommendations can be made.

Other Approaches

Self-help books ("bibliotherapy") are available. These include *Shopaholics: Serious Help for Addicted Spenders* (Damon 1988), *Born to Spend: How to Overcome Compulsive Spending* (Arenson 1991), *Women Who Shop Too Much: Overcoming the Urge to Splurge* (Wesson 1991), *Consuming Passions: Help for Compulsive Shoppers* (Catalano and Sonenberg 1993), *Addicted to Shopping . . . and Other Issues Women Have with Money* (O'Connor 2005), and *To Buy or Not to Buy: Why We Overshop and How to Stop* (Benson 2008). Each provides sensible recommendations that individuals can implement to help gain control over their inappropriate shopping and spending.

Debtors Anonymous, patterned after Alcoholics Anonymous, may also be helpful (Levine and Kellen 2000). This voluntary, lay-run group provides an atmosphere of mutual support and encouragement for those with substantial debts. Simplicity circles are available in some U.S. cities; these voluntary groups encourage people to adopt a simple lifestyle and to abandon their CBD (Andrews 2000). Marriage (or couples) counseling may be helpful, particularly when CBD in one member of the dyad is disrupting the relationship (Mellan 2000). Many individuals with CBD develop financial difficulties and can benefit from financial recovery counseling (McCall 2000). The author has seen cases in which appointing a financial conservator to control the patient's finances has been helpful. Although a conservator controls the patient's spending, this approach does not reverse the individual's preoccupation with shopping.

The author has developed a set of treatment recommendations (Kuzma and Black 2006) that his clinical experience suggests may be helpful to clinicians. First, because pharmacologic treatment trials provide little guidance, patients should be informed that they cannot rely only on medications. Second, patients should be encouraged to: (1) admit they have CBD; (2) get rid of credit cards and checkbooks because they are easy sources of funds that fuel the disorder; (3) shop with a friend or relative because the presence of a person without CBD may help curb the tendency to overspend; and (4) find meaningful ways to spend leisure time other than by shopping.

Summary

Interest in CBD has grown in the past two decades, leading to a greater understanding of its epidemiology, phenomenology, family history, and treatment. The disorder is common, associated with important comorbid psychiatric disorders, and can lead to serious functional impairment, financial problems, and legal entanglements. A great deal more work is needed to better understand the disorder and to develop effective treatments. First, although several definitions have been proposed, most prominently the criteria of McElroy et al. (1994), their reliability and validity have yet to be established. Although the MIDI (Christenson et al. 1994) shows promise as a diagnostic tool, its psychometric properties need further study. Compulsive buying disorder is likely chronic or intermittent, but at least one study (Aboujaoude, Gamel, and Koran 2003) shows that the course may be modified with treatment. Follow-up studies would be helpful in charting the course of the disorder, tracking its emergence or subsidence, and determining its relationship to other psychiatric disorders.

Whether gender differences exist is unsettled. The recent survey reported by Koran et al. (2006) suggests that CBD affects men and women equally, yet this conclusion conflicts with other surveys as well as nearly all data from clinical samples. Whether CBD represents a single construct or has multiple subtypes, each suggesting alternate etiologies or pathophysiologies, needs investigation. Some researchers suggest that CBD is related to OCD and others that it is related to the substance use disorders, the mood disorders, or the disorders of impulse control. Perhaps all are correct and subgroups of compulsive buyers are motivated by different underlying diatheses that correspond to these different diagnostic groups. Neurobiological and genetic studies would help clarify these links. Treatment studies suggest that CBD may respond to cognitive-behavioral strategies, yet which patients respond best to this treatment and whether the improvement persists are not clear. Medication studies are hampered by high placebo response rates, a confound that needs to be considered in planning future studies. Different subgroups of patients may respond preferentially to particular types of drugs, reflecting differences in underlying neurobiology. Finally, combined treatment strategies also deserve study.

References

Aboujaoude E, Gamel N, Koran, LM. A 1-year naturalistic follow-up of patients with compulsive shopping disorder. *J Clin Psychiatry* 64:946–950, 2003.

American Psychiatric Association. Diagnostic and Statistical Manual of Mental Disorders, 4th edition, text revision. Washington, DC: American Psychiatric Publishing, 2000.

Andrews C. Simplicity circles and the compulsive shopper, in *I Shop, Therefore I Am: Compulsive Buying and the Search for Self*. Edited by Benson A. New York: Aronson, 2000, pp. 484–496.

Arenson G. *Born to Spend: How to Overcome Compulsive Spending*. Blue Ridge Summit, PA: Tab Books, 1991.

Arnold LM, Auchenbach MB, McElroy SC. Psychogenic excoriations: Clinical features, proposed diagnostic criteria, epidemiology and approaches to treatment. *CNS Drugs* 15:351–359, 2001.

Baker JH. *Mary Todd Lincoln: A Biography*. New York: W.W. Norton, 1987.

Barratt E. Anxiety and impulsiveness related to psychomotor efficiency. *Percept Motor Skills* 9:191–198, 1959.

Benson A (Ed.): *I Shop, Therefore I Am: Compulsive Buying and the Search for Self*. New York: Aronson, 2000.

Benson A. *Stopping Overshopping: A Comprehensive Program to Help Eliminate Overshopping*. New York: Benson, 2006.

Benson A. *To Buy or Not to Buy: Why We Overshop and How to Stop*. Boston: Trumpeter Books, 2008.

Benson A, Gengler M. Treating compulsive buying, in *Addictive Disorders: A Practical Handbook*. Edited by Coombs R. New York: Wiley, 2004, pp. 451–491.

Bernik MA, Akerman D, Amaral JAMS et al. Cue exposure in compulsive buying (letter). *J Clin Psychiatry* 57:90, 1996.

Black DW. Compulsive buying: A review. *J Clin Psychiatry* 57(suppl 8): 50–55, 1996.

Black DW. Assessment of compulsive buying, in *I Shop, Therefore I Am: Compulsive Buying and the Search for Self*. Edited by Benson A. New York: Aronson, 2000, pp. 191–216.

Black DW. Compulsive buying disorder: Definition, assessment, epidemiology and clinical management. *CNS Drugs* 15:17–27, 2001.

Black DW. Compulsive buying disorder: A review of the evidence. *CNS Spectr* 12:124–132, 2007.

Black DW, Belsare G, Schlosser S. Clinical features, psychiatric comorbidity, and health-related quality of life in persons reporting compulsive computer use behavior. *J Clin Psychiatry* 60:839–844, 1999.

Black DW, Gabel J, Hansen J et al. A double-blind comparison of fluvoxamine versus placebo in the treatment of compulsive buying disorder. *Ann Clin Psychiatry* 12:205–211, 2000.

Black DW, Monahan P, Gabel J. Fluvoxamine in the treatment of compulsive buying. *J Clin Psychiatry* 58:159–163, 1997.

Black DW, Monahan P, Schlosser S et al. Compulsive buying severity: An analysis of compulsive buying scale results in 44 subjects. *J Nerv Ment Dis* 189:123–127, 2001.

Black DW, Moyer T. Clinical features and psychiatric comorbidity in 30 subjects reporting pathological gambling behavior. *Psychiatr Serv* 49:1434–1439, 1998.

Black DW, Repertinger S, Gaffney GR et al. Family history and psychiatric comorbidity in persons with compulsive buying: Preliminary findings. *Am J Psychiatry* 155:960–963, 1998.

Bleuler E. *Textbook of Psychiatry*. Translated by Brill AA. New York: Macmillan, 1930.

Budden MC, Griffin TF. Explorations and implications of aberrant consumer behavior. *Psychol Marketing* 13:739–740, 1996.

Burgard M, Mitchell JE. Group cognitive-behavioral therapy for buying disorders, in *I Shop, Therefore I Am: Compulsive Buying and the Search for Self*. Edited by Benson A. New York: Aronson, 2000, pp. 367–397.

Carmin CN. Addicted women: When your patient can't stop drinking, smoking, shopping, eating. *Int J Fertil Womens Med* 43(4): 170–185, 1998.

Castelot A. *Queen of France: A Biography of Marie Antoinette*. New York: Harper and Brothers, 1957.

Catalano EM, Sonenberg N. *Consuming Passions: Help for Compulsive Shoppers*. Oakland, CA: New Harbinger, 1993.

Christenson GA, Faber JR, de Zwann M et al. Compulsive buying: Descriptive characteristics and psychiatric comorbidity. *J Clin Psychiatry* 55:5–11, 1994.

Comings DE. The molecular genetics of pathological gambling. *CNS Spectr* 6:20–37, 1998.

Damon JE. *Shopaholics: Serious Help for Addicted Spenders*. Los Angeles: Price Stein Sloan, 1988.

Davies N. *Diana: The Lonely Princess*. New York: Birch Lane Press, 1996.

Devor EJ, Magee HJ, Dill-Devor RM et al. Serotonin transporter gene (5-HTT) polymorphisms and compulsive buying. *Am J Med Genet* 88:123–125, 1999.

Dittmar H. Understanding and diagnosing compulsive buying, in *Addictive Disorders: A Practical Handbook*. Edited by Coombs R. New York: Wiley, 2004, pp. 411–450.

Dittmar H. Compulsive buying – a growing concern? An examination of gender, age, and endorsement of materialistic values as predictors. *Br J Psychol* 96:467–491, 2005.

Dittmar H. When a better self is only a button click away: Associations between materialistic values, emotional and identity-related buying motives, and compulsive buying tendency online. *J Soc Clin Psychol* 26:334–361, 2007.

Dittmar H, Drury J. Self-image – is it in the bag? A qualitative comparison between "ordinary" and "excessive" consumers. *J Econ Psychol* 21:109–142, 2000.

du Toit PL, van Kradenburg J, Niehaus D et al. Comparison of obsessive-compulsive disorder patients with and without comorbid putative obsessive-compulsive spectrum disorders using a structured clinical interview. *Compr Psychiatry* 42:291–300, 2001.

Edwards EA. Development of a new scale to measure compulsive buying behavior. *Fin Counsel Plan* 4:67–84, 1993.

Elliott R. Addictive consumption: Function and fragmentation in post-modernity. *J Consumer Policy* 17:159–179, 1994.

Elliott R, Eccles S, Gournay K. Revenge, existential choice, and addictive consumption. *Psychol Marketing* 13:753–768, 1996.

Erickson C. *To the Scaffold: The Life of Marie Antoinette*. New York: Morrow, 1991.

Esquirol JED. *Des maladies mentales*. Paris: Baillière, 1838.

Faber RJ, Christenson GA. In the mood to buy: Differences in the mood states experienced by compulsive buyers and other consumers. *Psychol Marketing* 13:803–820, 1996.

Faber RJ, Christenson GA, de Zwaan M et al. Two forms of compulsive consumption: Comorbidity of compulsive buying and binge eating. *J Consumer Res* 22:296–304, 1995.

Faber RJ, O'Guinn TC. Classifying compulsive consumers: Advances in the development of a diagnostic tool. *Adv Consumer Res* 16:147–157, 1989.

Faber RJ, O'Guinn TC. A clinical screener for compulsive buying. *J Consumer Res* 19:459–469, 1992.

Farrell J. *One Nation Under Goods: Malls and the Seduction of the American Shopper*. Washington, DC: Smithsonian, 2003.

Frost RO, Kim HJ, Morris C et al. Hoarding, compulsive buying and reasons for saving. *Behav Res Ther* 36:657–664, 1998.

Glatt MM, Cook CC. Pathological spending as a form of psychological dependence. *Br J Addict* 82:1252–1258, 1987.

Goldman R. Compulsive buying as an addiction, in *I Shop, Therefore I Am: Compulsive Buying and the Search for Self*. Edited by Benson A. New York: Aronson, 2000, pp. 245–267.

Grant JE. Three cases of compulsive buying treated with naltrexone. *Int J Psychiatry Clin Pract* 7:223–225, 2003.

Grant JE, Levine L, Kim D et al. Impulse control disorders in adult psychiatric inpatients. *Am J Psychiatry* 162:2184–2188, 2005.

Hantouche EG, Bourgeois M, Bouhassira M et al. Clinical aspects of obsessive-compulsive syndromes: Results of phase 2 of a large French survey. *Encephale* 22:255–263, 1996.

Hantouche EG, Lancrenon S, Bouhassira M et al. Repeat evaluation of impulsiveness in a cohort of 155 patients with obsessive-compulsive disorder: 12 months prospective follow-up. *Encephale* 23:83–90, 1997.

Hassay DN, Smith CL. Compulsive buying: An examination of consumption motive. *Psychol Marketing* 13:741–752, 1996.

Heymann CD. *A Woman Named Jackie.* New York: Lyle Stuart, 1989.

Holden C. Behavioral addictions: Do they exist? *Science* 294:980–982, 2001.

Hollander E (Ed.). *Obsessive-Compulsive Related Disorders.* Washington, DC: American Psychiatric Press, 1993.

Hollander E, Allen A. Is compulsive buying a real disorder, and is it really compulsive? *Am J Psychiatry* 163:1670–1672, 2006.

Kim SW. Opioid antagonists in the treatment of impulse-control disorders. *J Clin Psychiatry* 59:159–164, 1998.

Knutson B, Rick S, Wimmer GE et al. Neural predictors of purchases. *Neuron* 53:147–153, 2007.

Koran LM, Aboujaoude EN, Solvason B et al. Escitalopram for compulsive buying disorder: A double-blind discontinuation study (letter). *J Clin Psychopharmacol* 27:225–227, 2007.

Koran LM, Bullock KD, Hartson HJ et al. Citalopram treatment of compulsive shopping: An open-label study. *J Clin Psychiatry* 63:704–708, 2002.

Koran LM, Chuong HW, Bullock KD et al. Citalopram for compulsive shopping disorder: An open-label study followed by a double-blind discontinuation. *J Clin Psychiatry* 64:793–798, 2003.

Koran LM, Faber RJ, Aboujaoude E et al. Estimated prevalence of compulsive buying in the United States. *Am J Psychiatry* 163:1806–1812, 2006.

Kowinski W. *The Malling of America.* New York: Morrow, 1985.

Kraepelin E. *Psychiatrie*, 8th edition. Leipzig: Verlag Von Johann Ambrosius Barth, 1915, pp. 408–409.

Krueger DW. On compulsive shopping and spending: A psychodynamic inquiry. *Am J Psychother* 42:574–584, 1988.

Krueger DW. The use of money as an action symptom, in *I Shop, Therefore I Am: Compulsive Buying and the Search for Self.* Edited by Benson A. New York: Aronson, 2000, pp. 288–310.

Krych R. Abnormal consumer behavior: A model of addictive behaviors. *Adv Consumer Res* 16:745–748, 1989.

Kuzma J, Black DW. Compulsive shopping: When spending begins to consume the consumer. *Curr Psychiatry* 7:27–40, 2006.

Kwak H, Zinkhan GM, Crask MR. Diagnostic screener for compulsive buying: Applications to the USA and South Korea. *J Consumer Affairs* 37:161–169, 2003.

Kyrios M, Steketee G, Frost RO et al. Cognitions in compulsive hoarding, in *Cognitive Approaches to Obsessions and Compulsions: Theory, Assessment, and Treatment.* Edited by Frost RO, Steketee, G. Oxford: Elsevier, 2002, pp. 269–289.

Lawrence L. The psychodynamics of the compulsive female shopper. *Am J Psychoanal* 50:67–70, 1990.

Lee S, Mysyk A. The medicalization of compulsive buying. *Soc Sci Med* 58:1709–1718, 2004.

Lejoyeux M, Andes J, Tassian V et al. Phenomenology and psychopathology of uncontrolled buying. *Am J Psychiatry* 152:1524–1529, 1996.

Lejoyeux M, Hourtane M, Ades J. Compulsive buying and depression (letter). *J Clin Psychiatry* 56:38, 1995.

Lejoyeux M, Tassian V, Solomon J et al. Study of compulsive buying in depressed persons. *J Clin Psychiatry* 58:169–173, 1997.

Levine B, Kellen B. Debtors Anonymous and psychotherapy, in *I Shop, Therefore I Am: Compulsive Buying and the Search for Self.* Edited by Benson A. New York: Aronson, 2000, pp. 431–454.

Magee A. Compulsive buying tendency as a predictor of attitudes and perceptions. *Adv Consumer Res* 21:590–594, 1994.

Maier T. Uncontrolled buying (letter). *Am J Psychiatry* 154:1477–1478, 1997.

Marks IM. Behavioral (non-chemical) addictions. *Br J Addict* 85:1389–1394, 1990.

McCall K. Financial recovery counseling, in *I Shop, Therefore I Am: Compulsive Buying and the Search for Self.* Edited by Benson A. New York: Aronson, 2000, pp. 457–483.

McElroy S, Keck PE, Pope HG Jr et al. Compulsive buying: A report of 20 cases. *J Clin Psychiatry* 55:242–248, 1994.

McElroy S, Satlin A, Pope HG Jr et al. Treatment of compulsive shopping with antidepressants: A report of three cases. *Ann Clin Psychiatry* 3:199–204, 1991.

Mellan O. Overcoming overspending in couples, in *I Shop, Therefore I Am: Compulsive Buying and the Search for Self.* Edited by Benson A. New York: Aronson, 2000, pp. 341–366.

Miltenberger RG, Redlin J, Crosby R et al. Direct and retrospective assessment of factors contributing to compulsive buying. *J Behav Ther Exp Psychiatry* 34:1–9, 2003.

Mitchell JE, Burgard M, Faber R et al. Cognitive behavioral therapy for compulsive buying disorder. *Behav Res Ther* 44:1859–1865, 2006.

Monahan P, Black DW, Gabel J. Reliability and validity of a scale to measure change in persons with compulsive buying. *Psychiatry Res* 64:59–67, 1995.

Natarajan R, Goff BG. Compulsive buying: Toward a reconceptualization. *J Soc Behav Pers* 6:307–328, 1991.

Neuner M, Raab G, Reisch L. Compulsive buying in maturing consumer societies: An empirical re-inquiry. *J Econ Psychol* 26:509–522, 2005.

Ninan PT, McElroy SL, Kane CP et al. Placebo-controlled study of fluvoxamine in the treatment of patients with compulsive buying. *J Clin Psychopharmacol* 20:362–366, 2000.

O'Connor K. *Addicted to Shopping . . . and Other Issues Women Have with Money.* Eugene, OR: Harvest House, 2005.

O'Guinn TC, Faber RJ. Compulsive buying: A phenomenological exploration. *J Consumer Res* 16:147–157, 1989.

Otter M, Black DW. Compulsive buying behavior in two mentally challenged persons. *Prim Care Companion J Clin Psychiatry* 9:469–470, 2007.

Richards AK. Ladies of fashion: Pleasure, perversion or paraphilia. *Int J Psychoanal* 77:337–351, 1996.

Ridgeway NM, Kubar-Kinney M, Monroe KB. An expanded conceptualization and a new measure of compulsive buying. *J Consumer Res* 35:622–639, 2008.

Roberts JA. Compulsive buying among college students: An investigation of its antecedents, consequences, and implications for public policy. *J Consumer Affairs* 32:295–319, 1998.

Roberts, JA, Sepulveda CJ. Money attitudes and compulsive buying: An exploratory investigation of the emerging consumer culture in Mexico. *J Int Consumer Marketing* 11:53–74, 1999.

Roberts JA, Tanner JF Jr. Compulsive buying and risky behavior among adolescents. *Psychol Rep* 86:763–770, 2000.

Roberts JA, Tanner JF Jr. Compulsive buying and sexual attitudes, intentions, and activity among adolescents: An extension of Roberts and Tanner. *Psychol Rep* 90:1259–1260, 2002.

Scherhorn G, Reisch LA, Raab G. Addictive buying in West Germany: An empirical study. *J Consumer Policy* 13:355–387, 1990.

Schlosser S, Black DW, Repertinger S et al. Compulsive buying: Demography, phenomenology, and comorbidity in 46 subjects. *Gen Hosp Psychiatry* 16:205–212, 1994.

Schwartz HJ. Psychoanalytic psychotherapy for a woman with diagnoses of kleptomania and bulimia. *Hosp Community Psychiatry* 43:109–110, 1992.

Stekel W. *Peculiarities of Behavior.* Translated by Van Teslaar JS. New York: Liveright, 1924.

Swanberg WA. *Citizen Hearst.* New York: Galahad, 1961.

Valence G, D'Astous A, Fortier L. Compulsive buying: Concept and measurement. *J Clin Policy* 11:419–433, 1988.

Villarino R, Otero-Lopez JL, Casto R. *Adicion a la compra: Analysis, evaluaction y tratamiento* [Buying addiction: Analysis, evaluation, and treatment]. Madrid: Ediciones Piramide, 2001.

Wesson C. *Women Who Shop Too Much: Overcoming the Urge to Splurge.* New York: St. Martin's Press, 1991.

Weun S, Jones MA, Beatty SE. Development and validation of the Impulse Buying Tendency Scale. *Psychol Rep* 82:1123–1133, 1998.

Winestine MC. Compulsive shopping as a derivative of childhood seduction. *Psychoanal Q* 54:70–72, 1985.

World Health Organization. *International Classification of Diseases,* 10th edition. Geneva: World Health Organization, 1992.

Yurchisin J, Johnson KKP. Compulsive buying behavior and its relationship to perceived social status associated with buying, materialism, self esteem, and apparel product involvement. *Fam Consumer Sci Res J* 32:291–314, 2004.

Zuckerman M. *Behavioral Expressions and Biosocial Bases of Sensation Seeking.* Cambridge: Cambridge University Press, 1994.

2

Compulsive Buying: Cultural Contributors and Consequences

April Lane Benson, PhD, Helga Dittmar, DPhil, and Reeta Wolfsohn, CMSW

Introduction

Affluenza, aspendicitis, luxury fever – these often-used, tongue-in-cheek disease names for our modern American plague of materialism and overconsumption boldly illustrate the fact that compulsive buying is trivialized by our culture. Amid this tendency to make light of the problem, a serious discussion of its social factors and social costs, and how to craft public (and private) policies to mitigate it, feels like swimming against a riptide. Yet, unless we focus more on what gives rise to this problem, what it costs us, and how we can keep ever more of it from developing, great numbers are likely to be washed away in a sea of dissatisfaction.

When we put less emphasis on the cultivation of what Paul Howchinsky (1992) persuasively called "true wealth" and more on monetary wealth and possessions, we sell ourselves the costliest and most debilitating bill of goods possible. For the sake of *things* (and our unrealizable hope of what they will do for us), we diminish what really matters: personal and spiritual development, quality time with family and friends, and involvement with community, nature, and the well-being of our planet. This is the devastation that the tide of compulsive buying leaves in its wake.

Social Factors

Although compulsive buying is a multidetermined disorder, social and cultural factors play a significant role in its onset and course. Typically reported only in societies with the mushrooming credit facilities and boundless buying opportunities that characterize a consumer culture (Dittmar 2007; Lee and Mysyk 2004), compulsive buying can be described as a culture-bound syndrome; and globalization is extending these boundaries. On a monthly basis, visitors from more than 60 foreign countries (and nearly all 50 U.S. states) visit stoppingovershopping.com, one of the few comprehensive Web sites for compulsive buyers and mental health professionals interested in this "addiction."

Not surprisingly, there is a strong relationship between the development of the core features of consumer culture – broad availability of credit, endless choice of purchases, and constant encouragement to buy – and professional interest in the problem of compulsive buying. Although *oniomania* (buying mania) was first described as early as 1915, research publications on the problem did not surface until the mid-1980s. Since then, more and more professional literature has appeared (Baker 2000; Benson 2000; Dittmar 2007; Kottler 1999) alongside a proliferation of mass-media attention, self-help books (Arenson 2003; Benson 2008; Catalano and Sonenberg 1993; O'Connor 2005), self-help and online support groups

(Debtors Anonymous; Shopping Addicts Only), and mixed-media programs (Benson 2006; Mitchell 2008).

Two simultaneous social factors have come into play. First is the disconnect that gradually emerged in the developed world (and now even in parts of the developing world) between large-scale *production* of goods and a genuine *need* for those goods. In ever more numerous parts of the globe, economic growth has become dependent on satisfying the new or invented needs of consumers whose essential needs have already been met. Put simply, we now produce such a galaxy of products – many of them nonessential – that in order to sell them, people must be convinced to buy things they do not really need.

To promote that goal, to cultivate in the general public a powerful desire for material goods, a formidable array of resources has been mounted. Advertising and the rise of the media gave the desire a shape, and the explosion of credit cards, combined with the rise in disposable personal incomes, made material dreams seem tantalizingly accessible. Today, in order to promote the ceaseless stoking of economic engines, every one of us is targeted as a consumer. We are pushed, prodded, and *programmed* to purchase. Shopping itself has become a leisure and lifestyle activity, perhaps as a response to the alienation and loss of community so many feel. Malls are the new town centers. All of us are immersed, cradle to grave, in "buy messages" that, with greater and greater psychological sophistication, mis-leadingly associate *products we do not need* with *feelings we deeply desire.* Because compulsive buyers tend to be insecure as well as materialistic (Dittmar 2005), they are particularly vul-nerable to the self-idealizing promises of advertising, promises only thinly disguised as products.

The second factor in the meteoric rise of compulsive buying involves the public's radical shift in reference group. Thirty years ago, the Joneses were the people who lived next door, and keeping up with them – attaining a lifestyle at approximately their level – was not too much of a problem. By the 1980s, the Joneses had become the people we saw on television. They lived farther away – and had a significantly more affluent lifestyle. Soon, everybody, no matter where they were on the economic spectrum or where they lived – but especially in the middle classes – began comparing themselves with the televised Joneses. Despite a marked rise in disposable personal income over the last 50 years, what people thought they needed – what seemed an acceptable lifestyle – shifted so sharply upward that they had to borrow money to achieve it (Schor 1998).

Certain social features are particularly noteworthy. "Neither a borrower nor a lender be," Polonius advised his son Laertes as he was going off to school. But this advice, particularly the first part of it, is largely ignored by both parents *and* children in today's consumer cultures (and even more insistently by governments). Attitudes toward debt have changed from the cautious thrift of our forefathers (there were, of course, exceptions) to today's buy now, pay later (Kahn 2000) mentality.

In an age when everything moves fast – aircraft, information, opportunity – gratifica-tion, too, gravitates toward the instantaneous. Furthering this mentality are today's vastly increased opportunities for credit, an infrastructure that makes it easy to spend money one does not have. Thus, financial constraint ceases to be a barrier to immediate gratification. With lending standards dramatically loosened, consumers have been led to make purchases and financial commitments they cannot afford, whether they have understood this reality or have been in denial about it.

One arena in which this drama is playing out is the mortgage meltdown of 2007–2008, where a slowing economy has collided head-on with a host of unrealistic homeowners. *Intending* to pay more later so they could have more now, these consumers are squeezed between the rising payments of their adjustable-rate mortgages and personal incomes that cannot keep up. A second arena – and one that affects far more people than the foreclosure crisis – is credit cards. In 2005, 2006, and 2007, an all-time high average of nearly *six billion credit card offers* went out to America's three hundred million people – *more than twenty offers per year* to every man, woman, and child (Credit Fact Sheet 2008; Synovate 2007)! By no means coincidentally, these are the only years, except for 1932 and 1933, in the belly of the Great Depression, when the collective American populace had a *negative* personal savings rate: when the average American spent all his or her after-tax income and then had to dip into savings or borrow to make ends meet. Today, the average credit-card-holding family carries a debt of more than $8000, at interest rates often in the teens or higher (Kahn 2008). The depth of the current recession, however, has led to the forecast that for the next several years, consumers, in order to dig themselves out of their deep financial holes, will be saving much more and spending much less. According to the Commerce Department, the savings rate has risen sharply in the recession from the negative rate previously mentioned to a current 5.2 percent of income (Andrews 2009). The Credit Card Accountability Responsibility and Disclosure Act of 2009, passed by Congress and signed by President Barack Obama in May 2009, has significantly impacted the amount of credit offered to consumers (Credit Card Accountability Responsibility and Disclosure Act of 2009). And the Federal Reserve reported on June 11 that household debt has fallen to a 3.5% annual rate, the largest recorded decline since 1980 (Nutting 2009). Consumers are seeing the high cost of credit card debt.

Current economic conditions notwithstanding, the profound shift toward the materialistic is particularly strong among young people, the first generation to have grown up in the full bloom of our pro-credit orientation. Wherever one looks, the under 30s are the most likely age group to be compulsive buyers: in the United States (e.g., Koran et al. 2006; O'Guinn and Faber 1989), in Canada (e.g., d'Astous 1990), in France (e.g., Lejoyeux et al. 1999), in Germany (e.g., Scherhorn, Reisch, and Raab 1990), and in the United Kingdom (e.g., Dittmar 2005, 2007). This age group has stronger pro-credit attitudes (e.g., Lea and Webley 1995) and higher levels of debt. In the United Kingdom, to cite a statistic that may well be typical, over 60% of insolvency cases involve young people under the age of 30 (Creditaction 2006).

In qualitative studies, individuals spontaneously comment on how the ready availability of credit fosters their behavior: "[Y]ou get a bank loan and pay off all your credit cards and then, of course, you've got nothing outstanding on all your credit cards, so you start again. . . . [F]or a person who's not strong-willed enough, it's terribly easy to get into debt" (Dittmar and Drury 2000).

Results from the Higher Education Research Institute, which has polled 12 million college freshmen over the last 40 years, corroborate the steady and profound shift of young people toward materialism. In the late 1960s, approximately 40% considered it "very important" or "essential" to be "very well off" financially. The percentage rose to 50% in the 1970s, well above 60% in the 1980s, and over 70% every year since 1990. Young people, it seems clear, have internalized the culture's materialism. Quite literally, they have bought into the notion that material goods are the way to achieve success, happiness, and a positive identity (Dittmar 2007; Kasser and Kanner 2004; Richins 2004).

As we noted earlier, this materialism is a carefully nurtured credo. A huge, psychologically sophisticated, and omnipresent advertising industry markets consumer items as bridges toward a happier and better self, an enhanced image, and a heightened popularity (Barber 2007). Compulsive buyers, who suffer from low self-esteem, are particularly susceptible to the ubiquitous subtext of most ads, with their purported self-image benefits (d'Astous and Bellemare 1989): buy this product and you can become whatever idealized self you aspire to; fail to buy, and you are an outcast at life's feast. It is no surprise, then, that compulsive buyers are four times less likely to pay their monthly credit card balances in full (Koran 2006). Compulsive buyers lead the charge, both literally and figuratively. Only time will tell what effect the recession, the recent reduced availability of credit, and the increased pressure to save will have on the prevalence of compulsive buying.

The pursuit of material goods, and the tendency toward compulsive buying that often accompanies it, has been accelerated by one more cultural wrinkle, the burgeoning of marketplaces. Augmenting traditional brick-and-mortar stores, powerful new venues have sprung up – catalog shopping, television shopping channels, and, above all, the Internet – and stretched the hand of commerce to wherever you are, however you are dressed, whenever you want. This omnipresence of buying opportunities lends fuel to the fire. Sheer repetitive exposure, both to advertising and to buying venues, makes it easy for anyone, and especially for overshoppers, to see the material ideal as normal, desirable, and achievable. As many as 75% of the buying motives given by QVC buyers are related to compulsive buying (Ridgway et al. 2005), and compulsive buying tendencies have also been demonstrated among online purchasers (Dittmar, Long, and Bond 2007).

As a culture, then, we have moved away from seeking usefulness and quality in what we buy and moved instead toward asking material goods to regulate our emotions, improve our social status, and transform us into our ideal selves (Dittmar 1992, 2004). This use of goods is doomed to failure – as study after study demonstrates. Though it is a particularly hard pill for overshoppers to swallow, the repeated conclusion of investigations into the relationship between materialism and happiness is that yes, there is a relationship – but it is an *inverse* one! Dozens of studies, both in the United States and elsewhere (for a review, see Kasser 2002), suggest that the more we pursue material goods and material gain and the more we invest things with the hope of making us happier (or more desirable, or more the person we wish we were), the *less* well-being we actually experience. And this leads us to a consideration of the social costs of compulsive buying.

Social Costs

The culture, communities, families, and individuals – compulsive buying hurts them all. At the scale of culture and communities, overshopping, as an extreme manifestation of our materialism, leaks away social coherence. Tim Kasser (2002) says it well: "[W]hen materialistic values dominate our society, we move farther and farther from what makes us civilized. We treat each other in less humane ways. We allow the pursuit of money to take precedence over equality, the human spirit, and respectful treatment of each other." More specifically, materially oriented people show a demonstrated detachment from civic concerns and activities. For example, environmental and ecological issues such as global warming and deforestation tend to be of little import to them (Richins and Dawson 1992; Saunders and Munro 2000).

It is at the smaller scale, however – families and individuals – that compulsive buying wreaks its most intense and visible havoc. Here, we see a host of ills: debilitating debt, familial friction, problems in the workplace, and numerous psychological difficulties, such as shame, guilt, depression, hopelessness, and anger (Benson 2004).

Most visible, of course – and it is often a trigger for the other problems – is debt. *Fifty million of us are three paychecks away from bankruptcy* (In Charge Institute, www.incharge.org). While the straws that break the camel's back are typically medical expenses, divorce, or job loss, compulsive spending plays a substantial role in overloading the beast to begin with. Just how bad is the situation? Foreclosure filings, default notices, auction sale notices, and bank repossessions in 2007 were up a staggering 75% from the year before. Americans falling more than 60 days behind on car payments spiked to a 10-year high. Credit card balances written off as uncollectible by banks jumped 24%, with late payments up 16% (Cho and Trejos 2008). During the first six months of 2008, the situation worsened; foreclosures were up 136% from the same period in 2007 (Christie 2008).

There can be little doubt that compulsive buying plays a significant role in all this. A recent prevalence study in the United States found that overshoppers in all income groups had higher credit card balances than normal buyers (Koran et al. 2006), which is no surprise. As far back as 2000, research showed that compulsive buying and the indiscriminate use of credit cards were playing a central role in the record number of personal bankruptcies

(Boss 2006; Morgenson 2008). In the years since then, that record has risen continuously, and today, in spite of recent legal reforms that have made the bankruptcy process more onerous, it continues to climb (Lawless 2008). Compulsive shopping is to bankruptcy as steroids are to home runs. What it compromises, though, is not "the integrity of the game" but "the integrity of the home," the capacity to own or take care of one, to have a financial safety net, to find resources to further education, to retire, or to properly take care of a spouse or partner, children, or parents.

Relationship costs, not the least of which is an individual's relationship with himself or herself, are significant, too. Lying to oneself about overshopping renders an individual isolated, guilty, and ashamed. Lying to others, and begging, borrowing, or stealing, often result in a compulsive buyer's diminished engagement at home, in neglecting or withdrawing from family and friends. Other frequent interpersonal consequences are loss of trust, hostility, estrangement, and divorce. Under the pressure of this compulsion, family and social life are seriously impacted; needs for intimacy, closeness, and connection are not sufficiently met. And compulsive buying – again, no surprise – plants poison seeds in the next generation. Compulsive buying in children is clearly associated with family histories of compulsive/addictive behaviors. It has also been shown to be associated among adolescents with eating disorders, drinking alcohol, smoking, and early life sexual experiences (Roberts and Tanner 2000).

Living with the financial and other stresses of their habit inclines overshoppers toward a raft of negative emotions – emptiness, inadequacy, depression, anxiety, anger, shame, guilt, overexcitement, helplessness, and hopelessness – and damages their health. In a series of studies, Tim Kasser (2000) has reported that overshoppers suffer substantially higher rates of insomnia, stomach problems, high blood pressure, backaches, headaches, and a wide variety of other mental and physical illnesses that inevitably bleed into all areas of their lives. Yet, they tend to forego regular physical exams, regular exercise, and proper nutrition.

Riding an emotional roller coaster diminishes their clear thinking and reduces decision-making and coping skills, leaving them overwhelmed and immobilized. They become increasingly vulnerable to predatory lenders and increasingly likely to steal, gamble, avoid creditors and collection calls, and incur additional debt (Boss 2006; Schulman 2003). The addictive "high of the buy" more and more quickly crashes to the "down of the debt."

People struggling with compulsive buying tend to become less productive at work; they are easily distracted, often irritable, and frequently impatient (Schwartz 2004). Some flirt with the risk of being fired for excessive shopping during work time, whether on the Internet or away from the office in stores. Some out-and-out steal from their employers, falsifying expense reports or worse (Moore 2001). The threat of being unable to meet financial obligations makes them more likely to be late or absent and leaves them increasingly prone to mistakes or accidents, telling lies, or arguing. Often, compulsive buyers work unhealthily long hours, sometimes in more than one job, trying to support a lifestyle they cannot afford.

What seems to get sacrificed in this tumult is personal development. The compulsive buyer generally cannot afford to go back to school or take classes, and a preoccupation with shopping may take the place of intellectual challenge. Hobbies and other ways to nurture creativity are sometimes abandoned. The routes to horizon-broadening travel may be blocked for lack of money. And worst of all, a form of spiritual emptiness may result – overshoppers regularly report feeling "hollow." They are at risk of losing their connection with family, community, and nature (Kasser 2002; Schwartz 2004). For many of them, awareness that growth is about *being* more, not *having* more, seems to have disappeared.

Public Policy

The toll is clear and unacceptable. But how are we to curtail this pernicious addiction, whose roots are woven deep into the fabric of consumer culture? How are we to stop the spread of affluenza, when from the highest levels of government we are told that buying is the patriotic thing to do? "We cannot let the terrorists achieve their objective of frightening our nation to the point where we don't conduct business, where people don't shop," President Bush told the nation in the aftermath of 9/11. "Mrs. Bush and I want to encourage Americans to go out shopping." How do we go about changing the insecurities that lead us to adopt a materialistic value orientation? How do we encourage people to instead begin adopting intrinsic values such as self-acceptance and personal growth, close interpersonal relationships, and contributions to the community and the planet?

Changing the status quo would threaten the present basis of our economy. It would topple a worldview we have been fed from infancy: that more is better, that happiness is the next purchase away or the following one, and that clothes (or shoes, toys, computers, TVs, boats, or automobiles) make the man (or woman or child). So formidable a transformation will not be easy. We can begin it, however, with education, legislation, and, above all, action at home.

On the educational front, every public and private school, elementary through high, should have financial and media literacy courses. These can give students the tools to become knowledgeable consumers who understand the basics about the creation and manipulation of desire and about money management. School districts need to do what they can to decrease the pressure on students to consume. For some districts, school uniforms are part of that consciousness; for others it is refusing to form financial alliances with corporations that want to sell their products on school grounds. Still other districts could discontinue their subscription to Channel One, the ad-studded news program that currently reaches over 8 million American schoolchildren, conveying its message that television and advertisements are more important than live pedagogy. The American Academy of Pediatrics has reported that children who watch it tend to remember the commercials better than the news (Miller 2007).

Research shows that college students and young adults are particularly vulnerable to compulsive buying (Barber 2007; Roberts and Jones 2001). The wide availability and aggressive marketing of credit cards on college campuses to students who often have no jobs, income, credit history, or financial education is a serious enabler of compulsive buying. Pending legislation would restrict this, but the universities themselves could do much more. For example, more college and university administrators could adopt policies to ban credit card companies from marketing on campuses. Also seriously needed on college campuses are more financial education programs for the students. As we have learned from recent disclosures about kickbacks on student loans, colleges are often only too eager for a piece of the financial pie, in direct contravention of their obligations to students.

Adult compulsive spenders, too, need help that addresses their behavior and supports their efforts to take back control of their money and their lives. Establishing targeted programs for them and the general public to make sure both understand the characteristics of compulsive buying and the problems it may cause would seem reasonable. One way to do this might be to use "public service announcements [to] lead consumers to helpful websites [that] provide links to compulsive buying chat rooms, to symptoms lists and outcomes, and to self-help books and free online content" (Ridgway, Kukar-Kinney, and Monroe 2008). Many books, online resources, nonprofit organizations, and adult education courses cater to adults and the problems they face regarding general financial issues. These can be useful when the timing is right, but compulsive buyers also need targeted, specialized help that both addresses the psychological issues underlying their compulsion and gives them the tools, skills, and strategies necessary to overcome it. Programs of this kind are beginning to appear. Some research on their efficacy has been reported (Mitchell 2006), and more is in process. A list of books and online resources that specifically address compulsive buying is available at www.stoppingovershopping.com/resources.

Like education, legislation cannot single-handedly stay the impending "shopocalypse," but it can have an impact. To begin with, the financial industry must be prevented from using practices that endanger the futures of Americans too naïve to comprehend the long-term consequences of their choices – offering credit cards to children, for example, and sometimes even to infants. The Credit Card Reform Act of 2009 will put into effect some extremely important changes, most notably the change in the age that one can get a credit card without a co-signer. As of February 2010, those under the age of 21 will need a co-signer for their credit cards. The only exceptions are for those applicants who can prove that they have an independent income and can make monthly payments (Credit Card Accountability Responsibility and Disclosure Act of 2009).

This same legislation has now made deceptive and predatory lending practices illegal, with severe penalties to thoroughly discourage them. This legislation is a huge advance; it offers protections to consumers including the requirement that consumers "opt in" for over-the-limit charges; full up-front disclosure by credit card companies of repayment information and possible interest rate hikes; and the elimination of universal default (Credit Card Accountability Responsibility and Disclosure Act of 2009).

Further steps are available. The placement or targeting of advertisements could be regulated, as some states and countries have already moved to do. Sweden and Norway, for example, do not allow advertising targeted at children under 12; Greece forbids advertising of toys to children between 7 a.m. and 10 p.m. (Linn 2004). Legislation could be drafted that views advertising as a form of pollution, with suitable penalties invoked against polluters (Kasser 2002). While it is unlikely that we will see *Beware: Shopping May Be Hazardous to Your Health* on price tags, the retail sector can, and in our view should, take proactive steps. A global marketplace such as Ebay, for example – fertile soil indeed for compulsive buyers – could initiate a Shop Responsibly campaign, an analogue to the Drink Responsibly campaigns of the beer companies.

For all that education and legislation can do, the most important bulwark against runaway materialism and the compulsive shopping that it spawns must be the home and family. Overshopping behavior is seeded very early, with infants as young as 18 months recognizing logos and children requesting brands as soon as they can speak (Linn 2004). Kids are assaulted by advertising, the average child seeing an almost unimaginable 40,000 commercials a year on TV alone (Linn 2004). Is there any wonder that children, on whom $15 billion a year is spent pitching products, want what they see there, and want it now?

We believe that the most effective counterstep that parents can take is a long, hard look at their own relationship with material goods, at the messages they are sending their children through their own shopping and buying behavior. Apples seldom fall very far from apple trees. And parents need to face what they already know at a gut level, that placating kids with material rewards is detrimental to their social and psychological development (Bee-Gates 2006).

These things are not academic niceties; they really matter. Some research suggests that, as opposed to their less-materialistic counterparts, materialistic youngsters report more insecurity and less happiness. They are more critical of other people and more likely to have difficulties with attention (Kasser 2002). They more frequently exhibit unusual thoughts and behaviors, isolate themselves socially, and ascribe malevolent intentions to others. They are more prone to difficulty with emotional expression and controlling impulses and more likely to either avoid or overdepend on others. They try to overcontrol many aspects of their environment and may more often relate to people in a passive-aggressive manner (Kasser 2002, p. 17). Their materialistic yearnings seem to overwhelm their desire for healthy social interactions.

Parents who express their love through things are teaching their children that love *means* things. When parents focus more on making and spending money than on being with their families, children learn that money and its trappings are more important than they are.

A healthier childhood is often a simpler childhood, one that puts good communication and quality time with family and friends far above engagement with the material world. We believe parents need to look beyond the traditional benchmarks of success and embrace the importance of passion, spirituality, relationships, and meaningful work in their children's lives (Bee-Gates 2006).

To help children resist the pressures to overshop, parents can apply the same tools and techniques they apply to themselves, identifying the ways that they are triggered and recognizing what overshopping is costing them. Helping children explore *why* they think they need a particular object, discern what they *really* need, and discover what underlying feelings might be triggering their wish for a desired object will pay off in spades. And parents need to talk to children about using money responsibly, about saving as well as spending: the stuff of piggy banks, allowances, and later savings accounts. Other concrete actions include reducing their children's exposure to shopping venues and to television, magazines, and Internet sites with overwhelmingly materialistic messages.

Parents who watch television and surf the Web with their children can use the opportunity to teach media literacy, helping them learn to think critically about the images and information presented by media. Together, the family can identify the often unspoken promises of advertising, then look at the product, and then examine the likelihood of the one leading to the other. Another important step parents can take is to help their children find alternative ways of handling the emotions and needs that propel them to buy unneeded things. They can look for, and enlist their children in looking for, healthy, constructive nonshopping activities, alternatives to consumerism that promote well-being rather than material wealth. Particularly worthwhile are alternatives that incorporate generosity. Overstuffed as many of us are in this life, we are at the same time starved for connection, vitality, and engagement. Generosity feeds these needs and in our view is far more satisfying than getting and spending.

Conclusion

Compulsive shopping is the dark underbelly of the American dream of prosperity. Overshoppers pursue a vanishing horizon, marching, purchase after purchase, to nowhere, becoming more and more miserable with each step. If we are to mitigate the sting and curtail the spread of this epidemic, we must focus on intrinsic values, on making time for mindful, meaningful engagement with ourselves, others, and our communities, on ideas and experiences rather than goods and services.

We end this discussion where we began, with *True Wealth* (1992), Paul Howchinsky's seminal look at materialism gone wild. Howchinsky urges us to leverage those nonfinancial assets, different for each person, that invigorate and vitalize – talents, hobbies, close connections with people and animals, communion with nature – food for our neglected spiritual and emotional appetites. Materialism, he notes, focuses on status, power, and control and cannot fulfill us. True wealth can and does by embracing self-acceptance, personal growth, intimacy, creativity, curiosity, courage, integrity, compassion, forgiveness, and community feeling. Howchinsky's arguments, strong when the book first appeared, seem more and more powerful with each passing year.

But making these changes will not be easy. Powerful forces feed luxury fever. To overcome them, the culture must back away from its fierce pursuit of excess. The legislative steps that have recently been taken, in combination with the educational and personal steps we have outlined, would be a more than respectable start. Above all, we must learn and teach proportion and perspective. *Enough* makes life rich. *Too much* impoverishes.

Perhaps we need to take a hint from the government of Bhutan, which some years ago threw out traditional economic progress indicators like the GNP and replaced them with a revolutionary instrument called the GNH, the gross national happiness. Embracing everything from the protection of natural resources to the promotion of a strong culture and ensuring democratic governance, the GNH puts the overall well-being of citizens at the forefront of national policy. No dark underbelly there!

References

Americans for Fairness in Lending, Inc. Credit Fact Sheet, 2008. Available atwww.affil.org/uploads/Mh/FL/MhFLKwsEfqDFFJKC0e9sRA/AFFILFact-Sheet.pdf. Accessed on July 28, 2008.

Andrews E. Obama Aides See Signs of Recovery but Say It Will Be Slow. *New York Times*, Business, August 3, 2009.

Arenson G. *Born to Spend*. Santa Barbara, CA: Brockart Books, 2003.

Baker A (Ed.). *Serious Shopping: Essays in Psychotherapy and Consumerism*. London: Free Association Books, 2000.

Barber B. *Consumed*. New York: W. W. Norton, 2007.

Bee-Gates D. *I Want It Now*. New York: Palgrave Macmillan, 2006.

Benson AL (Ed.). *I Shop Therefore I Am: Compulsive Buying and the Search for Self*. New York: Aronson, 2000.

Benson AL. Treating compulsive buying, in *Handbook of Addictive Disorders*. Edited by Coombs R. Hoboken, NJ: Wiley, 2004.

Benson AL. *Stopping Overshopping: A Comprehensive Program to Help Eliminate Compulsive Buying*. New York: Stopping Overshopping LLC, 2006. See also Web site at www.stoppingovershopping.com.

Benson AL. *To Buy or Not to Buy: Why We Overshop and How to Stop*. Boston: Trumpeter Books, 2008.

Boss S. *Green with Envy*. New York: Warner Business Books, 2006.

Catalano EM, Sonenberg N. *Consuming Passions: Help for Compulsive Shoppers*. Oakland, CA: New Harbinger, 1993.

Cho D, Trejos N. From Foreclosure Signs to Auto Repo Lots: Easy Credit Gives Way to High Consumer Debt and Defaults. *Washington Post*. February 18, 2008.

Christie, Les. Six months, 343,000 lost homes. *CNN Money*. July 10, 2008. Available at: http://money.cnn.com/2008/07/10/real_estate/foreclosures_no_break/index.htm. Accessed on August 2, 2009.

Credit Card Accountability Responsibility and Disclosure Act of 2009, H.R. 627, 111th Cong., 1st Sess. (2009).

Creditaction. Debt facts and figures, 2006.www.creditaction.org.uk/debstats.htm.

d'Astous A. An inquiry into the compulsive side of "normal" consumers. *J Consum Policy* 13:15–31, 1990.

d'Astous A, Bellemare Y. Contrasting compulsive and normal buyers' reactions to image versus product quality advertising, in *Proceedings of the Annual Conference of the Administrative Sciences Association of Canada – Marketing Division*. Edited by d'Astous A. Montreal: Administrative Sciences Association of Canada, 1989, pp. 82–91.

Debtors Anonymous. http://www.debtorsanonymous.org./ Accessed July 25, 2008.

Dittmar H. *The Social Psychology of Material Possessions: To Have Is to Be*. HemelHempstead: Harvester Wheatsheaf; New York: St. Martin's Press, 1992.

Dittmar H. Understanding and diagnosing compulsive buying, in *Handbook of Addictive Disorders*. Edited by Coombs R. New York: Wiley, 2004, pp. 411–450.

Dittmar H. Compulsive buying behavior – a growing concern? An empirical exploration of the role of gender, age, and materialism. *Br J Psychol* 96:467–491, 2005.

Dittmar H. *Consumer Society, Identity, and Well-Being: The Search for the 'Good Life' and the 'Body Perfect'*. European Monographs in Social Psychology Series. Edited by Brown R. London: Psychology Press, 2007.

Dittmar H, Drury J. Self-image – is it in the bag? A qualitative comparison between ordinary and "excessive" consumers. *J Econ Psychol* 21:109–142, 2000.

Dittmar H, Long K, Bond R. When a better self is only a button click away: Associations between materialistic values, emotional and identity-related buying motives, and compulsive buying tendency online. *J Soc Clin Psychol* 26:334–361, 2007.

Howchinsky P. *True Wealth*. Berkeley: Ten Speed Press, 1992.

In Charge Institute. Research available at http://inchargesystems.com/incharge_research.htm. Accessed March 30, 2008.

Kahn J. Generation Excess. *Boston Globe* magazine. January 30, 2000. Available at: http://graphics. boston.com/globe/magazine/1999/12–26/featurestory1.shtml Accessed July 24, 2008.

Kahn K. The basics: How does your debt compare? Available at http://moneycentral.msn.com/ content/SavingandDebt/P70581.asp. Accessed March 28, 2008.

Kasser T. *The High Price of Materialism.* Cambridge, MA: MIT Press, 2002.

Kasser T, Kanner AD (Eds.). *Psychology and Consumer Culture: The Struggle For a Good Life in a Materialistic World.* Washington, DC: American Psychological Association, 2004.

Koran LM, Faber RJ, Aboujaoude MA et al. Estimated prevalence of compulsive buying behavior in the United States. *Am J Psychiatry* 163:1806–1812, 2006.

Kottler JA. *Exploring and Treating Acquisitive Desire: Living in the Material World.* London: Sage Publications, 1999.

Lawless B. U.S. Bankruptcy Filing Rate Holding Steady. July 6, 2008. Available at http://www.creditslips. org/creditslips/2008/07/us-bankruptcy-f.html. Accessed July 25, 2008.

Lea SE, Webley P. Psychological factors in consumer debt: Money management, economic socialization, and credit use. *J Econ Psychol* 16:681–701, 1995.

Lee S, Mysyk M. The medicalization of compulsive buying. *Soc Sci Med* 58:1709–1718, 2004.

Lejoyeux M, Haberman N, Solomon J et al. Comparison of buying behavior in depressed patients presenting with and without compulsive buying. *Compr Psychiatry* 40:51–56, 1999.

Linn S. *Consuming Kids.* New York: Anchor Books, 2004.

Miller L. NBC News to Provide Content for Channel One. *New York Times* online, July 9, 2007. Available at www.nytimes.com/2007/07/09/business/media/09channel.html?partner=rssnyt&emc=rss. Accessed March 30, 2008.

Mitchell J. *Cognitive Behavioral Therapy for Compulsive Buying Disorder.* Behaviour Research and Therapy 44. *Science Direct,* 2006. Available at www.sciencedirect.com.

Mitchell J. *Compulsive Buying Self-Help Manual.* Fargo, ND: NRI Press, 2008.

Moore B. Out of the Mall and into Court: The 'Shopaholic Defense' Successful 'Retail Therapy' Argument Is a Wake-up Call for a Consumer-Driven Culture. *Los Angeles Times* home edition, July 6, 2001, p. E-1.

Morgenson G. Given a Shovel, Americans Dig Deeper into Debt. *New York Times,* Business, July 20, 2008.

Nutting, Rex. Household wealth drops for 7th straight quarter [Market Watch : The Wall Street Journal]. June 11, 2009. Available at: http://www.marketwatch.com/story/household-wealth-drops-for-7th-straight-quarter-200961112100. Accessed on July 31, 2009.

O'Connor K. *Addicted to Shopping and Other Issues Women Have with Money.* Eugene, OR: Harvest House, 2005.

O'Guinn TC, Faber RT. Compulsive buying: A phenomenological explanation. *J Consum Res* 16:147–157, 1989.

Richins M. The material values scale: Measurement properties and development of a short form. *J Consum Res* 31:209–219, 2004.

Richins M, Dawson S. Materialism as a consumer value: Measure development and validation. *J Consum Res* 19:303–318, 1992.

Ridgway NM, Kukar-Kinney M, Monroe K. An expanded conceptualization and a new measure of compulsive buying. *J Consum Res,* 2008.

Ridgway NM, Menon G, Akshay R et al. Hi, I'm a compulsive buyer: A content analysis of themes from testimonial telephone calls at QVC. *Adv Consum Res* 32:431–436, 2005.

Roberts J, Jones E. Money attitudes, credit card use, and compulsive buying among American college students. *J Consum Affairs* 35:213–240, 2001.

Roberts J, Tanner J. Compulsive buying a risky behavior among adolescents. *Psychol Rep* 86:763–770, 2000.

Saunders S, Munro D. The construction and validation of a consumer orientation questionnaire (SCOI) designed to measure Fromm's (1955) "Marketing Character" in Australia. *Soc Behavd Pers* 28:219–240, 2000.

Scherhorn G, Reisch LA, Raab G. Addictive buying in West Germany: An empirical investigation. *J Consum Policy* 13:155–189, 1990.

Schor J. *The Overspent American: Upscaling, Downshifting, and the New Consumer.* New York: Basic Books, 1998.

Schulman T. *Something for Nothing: Shoplifting Addiction and Recovery.* West Conshohocken, PA: Infinity, 2003.

Schwartz B. *The Paradox of Choice: Why More Is Less.* New York: Harper Collins, 2004.

Shopping Addicts Only. http://health.groups.yahoo.com/group/Shoppingaddictsonly/. Accessed July 25, 2008.

Synovate. U.S. Credit Card Mail Offers Expected to Reach 5.3 Billion in 2007: Synovate Mail Monitor Predicts Slight Dip in Overall Volume, Increased Response Rates. Market Research World. New York: Research Portals Ltd., October 12, 2007. Available at www.marketresearchworld.net/index.php?option=content&task=view&id=1667&Itemid=. Accessed on July 28, 2008.

3

Kleptomania: Clinical Aspects

Lorrin M. Koran, MD, Dana Bodnik, MD, and Pinhas N. Dannon, MD

Introduction

Kleptomania is characterized by recurrent, strong, sudden urges to steal items that one does not need and that have little value, or that one can afford to purchase. The word "kleptomania" is derived from two Greek words: κλέπτειν (kleptein, "to steal"), and μανία ("mania"). Although kleptomania was first described more than 170 years ago, no treatment has been demonstrated to be clearly and commonly effective.

History of Attention to the Disorder

Kleptomanic stealing has long been noted. In the eighteenth century, Franz Joseph Gall, a German neurophysiologist, pointed out that "Victor Amadis, the King of Sardinia, on all occasions appropriated trifling articles." Gall also described an educated Prussian officer who "had so decided a propensity to steal, that often on parade he took away the handkerchiefs of the officers" (Bucknill 1863). An early legal case involved Mrs. Jane Leigh-Perrot, Jane Austen's aunt, a wealthy woman who stole lace repeatedly (James 1977).

Fullerton and Punj (2004), Goldman (1991), and Murray (1992) provide detailed histories of the concepts and theories surrounding kleptomania. To summarize briefly, kleptomania was defined by Matthey (1816) as the act of compulsively stealing worthless or unneeded objects; he termed this behavior "klopemania," or stealing insanity (McElroy et al. 1991a). In 1838, Marc and Esquirol, in describing a case, coined the term "kleptomania" (Marc and Esquirol 1838). Esquirol reported that the individual with this disorder frequently tries to avoid the stealing behavior, which Esquirol postulated was by its nature irresistible. He wrote: "[V]oluntary control is deeply compromised: the patient is constrained to practice acts which are dictated neither by his reasoning, nor by his emotions, acts that his conscience condemns, but over which he has no conscious control" (Esquirol 1845). In the late 1800s, some writers attributed kleptomania to the intoxicating atmosphere of the newly invented urban department stores (Fullerton and Punj 2004). In the nineteenth and early twentieth centuries, the discussion of kleptomania became part of the ongoing medical debate about the relationship of insanity to the female reproductive system and the menstrual cycle. During the first half of the twentieth century, psychoanalytic writers asserted that kleptomania had roots in unconscious conflicts related to the Oedipus complex, penis envy, castration fear, or forced loss of mother's milk (via weaning). Psychoanalysts interpreted the syndrome as reflecting an unconscious ego defense against anxiety, forbidden instincts or wishes, unresolved conflicts, or sexual drives (Goldman 1991). In the early 1900s, the labeling of selected shoplifters as kleptomaniacs largely disappeared. This may have occurred in part because the scientific community was unable to prove that female reproductive issues caused shoplifting and because more men than women were being arrested for shoplifting (Murray 1992).

Kleptomania was included in the first *Diagnostic and Statistical Manual* of the American Psychiatric Association (DSM-I 1952) as a supplementary term, rather than as an official diagnosis, but was omitted from DSM-II (1968) entirely. In DSM-III (1980), it reappeared within the diagnostic category of impulse control disorders not elsewhere classified, where it remains in DSM-IV-TR (American Psychiatric Association 2000).

Diagnosis

The DSM-IV-TR gives the following diagnostic criteria for kleptomania (Code 312.32) (American Psychiatric Association 2000):

A. Recurrent failure to resist impulses to steal objects that are not needed for personal use or for their monetary value.
B. Increasing sense of tension immediately before committing the theft.
C. Pleasure, gratification, or relief at the time of committing the theft.
D. The stealing is not committed to express anger or revenge and is not in response to a delusion or a hallucination.
E. The stealing is not better accounted for by conduct disorder, a manic episode, or antisocial personality disorder.

Kleptomania is classified in the *International Classification of Diseases* of the World Health Organization (ICD-10) (Code F63.2) under the heading of habit and impulse disorders (World Health Organization 1992) together with pathological gambling, pyromania, and trichotillomania. Both DSM-IV-TR and ICD-10 specify the presence of a recurrent failure to resist the impulse to steal despite the ego-dystonic nature of the impulse and the awareness of the wrongfulness of the act. The ICD-10 describes as diagnostic indicators the absence of an accomplice; the presence of attempts at concealment; and the presence of associated anxiety, despondency, or guilt that do not prevent continued stealing. DSM-IV-TR considers these findings Diagnostic Features or Associated Features rather than Diagnostic Criteria. ICD-10 excludes a diagnosis of kleptomania "when the acts are more carefully planned, and there is an obvious motive of personal gain," as well as when stealing is related to an organic mental disorder (Codes F00–F09) or a depressive disorder (Codes F30–F33).

Individuals with kleptomania typically suffer from emotional distress and/or impaired functioning in social and occupational areas.

Within the legal system, kleptomania is not classified as a form of insanity (i.e., does not qualify as an insanity defense), and individuals are held responsible for stealing except when a complete lack of control over their actions can definitely be established (see Chapter 4).

Differential Diagnosis

Kleptomania must be distinguished from other forms of shoplifting, such as professional shoplifting (characterized by profit-seeking or stealing for personal use and lack of moral conflict); shoplifting by teenagers (motivated by a desire to impress peers); shoplifting by substance abusers (to support a drug habit); shoplifting by an absent-minded individual (inadvertent shoplifting [Murray 1992]); and shoplifting associated with mania, conduct disorder, and antisocial personality disorder.

Kleptomania has occasionally been reported to stem from neurological disorders. Aizer, Lowengrub, and Dannon (2004) reported two patients who developed kleptomania after closed head trauma, and other authors have demonstrated links with medical conditions such as frontal lobe damage (Kozian 2001), left temporal lobe epilepsy (Kaplan 2007), dementia (Mendez 1988), large sellar craniopharyngioma with right-sided extension (Nyffler and Regard 2001), carbon monoxide poisoning (Gürlek et al. 2007), and hypoglycemia secondary to an insulinoma (Segal 1976).

Clinical Picture

The clinical picture is derived from case reports and case series that, having been produced over more than a century, differ widely in methods and the information presented. Still, a consensus exists that the stealing behavior associated with kleptomania commonly leads to personal stress, social and marital dysfunction, and often to legal problems. The stealing usually occurs without premeditation or planning and without rationally weighing the risks and consequences of being apprehended (McElroy et al. 1991a). Triggers for stealing include seeing particular objects, sights and sounds within stores, depression, anxiety, boredom, anger, and awakening with stealing urges (Aboujaoude et al. 2004; Grant and Kim 2002a). Items are most frequently stolen from stores but may be taken also or instead from friends, relatives, or workplaces.

The person recognizes that the stealing is wrong but feels compelled or driven to take the item(s). Case reports indicate that the stealing behavior may be associated with a sense of relief of tension, with pleasure, or both (Goldman 1991). The stolen objects may be discarded, given away, hidden, hoarded, or returned (Grant and Kim 2002a; McElroy et al. 1991a). Many individuals who suffer from kleptomania develop self-control strategies in an effort to refrain from the act. They may avoid shopping malls, for instance, go shopping only when accompanied by others, or avoid going shopping altogether (Glover 1985; Gudjonsson 1987). They may socially isolate themselves in an attempt to eliminate the opportunities to steal (McElroy et al. 1991a, 1991b; McElroy, Keck, and Phillips 1995; Presta et al. 2002).

The syndrome appears to afflict women two to three times more often than men (Goldman 1991; Grant and Potenza 2008; McElroy et al. 1991a), and some researchers have posited an association between kleptomanic acts and menstruation or the premenstrual period (Bradford and Balmaceda 1983). But these gender differences may instead reflect differences in help-seeking behavior or in legal system labeling of women versus men apprehended for stealing (Goldman 1991). Examining a series of 95 consecutive adults with DSM-IV kleptomania recruited between 2001 and 2007 by means of advertisements and referrals for participation in research studies, Grant and Potenza (2008) found that women with kleptomania were significantly more likely to be married (47% vs. 26%), start shoplifting at a later age (21 vs. 14 years of age), steal items for the household, and hoard stolen goods. Men were more likely to steal electronic goods. In this series, subjects reported stealing a mean of 2.0 ± 1.8 times/week and experiencing urges to steal a mean of 3.8 ± 2.4 days/week.

Assessment Instruments

The Kleptomania Symptom Assessment Scale (K-SAS) is an 11-item self-rated scale, with each item scored from 0 to 4. The items ask the individual to consider the past 7 days and to rate the average severity, frequency, duration, and control over stealing urges; the average frequency, duration, and control over stealing thoughts; the degree of excitement before and during stealing; the distress caused by stealing; and the related life difficulties or consequences. In a small study ($n = 12$), the K-SAS showed reasonable test-retest reliability at one week ($r = 0.572$), good internal consistency (Cronbach's alpha $= 0.903$), and substantial convergent validity when compared with the Clinical Global Impressions-Improvement scale and Global Assessment of Functioning scores (Grant and Kim 2002b). The Structured Clinical Interview for Kleptomania (SCI-K) provides a reliable and valid means of establishing the presence of DSM-IV kleptomania and excludes stealing due to hypomania, mania, or antisocial personality disorder (Grant, Kim, and McCabe 2006; Grant and Potenza 2008). Its use would be appropriate for research studies but is not necessary in clinical practice.

Prevalence

The prevalence of kleptomania in the U.S. general population is unknown but has been estimated at 6 people per 1,000 (Goldman 1991). This estimate was made by multiplying the rate of DSM-III-R kleptomania among a group of patients with bulimia (24%) by the prevalence of bulimia in a large nonreferred adolescent population (2.5%). Kleptomania is thought to account for about 5% of shoplifting, which translated in 2002 into a $500 million annual loss for retail businesses, although this figure is uncertain because the percentage of shoplifters receiving a kleptomania diagnosis after court-ordered evaluations ranges from zero to as high as 10% (Goldman 1991). Kleptomania also creates costs for the legal system, accounting for about 5% of approximately 2 million Americans who are charged with shoplifting annually or, in other words, for the costs associated with about 100,000 arrests (Goldman 1998). In one series of 40 individuals recruited by means of radio and newspaper advertisements for participation in a medication study, 31 subjects (77.5%) had been arrested for shoplifting and 7 (17.5%) had served jail time (Aboujaoude, Gamel, and Koran 2004). The mean number of arrests for all 40 subjects was 2.4 (median 2, range 0 to 10). In a larger series ($n = 95$) of subjects recruited for research studies, 66% had been arrested and 33% had received jail or prison terms (Grant and Potenza 2008).

Age at Onset and Natural History

Symptoms may begin in childhood, adolescence, or even late life (McNeilly and Burke 1998), but the average age of onset was the mid-teens to the mid-20s in several studies (Goldman 1991; Grant and Potenza 2008; McElroy et al. 1991b; Presta et al. 2002). The kleptomania behavior may be episodic or continuous and chronic in nature. Some individuals experience long periods of remission between episodes. In five (25%) cases reported by McElroy et al. (1991b), kleptomania had stopped "permanently," but the disorder was continuous or characterized by only weeks or months of remission in ten (50%). The long-term natural history is not definitely known because no extended prospective studies have been conducted.

Effects on Quality of Life

The emotional distress, stress, potential marital conflict, arrests, and jail time associated with kleptomania undoubtedly diminish patients' quality of life (QOL). In a study of 30 patients with kleptomania, Grant and Kim (2005) found that their subjects' QOL was significantly lower than that of normal controls and did not differ from the poor QOL of a concurrently evaluated group of pathological gamblers. Quality of life was measured with the Quality of Life Inventory, a 16-item self-administred scale assessing health, work, recreation, friendships, love relationships, home, self-esteem, and standard of living. Individual item scores were not reported.

Biological Studies

We are unaware of any studies elucidating pathophysiological factors in kleptomania, but Baylé et al. (2003) found no abnormalities in the CT scans and EEGs of four patients.

Table 3.1 Lifetime prevalence of psychiatric conditions in subjects with DSM-IV kleptomania

Comorbid Condition	Grant & Potenza (2008) $n = 95$	Aboujaoude et al. (2004) $n = 40$	Dannon et al. (2004) $n = 21$	Presta et al. (2002) $n = 20$
Major depressive disorder	39%	35%	33%	15%
Bipolar I disorder	–	excluded	5%	20%
Bipolar II disorder	10% (I & II)	excluded	19%	40%
Generalized anxiety disorder	21% (any anxiety disorder)	5%	5%	5%
OCD	not reported	5%	9%	60%
Compulsive buying disorder	24% ($n = 68$ women)	3%	not reported	not reported
Anorexia nervosa	2%	3%	not reported	10%
Bulimia nervosa	12%	3%	not reported	25%
Cannabis abuse	16% (any drug)	5%	9% (any drug)	not reported
Methamphetamine abuse	not reported	3%	not reported	15% (stimulants)
Cocaine abuse	not reported	8%	not reported	–
Alcohol abuse/dependence	30%	8%	not reported	25%
Attention deficit hyperactivity disorder	6%	8%	9%	15%

Comorbid Conditions

Kleptomania patients are highly likely to suffer from comorbid psychiatric disorders, most notably mood disorders, anxiety disorders, eating disorders (among women patients), other impulse control disorders, and alcohol and other psychoactive substance abuse/dependence disorders (Aboujaoude, Gamel, and Koran 2004; Baylé et al. 2003; Dannon et al. 2004; Grant and Potenza 2008; McElroy et al. 1991b, 1996; McElroy, Keck, and Phillips 1995). Table 3.1 displays the lifetime prevalence of associated psychiatric disorders reported in the four largest studies. Because these rates describe individuals who are seeking treatment, the data may suffer from ascertainment bias; that is, these rates may not apply to kleptomaniacs in the community who have not sought treatment.

Despite the very high prevalence of comorbid mood disorders, depression may, in some cases, be a result of kleptomania rather than a cause. Many kleptomania patients suffering from anxiety and depression describe a gradually increasing experience of these mood states as a result of their feelings of guilt about stealing (Dannon et al. 2004; Presta et al. 2002). On the other hand, some patients with kleptomania describe depressed moods as motivating stealing episodes (Aboujaoude, Gamel, and Koran 2004; Grant and Kim 2002a).

With regard to gender-associated differences, in the largest published series ($n = 95$), current other impulse control disorders were significantly more common in men (52%) than in women (27%), primarily because of the greater frequency of intermittent explosive disorder and compulsive sexual behaviors in the men (Grant and Potenza 2008). Lifetime eating disorders were significantly more common in women (19%) than in men (0%), as were biploar spectrum disorders (13% vs. 0%). These significant gender differences in the bipolar disorder and impulse control disorder categories were also observed in a smaller series ($n = 20$) (Presta et al. 2002).

Kleptomania has been linked heuristically to three groups of disorders in efforts to explore potential treatment approaches: (1) the "affective" spectrum, (2) the "obsessive-compulsive" spectrum, and (3) the "impulse control" disorders. Hudson and Pope proposed the existence of "affective spectrum disorders" and asserted a relationship between mood disorders and kleptomania, OCD, eating disorders, and panic disorder (Hudson and Pope 1990; McElroy et al. 1992, 1996). A link between kleptomania and affective disorders was supported by the high rate of comorbid affective disorders in kleptomania patients. Joined by McElroy, these authors based their theory on: (1) phenomenological similarities, including harmful, dangerous, or pleasurable behaviors, impulsivity, and affective symptoms and dysregulation; (2) similar onset in adolescence or early adulthood and episodic and/or chronic course; (3) high comorbidity of kleptomania and mood disorders, and similar comorbidity with other psychiatric disorders; (4) elevated familial rates of mood disorder; (5) possible abnormalities in central serotonergic and noradrenergic neurotransmission; and (6) response to mood stabilizers and antidepressants (McElroy et al. 1996).

McElroy and colleagues (1991a, 1992, 1995) and Hollander and Wong (1995) suggested that kleptomania is associated with strong compulsive and impulsive features and hence should be considered as lying within the "obsessive-compulsive spectrum" along with pathological gambling, compulsive buying, pyromania, nail biting, and trichotillomania. Increased impulsivity compared with a control group has been reported in a study that utilized the Barratt Impulsiveness Scale (Baylé et al. 2003). On the other hand, kleptomania ideation can be viewed as involving obsessions (intrusive, repetitive thoughts or images that produce anxiety), and kleptomania stealing can be viewed as a compulsion, defined as an internally forced act designed to reduce anxiety or distress (Fontanelle, Mendlowicz, and Versiani 2005; McElroy et al. 1991b, 1992; McElroy, Keck, and Phillips 1995). In addition, some individuals with kleptomania exhibit hoarding symptoms that resemble those seen in OCD. Studies of co-occurence rates between the two disorders have produced inconsistent results, with some showing a relatively high co-occurrence (45%) (McElroy et al. 1991b), while others demonstrate low rates (5%) (Aboujaoude, Gamel, and Koran 2004). The OCD spectrum model suggests the use of SSRIs and cognitive behavioral therapy as treatments for kleptomania.

Grant (2006) has suggested that a "behavioral addiction" model may be appropriate. He notes that kleptomania urges share many characteristics with those seen in substance use disorders and that the rate of comorbid substance use disorders in kleptomania is high. This model suggests that kleptomania may respond to opioid antagonists, for which Grant cites supportive open-label treatment data (reviewed later in this chapter).

Controlled studies of personality disorders in kleptomania subjects are rare. Grant (2004) assessed 28 of his kleptomania patients by means of the Structured Clinical Interview for DSM-III-R Personality Disorders. He found that 12 (43%) patients met criteria for at least one personality disorder and 4 (14%) did for two such disorders. The most common disorders were paranoid (18%), schizoid (11%), and borderline personality disorders (11%), with only one (4%) patient manifesting antisocial personality disorder.

Family Studies

Data concerning the prevalence of psychiatric disorders in the family members of klep- tomanic patients are limited. Dannon et al. (2004) investigated the DSM-IV psychiatric comorbidities in 21 kleptomanic patients, 57 first-degree relatives (parents or siblings), and 64 demographically matched controls. Of the first-degree relatives, 21% had current major depression, 7% OCD, 5% bipolar II disorder, and 5% panic disorder. Mean anxiety, depres- sion, and OCD rating scale scores were significantly higher among the relatives compared with the control group, but disorder prevalence figures in this group were not provided. Using 31 kleptomania patients and 35 control subjects as informants, Grant (2003) found significantly higher rates of an alcohol use disorder and "any psychiatric disorder" in the patients' first-degree relatives than in those of the control group but no significant difference in the rates of depression, bipolar disorder, or drug use disorder. McElroy et al. (1991b) interviewed 20 patients with DSM-III-R kleptomania about first-degree relatives ($n = 103$), reporting lifetime experience of various disorders as follows: major depression 17%, bipolar disorder 5%, alcohol use disorder 14%, OCD 7%, panic disorder and/or agoraphobia 6%, bulimia 2%, and kleptomania 2%.

Treatment Strategies

Various therapeutic strategies have been applied to the treatment of kleptomania, including psychoanalytically oriented psychotherapy, behavioral therapy, and pharmacotherapies, including antidepressants (mainly selective serotonin reuptake inhibitors [SSRIs]), opioid antagonists, mood stabilizers, and anti-anxiety drugs. No treatment has been demonstrated effective in a large controlled trial, but case reports and case series describing successful treatment outcomes provide a realistic basis for providing the patient with hope. Selective serotonin reuptake inhibitors have become a treatment of choice, but substantial data support the use of the opioid antagonist naltrexone. The goal of treatment should be the sustained cessation of stealing. Arrest and incarceration only occasionally produce this result, at least in individuals who seek treatment (Grant and Kim 2002a; Koran, Aboujaoude, and Gamel 2007; McElroy et al. 1991b). No long-term studies are available to indicate how long a successful pharmacotherapy should be continued, but one study of 17 patients treated with naltrexone reported continued benefit from the drug over periods ranging from 7 months to somewhat more than 3 years (Grant 2005). Treatment planning will often have to take into account considerations raised by comorbid conditions, especially mood disorders and substance use disorders. In addition, legal, marital, and/or occupational problems related to the patient's kleptomania may require the assistance of professionals skilled in related interventions.

Psychological Interventions

Kleptomania has attracted the attention of two generations of psychoanalytic theorists. In its heyday, from the 1920s to the 1950s, psychoanalytic theory dominated all discussions of kleptomania, and psychoanalytic therapy was the preferred treatment for kleptomanics, whether referred by courts or their own families. A few successful applications of psychoanalytic and psychodynamic approaches have been reported (McElroy et al. 1991a), but patients volunteering for pharmacotherapeutic or descriptive studies nearly universally report that "psychotherapy," which, in view of the dominant mode of psychotherapeutic practice in the United States, was probably psychodynamic or eclectic, has not been effective (Aboujaoude, Gamel, and Koran 2004; McElroy et al. 1991b).

Several behavioral strategies have been reported effective in case reports, including covert sensitization using aversive imagery of nausea and vomiting (Glover 1985) or imagery of stealing and the adverse consequences of being apprehended (Gauthier and Pellerin 1982; Guidry 1969); aversion therapy (Warmann 1980) involving aversive breath holding (until mildly painful) whenever an urge to steal or an image of stealing is experienced (Keutzer 1972); systematic desensitization (Marzagao 1972); and imaginal desensitization involving relaxation training coupled with imagining a stealing scene and the adverse consequences while the therapist suggests that the patient can control the stealing urge (McConaghy and Blaszczynski 1988).

Gudjonsson (1987) claimed that the provision of alternative sources of satisfaction, rather than aversive conditioning, was more likely to help the patient overcome comorbid depression, the need for excitement, and the pleasure presumably achieved through stealing.

Educating patients and their families about kleptomania may be helpful. Useful information can be found via the Internet at www.mayoclinic.com/health/kleptomania/, www.shopliftersanonymous.com/, and www.shopliftingprevention.org.

Informational books and self-help guides include Goldman (1998), Shulman (2004), and Grant and Kim (2003).

Pharmacological Interventions

Antidepressants have been commonly used in attempts to treat kleptomania. Several SSRIs have been reported successful in cases and case series: fluoxetine in two of ten patients, with remissions of 3 and 11 months (McElroy et al. 1991b) and in four patients with remissions of 7, 12, 18, and 20 months (Lepkifker et al. 1999); fluvoxamine, with a remission of 9 months (Chong and Low 1996); and paroxetine, with a remission of 3 months (Krause 1999; Lepkifker et al. 1999). However, the highly positive result observed in the 7-week open-label phase of an escitalopram treatment trial (mean dose 18.6 mg/day, with 19/24 subjects [79%] responders) was not maintained in the 4-month double-blind discontinuation phase: three (43%) of seven escitalopram subjects relapsed, compared with four (50%) of eight placebo subjects (Koran et al. 2007). Moreover, unsuccessful cases of SSRI treatment of kleptomania are reported by others (Grant and Kim 2002a; McElroy et al. 1991b). In addition, three cases have been reported of kleptomania with onset during treatment of major depression with an SSRI (Kindler et al. 1997).

A few cases of success with other antidepressants (trazodone and nortriptyline) have been reported along with unsuccessful cases involving trazodone, desipramine, and imipramine (McElroy et al. 1991b). In our clinical experience, titrating SSRIs to the highest comfortably tolerated dose, as in treating OCD, may be helpful for those who do not respond to initial doses. Response to a given dose should be evident within 6 weeks.

Mono-amine-oxidase inhibitors have been suggested as a possible option for treating kleptomania (Priest et al. 1995). In one case series (McElroy et al. 1991b), tranylcypramine was beneficial in only one in five cases, and only when combined with trazodone.

Opioid antagonists are considered useful in reducing urge-related symptoms, a core element of impulse control disorders. The most commonly used drug is naltrexone, a long-acting competitive opioid antagonist principally of mu, but also of kappa and lambda, opioid receptors. Open-label data strongly suggest the efficacy of naltrexone for some patients with kleptomania. Grant and Kim (2002b), in a 12-week open-label study completed by 10 of 13 patients, found that 7 were very much improved and 2 much improved at a mean ($\pm$SD) endpoint naltrexone dose of 145 $\pm$ 50 mg/day. Nausea during the first week of treatment was the most bothersome side effect. Liver function tests were monitored and remained stable throughout the study. In a chart-review study evaluating response after from 7 to 40 months of treatment, Grant (2005) found that 13 (77%) of 17 patients receiving naltrexone monotherapy, with mean ($\pm$SD) dose 135 $\pm$ 39 mg/day, reported reduced urges to steal, and 7 (41%) of these reported no stealing behavior. A few additional case reports of successful naltrexone treatment have been published (Dannon, Iancu, and Grunhaus 1999; Kim 1998).

These suggestions of naltrexone's efficacy have recently been confirmed in an 8-week, double-blind, placebo-controlled trial (Grant, Kim, and Odlaug 2009). Eight of 12 subjects assigned to naltrexone (50–150 mg/day, mean effective dose 116.7 mg/day) achieved remission of symptoms versus only one of 13 subjects assigned a placebo. Most subjects in both groups entered the study taking a stable dose of an antidepressant, which was continued. Statistically significant rating-scale score differences between the treatment groups first occurred after 6 weeks of treatment.

Grant and Kim (2002c) recommend starting naltrexone at 25 mg/day for 3 to 4 days to minimize nausea, and then raising the dose to 50 mg/day. A clinical response is expected within 2 weeks. If higher doses are needed, these authors recommend that liver function tests be obtained 3 to 4 weeks after starting naltrexone, at 2- to 4-week intervals for 2 months, once a month for 3 months, and then 3 to 4 times per year. By avoiding concomitant use of nonsteroidal analgesics, patients may reduce the risk of hepatic transaminase elevation, which, if it occurs, will abate if naltrexone is discontinued (Grant and Kim 2002b).

Naltrexone is thought to exert its therapeutic effect via the inhibition of dopamine release in the ventral tegmental (VTA) area of the prefrontal cortex (Grant 2005; Kim 1998). The VTA is considered to be the brain reward center, and according to animal studies, stimulation of this area is associated with the subjective experience of pleasure as well as cravings and urges (Anton 2001).

Case reports also support therapeutic trials of mood stabilizers in patients with kleptomania. Lithium was beneficial in one of four cases, and lithium combined with fluoxetine resulted in improvement in two of three cases (Burstein 1992; McElroy et al. 1991b). Kmetz et al. (1997) reported that valproic acid in combination with fluvoxamine was effective in treating a patient suffering from kleptomania with comorbid mixed mania. Topiramate at doses of 100 to 150 mg/day was effective in the treatment of three patients, with full remission after 4 to 8 weeks (Dannon 2003). One patient was treated with a combination of paroxetine and topiramate. In another case report, topiramate was effective in a patient with left temporal lobe epilepsy (Kaplan 2007).

Clonazepam and alprazolam have been reported to produce partial success in treating kleptomania (McElroy et al. 1991b).

Electroconvulsive therapy (ECT) has no demonstrated efficacy in treating kleptomania and should be reserved for treating resistant comorbid depression.

Conclusion

Kleptomania is probably more common than is generally believed. It seems to be more common in women than in men and is usually accompanied by other psychiatric disorders. Like major depression, kleptomania may not be a biologically homogeneous disorder but rather a pathological behavior with various causes and thus a condition for which different treatments will be needed for different individuals. Attention to comorbid psychiatric conditions and to associated legal, marital, and occupational problems will usually be required. Over the past 50 years, the treatment approach toward kleptomania has shifted away from psychodynamic therapy. Cognitive-behavioral interventions have been reported to help in individual cases. An SSRI may be effective for some individuals and should be seriously considered as a first treatment option in new cases. Naltrexone, alone or in combination with a stable dose of an antidepressant, represents another first-line treatment option. Mood stabilizers, alone or combined with an SSRI, can be considered as secondary options. Controlled trials of pharmacotherapies for kleptomania are needed to determine effective drugs, optimal dosing, duration of treatment, and augmentation strategies, as well as to provide some understanding of the underlying etiopathology of this disorder. Controlled studies of psychotherapeutic interventions are also urgently needed.

References

Aboujaoude E, Gamel N, Koran LM. Overview of kleptomania and phenomenological description of 40 patients. *Prim Care Companion J Clin Psychiatry* 6:244–247, 2004.

Aizer A, Lowengrub K, Dannon PN. Kleptomania after head trauma: Two case reports and combination treatment strategies. *Clin Neuropharmacol* 27:211–218, 2004.

American Psychiatric Association. *Diagnostic and Statistical Manual of Mental Disorders*, 4th edition, text-revision. Washington, DC: American Psychiatric Association, 2000.

Anton RF. Pharmacological approaches to the management of alcoholism. *J Clin Psychiatry* 62(suppl 20): 11–17, 2001.

Baylé FJ, Caci H, Millet B et al. Psychopathology and comorbidity of psychiatric disorders in patients with kleptomania. *Am J Psychiatry* 160:1509–1513, 2003.

Bradford J, Balmaceda R. Shoplifting: Is there a specific psychiatric syndrome? *Can J Psychiatry* 28:248–254, 1983.

Bucknill JC. Kleptomania. *J Med Sci* 8:262–275, 1863.

Burstein A. Fluoxetine-lithium treatment for kleptomania. *J Clin Psychiatry* 53:28–29, 1992.

Chong SA, Low BL. Treatment of kleptomania with fluvoxamine. *Acta Psychiatr Scand* 93:314–315, 1996.

Dannon PN. Topiramate for the treatment of kleptomania: A case series and review of the literature. *Clin Neuropharmacol* 26:1–4, 2003.

Dannon PN, Aizer A, Lowengrub K. Kleptomania: Differential diagnosis and treatment modalities. *Curr Psychiatry Rev* 2:281–283, 2006.

Dannon PN, Iancu I, Grunhaus L. Naltrexone treatment in kleptomanic patients. *Hum Psychopharmacol* 14:583–585, 1999.

Dannon PN, Lowengrub KM, Iancu I et al. Kleptomania: Comorbid psychiatric diagnosis in patients and their families. *Psychopathology* 37:76–80, 2004.

Esquirol E. *Mental Maladies: A Treatise on Insanity.* Philadelphia: Lea and Blanchard, 1845.

Fontenelle LF, Mendlowicz MV, Versiani M. Impulse control disorders in patients with obsessive-compulsive disorder. *Psychiatry Clin Neurosci* 59:30–37, 2005.

Fullerton RA, Punj GN. Shoplifting as moral insanity: Historical perspectives on kleptomania. *J Macromarketing* 24:8–16, 2004.

Gauthier J, Pellerin D. Management of compulsive shoplifting through covert sensitization. *J Behav Ther Exp Psychiatry* 13:73–75, 1982.

Glover JH. A case of kleptomania treated by covert sensitization. *Br J Clin Psychol* 24:213–214, 1985.

Goldman MJ. Kleptomania: Making sense of the nonsensical. *Am J Psychiatry* 148:986–996, 1991.

Goldman MJ. Kleptomania: The Compulsion to Steal – What Can Be Done. Far Hills, NJ: New Horizon Press, 1998.

Grant JE. Family history and psychiatric comorbidity in persons with kleptomania. *Compr Psychiatry* 44:437–441, 2003.

Grant JE. Co-occurrence of personality disorders in persons with kleptomania: A preliminary investigation. *J Am Acad Psychiatry Law* 32:395–398, 2004.

Grant JE. Outcome study of kleptomania patients treated with naltrexone: A chart review. *Clin Neuropharmacol* 28:11–14, 2005.

Grant JE. Understanding and treating kleptomania: New models and new treatments. *Isr J Psychiatry Relat Sci* 43:81–87, 2006.

Grant JE, Kim SW. Clinical characteristic and associated psychopathology of 22 patients with kleptomania. *Compr Psychiatry* 43:378–384, 2002a.

Grant JE, Kim SW. An open-label study of naltrexone in the treatment of kleptomania. *J Clin Psychiatry* 63:349–356, 2002b.

Grant JE, Kim SW. Kleptomania: Emerging therapies target mood, impulsive behavior. *Curr Psychiatry* 1:45–49, 2002c.

Grant JE, Kim SW. *Stop Me Because I Can't Stop Myself.* New York: McGraw-Hill, 2003.

Grant JE, Kim SW. Quality of life in kleptomania and pathological gambling. *Compr Psychiatry* 46:34–37, 2005.

Grant JE, Kim SW, McCabe J. A Structured Clinical Interview for Kleptomania (SCI-K): Preliminary validity and reliability testing. *Int J Methods Psychiatr Res* 15:83–94, 2006.

Grant JE, Kim SW, Odlaug BL. A double-blind, placebo-controlled study of the opiate antagonist, naltrexone, in the treatment of kleptomania. *Biol Psychiatry* 65:600–606, 2009.

Grant JE, Potenza MN. Gender-related differences in individuals seeking treatment for kleptomania. *CNS Spectr* 13:235–245, 2008.

Gudjonsson GH. The significance of depression in the mechanism of "compulsive" shoplifting. *Med Sci Law* 27:171–176, 1987.

Guidry LS. Use of covert punishing contingency in compulsive stealing. *J Behav Ther Exp Psychiatry* 6:169, 1969.

Gürlek Yüksel E, Taşkin EO, Yilmaz Ovali G et al. Case report: Kleptomania and other psychiatric symptoms after carbon monoxide intoxication. *Turk Psikiyatri Derg* 18:80–86, 2007.

Hollander E, Wong CM. Obsessive-compulsive spectrum disorders. *J Clin Psychiatry* 56(suppl 4): 3–6, 1995.

Hudson JL, Pope HG. An affective spectrum disorder. *Am J Psychiatry* 147:552–556, 1990.

James IP. A case of shoplifting in the eighteenth century. *Med Sci Law* 17:200–202, 1977.

Kaplan Y. Epilepsy and kleptomania. *Epilepsy Behav* 11:474–475, 2007.

Keutzer C. Kleptomania: A direct approach to treatment. *Br J Med Psychol* 45:159–163, 1972.

Kim SW. Opioid antagonists in the treatment of impulse-control disorders. *J Clin Psychiatry* 59:159–164, 1998.

Kindler S, Dannon PN, Iancu I et al. Emergence of kleptomania during treatment for depression with serotonin selective reuptake inhibitors. *Clin Neuropharmacol* 20:126–129, 1997.

Kmetz GF, McElroy SL, Collins DJ. Response of kleptomania and mixed mania to valproate. *Am J Psychiatry* 154:580–581, 1997.

Koran LM, Aboujaoude EN, Gamel NN. Escitalopram treatment of kleptomania: An open label trial followed by double blind discontinuation. *J Clin Psychiatry* 68:422–427, 2007.

Kozian R. Kleptomania in frontal lobe lesion. *Psychiatr Prax* 28:98–99, 2001.

Krause JE. Treatment of kleptomania with paroxetine. *J Clin Psychiatry* 60:793, 1999.

Lepkifker E, Dannon PN, Ziv R et al. The treatment of kleptomania with serotonine reuptake inhibitors. *Clin Neuropharmacol* 22:40–43, 1999.

Marc CCH, Esquirol E. Consultation sur un cas de suspicion de folie, chez une feme inculpee de vol. *Ann Hyg Publique Ind Soc* 40:435–460, 1838.

Marzagao LR. Systematic desensitization treatment of kleptomania. *J Behav Ther Exp Psychiatry* 3:327–328, 1972.

Matthey A. Nouvelles Recherches sur les maladies de l'espirit. Paris: Paschoud, 1816.

McConaghy N, Blaszczynski A. Imaginal desensitization: A cost-effective treatment in two shop-lifters and a binge-eater resistant to previous therapy. *Aust N Z J Psychiatry* 22:78–82, 1988.

McElroy SL, Hudson JL, Pope HG et al. The DSM-III-R impulse control disorders not elsewhere classified: Clinical characteristics and relationships to other psychiatric disorders. *Am J Psychiatry* 149:318–327, 1992.

McElroy SL, Hudson JI, Pope HG et al. Kleptomania: Clinical characteristics and associated psychopathology. *Psychol Med* 21:93–108, 1991a.

McElroy SL, Keck PE Jr, Phillips KA. Kleptomania, compulsive buying, and binge-eating disorder. *J Clin Psychiatry* 56(suppl 4): 14–26, 1995.

McElroy SL, Pope HG, Hudson JL et al. Kleptomania: A report of 20 cases. *Am J Psychiatry* 148:652–657, 1991b.

McElroy SL, Pope HG, Keck PE Jr et al. Are impulse control disorders related to bipolar disorder? *Compr Psychiatry* 37:229–240, 1996.

McNeilly DP, Burke WJ. Stealing lately: A case of late-onset kleptomania. *Int J Geriatr Psychiatry* 13:116–121, 1998.

Mendez MF. Pathological stealing in dementia. *J Am Geriatr Soc* 36:825–826, 1988.

Murray JB. Kleptomania: A review of the research. *J Psychol* 126:131–138, 1992.

Nyffeler T, Regard M. Kleptomania in a patient with a right frontolimbic lesion. *Neuropsychiatry Neuropsychol Behav Neurol* 14:73–76, 2001.

Presta S, Marazziti D, Dell'Osso L et al. Kleptomania: Clinical features and comorbidity in an Italian sample. *Compr Psychiatry* 43:7–12, 2002.

Priest RG, Gimbrett R, Roberts M et al. Reversible and selective inhibitors of monoamine oxidase A in mental and other disorders. *Acta Psychiatr Scand Suppl* 386:40–43, 1995.

Segal M. Shoplifting [letter]. *Br Med J* 1:960, 1976.

Shulman TD. *Something for Nothing: Shoplifting Addiction and Recovery.* Haverford, PA: Infinity, 2004.

Warmann WA. The use of aversion therapy to treat kleptomania. *Psychopathol Afr* 16:77–82, 1980.

World Health Organization. *The ICD-10 Classification of Mental and Behavioural Disorders: Clinical Descriptions and Diagnostic Guidelines.* Geneva: World Health Organization, 1992.

4

Kleptomania and the Law

Brad Novak, MD

Theft is a major problem facing the American justice system. According to the U.S. Department of Justice, there were 13,605,590 thefts reported in 2005, accounting for $5.3 billion in economic loss (U.S. Department of Justice 2005). Given the common nature of this crime, forensic psychiatrists and psychologists can expect to be called on to evaluate defendants with theft-related criminal charges. Forensic research to guide the expert in such evaluations is notably lacking. Nevertheless, the forensic expert may be faced with determining whether a mental illness such as kleptomania played a significant role in the commission of the theft.

A brief review of criminal forensic psychiatry is needed to demonstrate the legal issues that an expert may encounter when evaluating a defendant who may be suffering from kleptomania. In order for a defendant to be found guilty of a crime, the state must prove, beyond a reasonable doubt, that he committed an illegal act (actus reus) and that he had intent to commit the crime (mens rea). The act must be voluntary and carried out consciously. Examples in which the act may not be voluntary and conscious include crimes committed during seizures, somnambulism, hypnotic states, metabolic disorders, and fugue states (Resnick 2006). Although cases of medical and neurological disorders acting as significant causative factors in theft are probably rare, there are case reports of kleptomania associated with disorders such as epilepsy, normal pressure hydrocephalus, head injury, and carbon monoxide intoxication (Aizer, Lowengrub, and Dannon 2004; Gürlek Yüksel et al. 2007; Kaplan 2007; McIntyre and Emsley 1990).

In cases where both actus reus and mens rea can be proven, defendants with mental illness may have their degree of criminal responsibility reduced because of the mental illness. Most states, as well as the federal legal system, provide for a not guilty by reason of insanity (NGRI) defense. Defendants found NGRI are free from criminal liability but are typically committed to a mental health facility. Even if the mental illness does not cause impairment that is significant enough to meet the insanity criteria, it may play a part in sentencing or disposition of the defendant by underpinning a diminished capacity defense, by serving as a mitigating factor, or by leading the defendant to be found guilty but mentally ill (Miller 1999).

Kleptomania provides an interesting example in the study of insanity in that the disorder could lead to enough impairment to qualify for an insanity defense under a volitional test but arguably not under a cognitive test for insanity. Early concepts of criminal responsibility can be traced back to the Greeks. Aristotle argued that behavior caused by compulsion was less blameworthy than if it were carried out by a person who deliberately chose to commit the act. In Western jurisprudence, the most significant impact on the modern-day insanity defense was the 1843 English case of Daniel M'Naghten. M'Naghten suffered from a persecutory delusion and stalked the prime minister, Sir Robert Peel, but he mistook his secretary for Peel and shot and killed the secretary. The outcome of the case was a new insanity standard that was a cognitive test in nature: a defendant was insane if, due to a disease of the mind, he did not know the nature and quality of the act he was doing or did not know that what he was doing was wrong (*M'Naghten* 1843).

The M'Naghten test was initially adopted by most U.S. jurisdictions, but it was criticized as being too strict a standard. The outcome of this criticism was the formation of the product or Durham test, which stated: "An accused is not criminally responsible if his unlawful act was the product of mental disease or defect" (*Durham v. U.S.* 1954). Because it was less strict, the product test led to a marked increase in NGRI acquittals. Accordingly, the majority of states abandoned the Durham test and replaced it with the American Law Institute (ALI) test, which contained both a cognitive and a volitional prong. This test stated that a defendant is insane if he "lacks substantial capacity to appreciate the criminality of his conduct or to conform his conduct to the requirements of the law" (Robinson and Dubber 2009). The ALI test may be viewed as combining the cognitive test of M'Naghten with the irresistible-impulse test. However, following the public outcry over the insanity finding regarding John Hinckley after his attempted assassination of President Reagan, many states, as well as the federal system, did away with the volitional arm of the insanity defense and returned to a strict cognitive test based on M'Naghten.

One may hypothesize that a person suffering from kleptomania could be found insane based on the irresistible-impulse test but would be unlikely to be found NGRI based on a strict M'Naghten cognitive test. Although cases in which a defendant enters an NGRI plea due to kleptomania seem to be rare in the United States, there have been examples that are interesting forensic case studies. Long before the Hinckley case, courts were faced with the dilemma of choosing the appropriate test of insanity. In 1902, an appeals court in Texas upheld the conviction of a man sentenced to 5 years in prison for horse theft despite his kleptomania "insanity" defense. The court rejected his argument that his kleptomania insanity defense should have been based on the irresistible-impulse test and not on the cognitive right and wrong test (*Lowe v. State* 1902).

In jurisdictions where irresistible impulse is still part of the insanity defense, the expert must first determine if kleptomania is allowed as a potential qualifying mental illness for this defense. The *Diagnostic and Statistical Manual of Mental Disorders*, 4th edition (DSM-IV), includes a cautionary statement regarding certain clinical disorders such as pathological gambling and pedophilia, whose inclusion in the DSM is not meant to imply that the condition meets legal criteria for a mental disease, disorder, or disability. In a U.S. Court of Appeals for the 2nd Circuit case involving pathological gambling as a potential qualifying mental illness for insanity, the court heard testimony by Dr. Ames Robey, who helped draft the DSM-III criteria. He testified that the clinical definition of compulsive gambling as a "failure to resist" rather than an "inability to resist" the urge to wager was a deliberate effort to distinguish this disorder from those defects of the mind appropriate for an insanity defense (*U.S. v. Torniero* 1984). Similarly, kleptomania is defined as a "failure to resist" and not as an "inability to resist" (DSM-IV-TR 2000). Thus, when assessing a defendant with kleptomania for a volitional component of the insanity defense, an expert may need to differentiate an "irresistible impulse" from an "impulse not resisted."

Courts have historically viewed the use of impulse control deficits as a defense with a degree of skepticism. *The Washington Post* published an account of the Charles Guiteau insanity trial in the nineteenth century after Guiteau assassinated President Garfield. Dr. John Gray, superintendent of the lunatic asylum at Utica, New York, testified during the Guiteau trial that kleptomania is: "A word to express thieving. I don't believe in it. I don't believe many of the so called moral insanities. I believe they are crimes" (*State of West Virginia v. Robinson* 1882). Courts have sometimes reasoned that kleptomania is similar to such diverse conditions as alcoholism and child molestation: "A plea of chronic alcoholism is not available as a defense to a charge of drunkenness.... Why not accept a plea of pyromania by an arsonist, or kleptomania by a thief, or nymphomania by a prostitute, or a similar plea of impulse and non-volitional action by the child molester?... This Pandora's box had best be left alone for now" (*Burger v. State* 1968). The 5th Circuit added: "A person is not to be excused for criminally offending simply because he wanted to very, very badly" (*U.S. v. Lyons* 1984).

A 1999 case in Ohio demonstrates the possible complexity facing a forensic expert evaluating a defendant accused of theft who is entering an NGRI plea related to alleged or actual kleptomania. The defendant reportedly entered a store and was observed by a security officer placing six items inside a girdle she was wearing under her dress. She was approached by the security officers, who discovered she had concealed a jacket, a dress, two pairs of pants, and two tank tops in her girdle, as well as other merchandise in her purse. Two forensic experts testified on behalf of the defense. One expert opined that the defendant was unable to refrain from doing the act because of kleptomania. The expert explained that the defendant was not stealing for monetary value and the nonselective and random quality of what she stole was consistent with a diagnosis of kleptomania. The other expert testified that the defendant was suffering from "obsessions and compulsions" and that individuals with mental illness take items without a preplan, without intent for personal use, and without regard for monetary value. The jury rejected the experts' opinions and returned a guilty verdict.

On appeal, the verdict was upheld. The justices reasoned that the jury was justified in rejecting the experts' opinions. The justices noted that the doctors relied on personal interviews of the defendant in reaching their conclusions; however, the facts of the case suggested a different set of facts than the defendant alleged. The appeals court reasoned that the defendant's wearing of an "altered booster girdle" that allowed her to conceal the items was evidence against a lack of preplanning and was inconsistent with a diagnosis of kleptomania. Moreover, the fact that she had stolen from a department store earlier in the day contradicted the defendant's statements that she felt an incredible urge to escape after stealing. In addition, the appeals court reasoned that the defendant may not have stolen random items but rather brand-name clothing for her 11-year-old daughter (*State v. Weber* 1999).

As this case demonstrates, when evaluating a defendant entering an NGRI plea by virtue of kleptomania, the expert may need to rely on objective evidence in addition to the defendant's subjective statements. It may be necessary to determine whether there is a motive other than an irresistible impulse to steal, such as personal use of the items or their monetary value. Moreover, to diagnose kleptomania, one must rule out theft as an expression of anger, vengeance, or stealing in the context of antisocial personality disorder. When possible, an expert should carefully review police reports and witnesses' statements in an attempt to find evidence for a motive for the theft other than kleptomania. Likewise, an expert should request a criminal history transcript to determine whether the defendant has a history of nontheft crimes. Such a history may be more consistent with antisocial behavior than with a diagnosis of kleptomania. Finally, when interviewing the defendant, an expert may wish to evaluate him or her for the presence of psychopathic traits such as pathological lying, superficial charm, lack of empathy, and callousness. These traits may be more indicative of stealing for profit than stealing symptomatic of kleptomania.

Even if a defendant is found guilty of theft, mental illness may lead to mitigation of the sentence. Historically, a diminished-capacity defense was based on the difference between general and specific intent. The diminished-capacity defense was significantly weakened in the early 1980s after the Dan White case in California (Miller 1999). In the "Twinkie defense," White's lawyers argued their client was depressed, as evidenced in part by the typically health-conscious White eating junk food in the days leading up to the shooting deaths of San Francisco Mayor George Moscone and supervisor Harvey Milk. Many members of the public were outraged when White, based on a diminished-capacity defense, received a sentence of less than 8 years for voluntary manslaughter.

Despite the weakening of the diminished-capacity defense, mental illness may be considered by the court as a mitigating factor at the time of sentencing. However, as a review of legal cases reveals, a defendant attempting to introduce evidence of kleptomania at the time of sentencing does so with a degree of risk. Judges may view kleptomania as a mental illness and hence a mitigating factor, or the introduced evidence may lead to increased punishment as an enhancement factor if it reveals a history of repeated criminal behavior. Moreover, courts do not necessarily display leniency even to the seemingly most sympathetic defendants suffering from kleptomania. In 2005, a New York court refused to dismiss the case of a 66-year-old female Holocaust survivor with kleptomania, reasoning: "While [a] defendant may steal due to motivations that may be alleviated or controlled through treatment, it can as readily be argued that individuals who use illegal drugs or who steal to support such addiction are also motivated by such factors as illness.... In a deterministic sense, all criminals commit the crimes they do because they must" (*People v. Meyers* 2005).

A Tennessee court of appeals case in 1997 serves as an example of a defendant attempting to have her diagnosis of kleptomania considered as a mitigating factor. The defendant pled guilty after being accused of stealing $24.41 worth of merchandise from a department store. She was sentenced to 11 months 29 days in county jail. She appealed, alleging the sentence was excessive. She was a 47-year-old, twice-divorced woman with a history of sexual abuse. Her father had died 2 weeks before her arrest, and her elderly mother was in poor health. The defendant's treating doctors diagnosed her with kleptomania, mixed-personality disorder, recurrent depression, and alcohol dependence in remission. According to her medical records, she told her psychiatrist she had probably shoplifted 1,000 or 1,500 times – a statement she denied making at her sentencing hearing. The trial judge found two enhancement factors and five mitigating factors. One enhancement factor, which was upheld by the appeals court, was her history of criminal behavior. The mitigating factors included her diagnosis of kleptomania. The appeals court reasoned that although her instant offense did not involve a large amount of money, her lengthy history of shoplifting rightly led the trial court to attempt to protect the public from these criminal acts (*State v. Downey* 1997). The appeals court upheld her sentence but modified it so she could serve the entire period on probation.

The Downey case demonstrates how past criminal behavior can be used as both an enhancement and a mitigating factor when interpreted as evidence of a mental illness such as kleptomania. A forensic expert may become involved in such a case to help the court determine how much consideration to give such potential mitigating or enhancement factors. Moreover, a court may be interested in a more in-depth understanding of the defendant's behavior in order to determine proper punishment and disposition. For instance, a court may be faced with determining if a person suffering from kleptomania should be incarcerated or placed on probation and encouraged or required to receive treatment. An expert familiar with the literature on kleptomania is more likely to be able to educate the court on these issues.

Patients with kleptomania have significant impulsivity and may have high rates of comorbid mood disorders, anxiety disorders, eating disorders, and personality disorders (Baylé et al. 2003; Dannon et al. 2004; Grant 2004; McElroy et al. 1991; Sarasalo et al. 1996) (see also Chapter 3, this volume). Although there are not enough studies of kleptomania to clearly and reliably define the profile of the typical defendant suffering from this disorder, the existing literature suggests some commonly occurring psychological characteristics and psychiatric comorbidities. One review article concluded that the average person suffering from kleptomania is a 35-year-old married woman who can afford the items she steals and began stealing at age 20. She almost never seeks treatment on her own. A personal history reveals she is unhappily married, may have sexual difficulties, and has been dysphoric and moody for many years. She likely had a stressful childhood and may have a personality disorder (Goldman 1991). Additional literature regarding common findings in kleptomania patients is summarized in Chapter 3 of this volume.

When using a profiling technique in an attempt to determine if a defendant accused of theft suffers from kleptomania, the expert must use caution. Not every kleptomaniac will fit the "typical" psychological profile, and not every shoplifter who seems to meet the profile will have kleptomania. Moreover, as one study suggests, there may be significant similarities between kleptomaniacs and other shoplifters (Sarasalo et al. 1997). This study found that the two groups did not differ significantly in the degree of planning, psychological imbalance, or need for the stolen item in question. The kleptomaniacs did rate higher than the shoplifters on the feeling of inner tension before the theft.

In summary, a forensic expert dealing with a defendant who may be suffering from kleptomania may be asked to offer an opinion regarding sanity at the time of the theft or to educate the court about the defendant's mental illness to help the court consider kleptomania as a mitigating factor. The existing literature suggests it is important to consider comorbid psychiatric diagnoses in these individuals. Moreover, the literature suggests it may be a challenge to differentiate between individuals suffering from kleptomania and other shoplifters. The expert is advised to consider carefully police reports, witness statements, past psychiatric records, and an interview with the client in forming his or her opinion. Finally, in order to be an effective witness, the expert should not simply accept the defendant's allegation that the theft was committed because of kleptomania but instead carefully consider the possibility of an alternative motive for the crime as well as evaluate evidence for psychopathic traits and malingering.

References

Aizer A, Lowengrub K, Dannon P. Kleptomania after head trauma: Two case reports and combination treatment strategies. *Clin Neuropharmacol* 27 (5): 211–215, 2004.

Baylé FJ, Caci H, Millet B et al. Psychopathology and comorbidity of psychiatric disorders in patients with kleptomania. *Am J Psychiatry* 160:1509–1513, 2003.

Burger v. State, 118 Ga. App. 328; 163 S.E. 2d 333 (1968).

Dannon PN, Lowengrub KM, Iancu J et al. Kleptomania: Comorbid psychiatric diagnosis in patients and their families. *Psychopathology* 37:76–80, 2004.

Durham v. U.S. (D.C. Cir. 1954).

Goldman MJ. Kleptomania: Making sense of the nonsensical. *Am J Psychiatry* 148:986–996, 1991.

Grant JE. Co-occurrence of personality disorders in persons with kleptomania: A preliminary investigation. *J Am Acad Psychiatry Law* 32:395–398, 2004.

Gürlek Yüksel E, Taşkin EO, Yilmaz Ovali G et al. Case report: Kleptomania and other psychiatric symptoms after carbon monoxide intoxication. *Turk Psikiyatri Derg* 18:80–86, 2007.

Kaplan Y. Epilepsy and kleptomania. *Epilepsy Behav* 11:474–475, 2007.

Lowe v. State, 44 Tex. Crim; 70 S.W. 206 (1902).

McElroy SL, Pope HG, Hudson JL et al. Kleptomania: A report of 20 cases. *Am J Psychiatry* 148:652–657, 1991.

McIntyre AW, Emsley RA. Shoplifting associated with normal-pressure hydrocephalus: Report of a case. *J Geriatr Psychiatry Neurol* 3:229–230, 1990.

Daniel M'Naghten case, England, 1843.

Miller RD. Criminal responsibility, in *Principles and Practice of Forensic Psychiatry*. Edited by Rosner R. London: Chapman & Hall, 1999.

People v. Meyers, 234 *NY Law J* 2005.

Resnick P. The insanity defense: A historical perspective and modern application. Outline of lecture presented at the Forensic Psychiatry Review Course, American Academy of Psychiatry and the Law, October 2006.

Robinson P, Dubber M. An Introduction to the Model Penal Code. Available at http://www.law.upenn.edu/fac/phrobins/intromodpencode.pdf. Accessed May 23, 2009.

Sarasalo E, Bergman B, Toth J. Personality traits and psychiatric and somatic morbidity among kleptomaniacs. *Acta Psychiatr Scand* 94:358–364, 1996.

Sarasalo E, Bergman B, Toth J. Theft behaviour and its consequences among kleptomaniacs and shoplifters: A comparative study. *Forensic Sci Int* 86:193–205, 1997.

State v. Downey, No. 03C01–9611-CR-00416, Tenn. Crim. App. (1997).

State v. Robinson, 20 W. Va. 713 (1882).

State v. Weber, No. 98AP-1230, Ohio App. (1999).

U.S. v. Lyons, 731 F. 2d 243 (5th Cir. 1984).

U.S. v. Torniero, 735 F.2d 725 (1984).

U.S. Department of Justice, Department of Justice Bureau of Justice Statistics. *Criminal Victimization in the United States, 2005 Statistical Tables.* Web site http://www.ojp.usdoj.gov/bis/cvict.htm. Accessed January 1, 2008.

5

Pathological Gambling: Clinical Aspects

Jon E. Grant, MD, JD, MPH, and Brian L. Odlaug, BA

Introduction

Pathological gambling (PG) is a psychiatric disorder characterized by persistent and recurrent maladaptive patterns of gambling behavior and by a chronic, relapsing course (Custer 1984; Hollander et al. 2000; National Opinion Research Center 1999; Rosenthal 1992). Psychosocial problems are common among pathological gamblers and include significant financial and marital problems, reduced quality of life, bankruptcy, divorce, incarceration, and impaired functioning (Blaszczynski and McConaghy 1989; Grant and Kim 2001; Petry 2005; Potenza et al. 2000; Rosenthal and Lorenz 1992; Wildman 1989). In order to fund the gambling addiction or to atone for losses resulting from past gambling, many pathological gamblers resort to illegal behavior (Blaszczynski and McConaghy 1989; Ledgerwood et al. 2007; Lesieur 1979; Meyer and Stadler, 1999; Potenza et al. 2000). Suicide attempts are also common (Ledgerwood and Petry 2004; Petry and Kiluk 2002).

Diagnosis

Pathological gambling was first recognized as an official psychiatric disorder in the ninth edition of the *International Classification of Diseases* (World Health Organization 1977). It was first included in official U.S. diagnostic coding three years later, in the *Diagnostic and Statistical Manual of Mental Disorders*, 3rd edition (DSM-III) (American Psychiatric Association 1980), where it was grouped with Disorders of Impulse Control (Not Elsewhere Classified) and remains today in DSM-IV-TR (text revision) (American Psychiatric Association 2000). The diagnostic criteria for PG were modeled on those for substance dependence. The evidence supporting this choice and lending validity to the criteria selected has been reviewed by Lesieur and Rosenthal (1991).

DSM-IV-TR requires five or more of the following criteria (Table 5.1) in order to meet the diagnostic threshold for PG (Code 312.31). In addition, DSM-IV-TR requires that the gambling behavior not be better accounted for by a manic episode (American Psychiatric Association 2000).

The DSM-IV diagnostic criteria are more detailed than those in the tenth edition of the *International Classification of Mental and Behavioral Disorders* (ICD-10) (World Health Organization 1992), which requires only that gambling behaviors persist despite adverse social consequences. The ICD diagnostic criteria require only two or more episodes of gambling over a period of 1 year; poor financial outcomes and continued gambling despite problems; an intense urge to gamble that is difficult to control or stop; and a preoccupation with gambling. The ICD-10 description of PG mentions the possibility of associated lying, breaking the law to obtain gambling money, and jeopardizing work and family relationships, and notes that gambling may be exacerbated by stress. Those writing the DSM-IV were careful to state that the essential feature of the impulse control disorders is "the failure to resist" an impulse, urge, or temptation (to do something harmful either to oneself

Table 5.1 DSM-IV-TR diagnostic criteria for pathological gambling

The person is:

1. preoccupied with gambling;
2. needs to gamble with increasing amounts of money in order to achieve the desired excitement;
3. has had repeated unsuccessful attempts to control, cut back, or stop gambling;
4. becomes restless or irritable when attempting to cut back or stop;
5. gambles as a way of escaping from problems or relieving a dysphoric mood;
6. returns often to gambling to "get even" after losing money;
7. lies to family members, therapists, or close friends to conceal the extent of gambling;
8. has committed illegal acts to finance gambling;
9. has jeopardized or lost a significant relationship or opportunity because of gambling; and
10. relies on others to provide money to relieve a desperate financial situation.

or others), thus abandoning the language of DSM-III, which had spoken of "irresistible impulse." The DSM-III formulation was abandoned because it had been used to justify pleas of diminished legal responsibility (Blaszczynski and Silove, 1996). ICD-10 has not taken this step and speaks of impulses "that cannot be controlled."

Differential Diagnosis

Pathological gambling is distinguished in both DSM-IV and ICD-10 from gambling secondary to mania and from social gambling, which does not persist when adverse events occur. Pathological gambling (and other impulse control disorders such as hypersexuality and compulsive shopping) may be associated with dopamine agonist treatments for Parkinson's disease (Voon, Potenza, and Thomsen 2007).

Prevalence

A range of prevalence rates have been reported for PG depending on the study's time frame and the instruments used to diagnose the disorder. Only four national studies and one meta-analysis of state and regional surveys have examined prevalence rates of PG in the general population. The first national study, in 1976, noted that 0.8% of 1,749 adults contacted via a telephone survey had a significant gambling problem (Kallick et al. 1979). Twenty years later, the National Opinion Research Center at the University of Chicago conducted a national telephone survey (requested by the National Gambling Impact Study Commission) of 2,417 adults and found a lifetime prevalence rate of PG of 0.8% (defined as meeting $\geq$ 5 DSM-IV criteria) and a 1.3% prevalence for problematic gambling behavior (meeting 3 or 4 DSM-IV criteria) (Gerstein et al. 1999). Another national telephone survey, of 2,628 adults, used the Diagnostic Interview Schedule (DIS) and the South Oaks Gambling Screen (SOGS). This survey found that 1.3% of respondents had current PG as measured by the DIS (met $\geq$ 5 criteria for PG) and 1.9% according to the SOGC (score $\geq$ 5 endorsed items, or 20). Another 2.8%–7.5% had problematic gambling behavior (3 or 4 DIS criteria and an SOGS score of 3 or 4) (Welte, Barnes, and Wieczorek 2001). The National Epidemiologic Survey on Alcohol and Related Conditions, a recent study of 43,093 noninstitutionalized U.S. adults (with oversampling of young adults and ethnic minorities), however, found that only 0.42% of adults met lifetime criteria for PG (Petry, Stinson, and Grant 2005). A meta-analysis of 120 prevalence-estimate surveys completed in North America over the past 30 years found a mean lifetime rate of 1.6% for PG and 3.85% for problem gambling (i.e., creating life problems but not meeting diagnostic criteria), for a combined rate of 5.45% of individuals exhibiting some sort of disordered gambling (Shaffer, Hall, and Vander Bilt 1999).

Clinical Picture

Pathological gambling usually begins in adolescence or early adulthood, with men tending to develop the disorder at an earlier age (Ibáñez et al. 2003; Shaffer, Hall, and Vander Bilt

1999). Although prospective studies are largely lacking, PG appears to follow a trajectory resembling that of substance dependence, with high rates in adolescent and young adult groups, lower rates in older adults, and periods of abstinence and relapse (Grant and Potenza 2004). But recent evidence suggests that approximately one-third of individuals with PG experience natural recovery (i.e., without treatment) (Slutske 2006).

Significant clinical differences have been observed between male and female pathological gamblers. Male gamblers are more likely to be single and live alone compared with females with PG (Crisp et al. 2004). Male pathological gamblers are also more likely to have sought treatment for substance abuse (Ladd and Petry 2002), may have higher rates of antisocial personality traits (Ibáñez et al. 2003), and more often experience marital consequences as a result of gambling (Ibáñez et al. 2003). Although men seem to start gambling at an earlier age and have higher rates of PG, women, who constitute approximately 32% of pathological gamblers in the United States, seem to progress more quickly from the start of gambling to a pathological state (National Opinion Research Center 1999; Potenza et al. 2001).

Men and women also differ in the type of gambling preferred. Men with PG are more likely to pursue "strategic" forms of gambling (for example, sports betting, dice, and blackjack), whereas women tend to prefer "nonstrategic" gambling (for example, slot machines or bingo) (Potenza et al. 2001). Higher rates of sensation-seeking or "action"-seeking behavior in men have been implicated as a possible reason for this difference in gambling preference (Potenza et al. 2001; Vitaro, Arseneault, and Tremblay 1997). With regard to gambling triggers, both men and women report that advertisements trigger their urges, but men tend to report gambling for reasons unrelated to their emotional state, whereas women report gambling to escape from stress or due to depressive states (Grant and Kim 2001; Ladd and Petry 2002; Petry and Kiluk 2002; Potenza et al. 2001).

The assessment instrument most widely used in epidemiological studies is the South Oaks Gambling Screen (SOGS), a 20-item questionnaire that can be self-administered or administered by a rater (Lesieur and Blume 1987). The SOGS incorporates DSM-III diagnostic criteria and assesses the types of gambling, largest amount gambled in a single day, parental history of problematic gambling, and whether the respondent thinks his or her gambling is problematic. Probable PG is indicated by a score of ≥ 5 and probable problematic gambling by a score of 3 or 4. The SOGS appears to have high sensitivity and low false-positive and false-negative rates (Lesieur and Blume 1987) but may nonetheless overestimate the prevalence of PG when the true population prevalence is in the low single digits (Westphal and Rush 1996).

The National Gambling Impact Study Commission developed the NODS (NORC DSM Screen for Gambling Problems), which is composed of 17 lifetime and 17 corresponding past-year items designed to evaluate the presence or absence of each of the DSM-IV diagnostic criteria (National Opinion Research Center 1999). Scores range from zero to 10, with a score of ≥ 5 indicating PG and a score of 3 or 4 problematic gambling. In epidemiological research, the NODS has several advantages over the SOGS, including mapping to DSM-IV rather than DSM-III diagnostic criteria and producing lower false-positive rates. In 44 individuals with PG, the test–retest reliability of the NODS over 2 to 4 weeks was $r = 0.99$ for lifetime and $r = 0.98$ for past-year diagnoses. A small study supported the validity of the NODS: in a sample of 40 individuals in outpatient gambling treatment programs, 38 (95%) scored ≥ 5 on the lifetime NODS and 34 (75%) on the past-year NODS. Because the DSM-IV criteria are meant to apply over a lifetime rather than a 1-year period and some individuals may have entered treatment to prevent relapse or may have responded to treatment, these results appear quite satisfactory (National Opinion Research Center 1999). Nonetheless, in clinical practice application, the SOGS has the advantage that it can be self-administered.

The 20-question screening instrument available from Gamblers Anonymous generates a high proportion of false negatives (Lesieur and Blume 1987).

Functional Impairment, Health Problems, and Quality of Life

Individuals with PG suffer significant impairment in their ability to function socially and within their occupations. Many individuals report intrusive thoughts and urges related to gambling that interfere with their concentration at home and at work (Grant and Kim 2001). Work-related problems such as absenteeism, poor performance, and job loss are common (National Opinion Research Center 1999). The inability to control unwanted behavior may lead to feelings of shame and guilt (Grant and Kim 2001). Pathological gambling is also frequently associated with marital problems (National Opinion Research Center 1999) and diminished intimacy and trust within the family (Pallanti et al. 2006). Financial difficulties often exacerbate the personal and family problems (Grant and Kim 2001). Pathological gambling is also associated with greater health problems (for example, cardiac problems and liver disease) and increased use of medical services (Morasco and Petry 2006; Morasco, Vom Eigen, and Petry 2006).

Given the functional impairment and health problems experienced by individuals with PG, it is not surprising that they also report poor quality of life. In two studies systematically evaluating quality of life, individuals with PG reported significantly poorer life satisfaction compared with general, nonclinical adult samples (Black et al. 2003; Grant and Kim 2005). Pathological gambling can also lead to attempted or completed suicide (Ledgerwood and Petry 2004; Petry and Kiluk 2002). One study of treatment-seeking pathological gamblers found that 48% had gambling-related suicidal ideation and 12% reported a gambling-related suicide attempt (Ledgerwood and Petry 2004).

Legal Problems Associated with Pathological Gambling

Many individuals with PG have faced legal difficulties associated with the disorder. One study ($n = 231$) found that 27.3% ($n = 63$) of pathological gamblers had committed at least one gambling-related illegal act, but only 5 of the 63 subjects had ever been arrested for the illegal behavior (Ledgerwood et al. 2007). Gambling addiction motivates some people to engage in illegal behavior, including embezzlement, stealing, and writing bad checks, in order either to finance the gambling or to recover past gambling losses (Potenza et al. 2000). One study showed high rates of embezzlement (31%) and robbery (14%) (Blaszczynski and Silove 1996). In a study of gamblers calling a helpline, those who reported gambling-related illegal behaviors were more likely to have a severe gambling problem, owe debts to acquaintances, have received mental health treatment, have a substance use disorder, and have features of antisocial personality disorder (Potenza et al. 2000). Whether the illegal acts are neurobiologically related to PG (Grant and Potenza 2007), caused by the need for money to maintain the gambling behavior (Lesieur 1979), or simply secondary to sociopathy is still open to debate.

Developmental Issues

Whether the development of PG is associated with early life losses or childhood trauma or abuse is uncertain (Niederland 1967; Whitman-Raymond 1988). Some regard excessive gambling as a means of coping with trauma or abuse (Jacobs 1989). Although one study found that 23% of pathological gamblers ($n = 44$) had experienced sexual or physical traumas (Taber, McCormick, and Ramirez 1987), this rate mirrors the estimated general population rate (20%–24%) (National Research Council 1993). A more recent study found that pathological gamblers, particularly females, reported more incidents than control subjects on questionnaires inquiring about childhood maltreatment (Petry and Steinberg 2005). In addition, one study assessing bonding between parents and children found that pathological gamblers perceived their early relationships with their parents as being marked by low parental care, affection, and protection, which suggests neglectful parenting (Grant and Kim 2002). Although retrospective studies have found associations between PG and early maltreatment and trauma, prospective studies remain to be done.

Co-occurring Psychiatric Disorders

Psychiatric comorbidity is quite common in individuals with PG. High rates of co-occurrence have been reported for substance use disorders (including nicotine dependence) and PG, with the highest odds ratios generally observed between gambling and alcohol use disorders (Cunningham-Williams et al. 1998; Gerstein et al. 1999; Petry, Stinson, and Grant 2005; Welte, Barnes, and Wieczorek 2001). A Canadian epidemiological survey estimated that the relative risk for an alcohol use disorder is 3.8 times higher when disordered gambling is present (Bland et al. 1993), and odds ratios ranging from 3.3 to 23.1 have been reported between PG and alcohol abuse/dependence in U.S. population-based studies (Cunningham-Williams et al. 1998; Welte, Barnes, and Wieczorek 2001). In addition, rates of drug use disorders appear to be four times higher among pathological gamblers than nongamblers (23.2% vs. 6.3%) (Bland et al. 1993).

Estimates of daily tobacco use among problem or pathological gamblers have varied from 41% to 69% (Crockford and el-Guebaly 1998; Potenza et al. 2004). These rates are notably higher than daily tobacco use among U.S. adults in general (16.7% to 22.4%) (Fagan et al. 2007; Falk, Yi, and Hiller-Sturmhöfel 2006). Research has also suggested that tobacco use is associated with more severe gambling problems and depressive symptoms (Grant and Potenza 2005; Petry and Oncken 2002).

Other studies examining the rates of co-occurring disorders in pathological gamblers have noted high rates of mood (34%–78%) (Black and Moyer 1998; Grant and Kim 2001; McCormick et al. 1984; Petry, Stinson, and Grant 2005; Specker et al. 1995) and anxiety (28%–41%) (Black and Moyer 1998; Linden, Pope, and Jonas 1986; Petry, Stinson, and Grant 2005) disorders. McCormick et al. (1984) studied 38 treatment-seeking pathological gamblers with major depressive disorder and found that in 86% of cases the gambling problem preceded the onset of depression. This raises the question as to whether co-occurring mood disorders are in many cases secondary to PG (McCormick et al. 1984).

Significantly less information is available regarding the rates of Axis II personality disorders among pathological gamblers. Studies have reported rates of any personality disorder ranging from 25% to 93% (Black and Moyer 1998; Blaszczynski and Steel 1998; Petry, Stinson, and Grant 2005; Specker et al. 1996), with obsessive-compulsive, paranoid, and antisocial personality disorders the most commonly reported (Petry, Stinson, and Grant 2005).

Family History and Genetics

High rates of psychiatric disorders are seen in the first-degree relatives of individuals with PG, including mood, anxiety, substance use, and antisocial personality disorders (Black et al. 2003; Ramirez et al. 1983; Roy et al. 1988). One study found that 20% of the first-degree relatives of pathological gamblers also have PG (Ibáñez et al. 2002). In another study, Black et al. (2006) examined 31 PG probands and 31 control probands. Lifetime rates of PG were significantly higher in family members of pathological gamblers (8.3%) than in those of controls (2.1%) (odds ratio of 4.49; $p = .018$), as were substance use disorders (odds ratio of 4.21) and antisocial personality disorder (odds ratio of 7.73) (Black et al. 2006). Problem gamblers at a Veteran's Hospital were up to 8 times more likely to have a parent with a gambling problem than were nonproblem gamblers (Gambino et al. 1993).

With regard to the genetics of PG, one study examining "high-action" forms of gambling (lottery, gambling machines, casino cards) found significantly higher concordance in male monozygotic (MZ) than dizygotic (DZ) twins (Winters and Rich 1998). In data from the Vietnam Era Twin (VET) registry, genetic factors were estimated to account for between 35% and 54% of the risk for DSM-III-R PG (Eisen et al. 1998). Additional studies of the VET sample have identified common genetic and environmental contributions to PG and alcohol dependence (Slutske et al. 2000), PG and antisocial behaviors (Slutske et al. 2001), and PG and major depression (Potenza et al. 2005). Interestingly, the shared genetic contribution to PG and major depression was as large as or larger than those for alcohol dependence and antisocial behaviors.

Neurobiology

Neuroimaging

There are few imaging studies of pathological gamblers. In one investigation, two gambling scenarios and two emotional scenarios were presented to men with PG and control subjects (Potenza et al. 2003a). Compared with control subjects, PG subjects reported stronger gambling urges after viewing gambling scenarios. The most pronounced between-group differences in brain activations were observed during the initial viewing of the gambling scenarios: PG subjects displayed decreased activity in frontal and orbitofrontal cortex, caudate/basal ganglia, and thalamus. During the period of videotape viewing corresponding to the most intense gambling cues, individuals with PG showed diminished activation in the ventromedial prefrontal cortex (vmPFC). The data suggest that activity in a complex network of brain regions distinguishes PG and control subjects during gambling-related motivational states and that these neural processes change over time.

The neural correlates of cognitive control in men with and without PG were examined via fMRI coupled with an event-related Stroop paradigm (Potenza et al. 2003b). Compared with control subjects, those with PG demonstrated greater deactivation of the left vmPFC.

Another study examined 12 subjects with PG and matched controls without PG using an fMRI task that simulates gambling and involves monetary rewards and losses (Reuter et al. 2005). Significantly lower activation of the right ventral striatum in winning versus losing contrasts was observed in PG subjects compared with controls. Consistent with prior studies (Potenza et al. 2003a, 2003b), the PG cohort also showed relatively diminished activation in the vmPFC. Severity of gambling exhibited significant negative correlations with both the ventral striatal and vmPFC activations.

In an fMRI study examining whether PG subjects exhibited differential brain activity when exposed to gambling cues (Crockford et al. 2005), these subjects had greater activity in the right dorsolateral prefrontal cortex, right parahippocampal gyrus, and left occipital cortex. They also experienced a significant increase in craving for gambling after the study.

Hollander et al. (2005a) performed two [^{18}F]FDG PET scans seven days apart on subjects with PG while they played computerized blackjack under two different reward conditions: monetary reward and computer game points only. The investigators observed a significantly higher relative metabolic rate in the primary visual cortex, the cingulate gryus, the putamen, and prefrontal areas during the monetary reward condition versus the point reward condition. The data highlight the salience of monetary reward in PG (Hollander et al. 2005a).

Although the neuroimaging data for PG are still relatively limited, imaging studies may ultimately allow for more targeted investigations into safe and effective treatments for PG.

Cognitive Functioning

Deficits in inhibition, working memory, planning, cognitive flexibility, and time management/estimation have been found to be common in pathological gamblers. These deficits are important for many reasons. Social, occupational, and marital functioning may be impaired as well as the ability to successfully undertake treatment for PG. Several studies have examined the cognitive processes in pathological gamblers (Table 5.2): (Brand et al. 2005; Cavedini et al. 2002; Fuentes et al. 2006; Goudriaan et al. 2006; Kalechstein et al. 2007; Kertzman et al. 2006; Marazziti et al. 2008; Patterson, Holland, and Middleton 2006; Petry 2001; Regard et al. 2003; Rugle and Melamed 1993). Some of these studies included individuals with comorbid psychiatric conditions such as substance dependence, which is important given the high rates of comorbid alcohol and substance abuse among pathological gamblers (Ramirez et al. 1983). Like comorbid conditions, the presence of psychotropic medication or current therapy must be noted as potentially confounding variables.

One of the first published examinations of pathological gamblers' neurocognition was conducted by Rugle and Melamed (1993), who compared 33 pathological gamblers with 33 controls using nine different measures of the executive functions of attention, learning, and memory. Pathological gamblers demonstrated significant cognitive impairment on the three tests (Wisconsin Card Sorting, Embedded Figures, and Porteus Maze Tests), which are particularly sensitive to attentional problems.

The Wisconsin Card Sorting Test (WCST) is a test of frontal (especially dorsolateral) cortex integrity and measures rule learning and cognitive flexibility. Based upon auditory feedback, subjects attempt to learn a rule about which of two cards is correct. Once the subject has clearly learned this rule, the examiner or computer changes the rule and the subject attempts to learn the new rule based on trial and error (feedback). The three other studies that used the WCST in PG subjects have produced mixed findings. Goudriaan et al. (2006) and Marazziti et al. (2008) have reported similar cognitive flexibility problems in pathological gamblers on the WCST, but Cavedini et al. (2002) found no significant differences between PG and controls.

Pathological gamblers tend to place a greater value on immediate rewards than on delayed ones, as assessed by measures of temporal discounting or by a gambling task (Cavedini et al. 2002; Patterson, Holland, and Middleton 2006; Petry 2001). The Iowa Gambling Task simulates real-life decision making and tests the ability to make advantageous decisions by balancing immediate and delayed rewards and punishments (Bechara et al. 1994). The disadvantageous decision making is thought to involve ventromedial prefrontal cortical function. In one study using this task, pathological gamblers made significantly more choices from the disadvantageous deck than did the control group, suggesting possible orbito-frontal cortex dysfunction.

Regard et al. (2003) compared 21 non–substance-abusing pathological gamblers, 81% of whom had a history of traumatic brain injury, with 19 control subjects, using neuropsychological tests that measure frontal lobe dysfunction. The PG group performed significantly worse than the control group on measures of executive functioning. Concentration levels, memory recall, and language dominance were all significantly worse in the PG group. In addition, 65% of the PG group demonstrated abnormal EEG activity compared with 26% of controls.

Using the Game of Dice Task, Brand et al. (2005) assessed risky decision making by asking subjects to guess which number on a single die will be displayed on a computer screen. Subjects can choose to have displayed one die or a combination of two, three, or four dice. The probability of correctly guessing which number will be displayed obviously increases with the number of dice chosen; however, the amount of possible gain or loss increases when fewer dice are chosen. The subject starts with a set amount of money and is told to maximize his or her capital within 18 throws of the dice. The PG group demonstrated a significant preference for disadvantageous choices (i.e., one or two dice) compared with controls. The researchers also found that negative feedback (losing $1,000 or $500) following a disadvantageous decision did not impact the next decision made by the PG subjects, suggesting problems with the executive functions of cognitive flexibility, set shifting, and categorization (Brand et al. 2005).

Table 5.2 Neurocognitive studies of pathological gambling

Study	Sample Size	PG Subjects – % Male; Age (± SD)	Psychiatric Comorbidity (in PG Subjects)	Treatment Status	Methodology	Key Findings in PG Subjects
Rugle & Melamed 1993	33PG; 33C	100% M; 41.4 (9.5)	Subjects with any lifetime Axis I psychiatric diagnosis were excluded	Never had taken psychotropic medications; ? therapy	9 tests, including the Wisconsin Card Sorting Test (WCST), Embedded Figures Test (EFT), Trail-Making Test, part B, List Learning with Categorical Clustering, Symbol Digit Substitution Test, Knox Cube Test, Primary Memory with Interference Test, Seashore Rhythm Test, and Porteus Maze Test	PG subjects showed significant impairment on the WCST, EFT, and Porteus Mazes compared to controls indicating frontally mediated activity impairment in PG
Petry 2001	21SDPG; 39PG; 26C	67% M; 43 (11)	n = 37 nicotine use; SDPG group, 71% alcohol use; 62% marijuana; 33% cocaine	66% of SDPG received treatment for substance use disorder	A delayed discounting procedure with four counterbalanced ascending or descending orders (rewards ascending/rewards descending, delays ascending/delays descending).	Both SDPG and PG groups discounted at higher rates than controls; SDPG group discounted at higher rate than PG alone group
Cavedini et al. 2002	20PG; 40C	95% M; 38.5 (7.6)	n = 13 nicotine dependent; n = 3 alcohol abuse; n = 1 panic disorder; n = 1 social phobia	Free from medication for >2 weeks; no current therapy	Iowa Gambling Task (IGT), Weigl's Sorting Test (WST), and Wisconsin Card Sorting Test (WCST)	No significant differences on WST or WCST. PG subjects performed significantly worse on IGT, indicating orbitofrontal cortex dysfunction
Regard et al. 2003	21PG; 19C	95% M; 33.6 (range 17–59)	n = 3 major depression; n = 5 past suicide attempt; n = 1 bulimia; n = 17 history of brain injury	Current psychotropic medication use allowed; question re therapy; no substance abuse was allowed	Measures of concentration, executive functioning, and memory; Rey Auditory Verbal Learning and Figural Learning Test, Stroop Interference Test, Word-Fluency and Five-Point Test, Goldenberg Association Learning and Concept Identification Test, and EEG	Significant impairment in concentration, executive functioning, language dominance, and memory in PG sample compared to controls; abnormal EEG findings in PG
Brand et al. 2005	25PG; 25C	100% M; 40.08 (10.12)	n = 21 nicotine use; n = 3 mild depression; no substance use was allowed.	No subjects with current or lifetime disorders	Modified Card Sorting Test (MCST), Word-Color Interference Test, and the Game of Dice Test	PG had significantly greater impairment on Game of Dice Test and MCST suggesting decision-making impairment

Study	Sample	% M; Age	Psychiatric comorbidity	Medication/treatment	Tests	Findings
Fuentes et al. 2006	214 PG (162CPG, 52NCPG); 82C	50% M; 42.7	$n = 133$ depressive disorder; $n = 77$ anxiety disorder; $n = 45$ substance use disorder; $n = 147$ nicotine dependence	No current psychiatric medications allowed	Auditory and visual reaction Go/No-Go Tasks	Both CPG and NCPG groups performed significantly worse on both the auditory and visual Go/No-Go than controls suggesting poor information processing
Kertzman et al. 2006	62PG; 83C	71% M; 40.59 (13.21)	No comorbid Axis I psychiatric conditions	Free from psychotropic medications >4 weeks	Reverse version of the Stroop Color-Word Test	PG subjects were significantly slower and less accurate than controls
Patterson et al. 2006	18PG; 23C	56% M; 45 (13)	$n = 15$ mood disorder; $n = 17$ anxiety disorder; $n = 5$ current alcohol use disorder; $n = 9$ nicotine use	Inpatient PG treatment facility sample – current medications and therapy allowed	Reversal Learning (RL) and Iowa Gambling Task	PG subjects performed significantly worse on RL and Iowa Gambling Task
Goudriaan et al. 2006	49PG; 48AA; 46T; 49C	81.6% M; 37.3 (9.5)	$n = 4$ ADHD; $n = 2$ antisocial personality disorder	No psychotropic medications or therapy	Stop Signal Task, Circle Tracing Task, Stroop Color-Word Test, Wisconsin Card Sorting Test, Tower of London, Controlled Oral Word Association Test and Self-Ordered Pointing task	Executive function deficits, including planning, cognitive flexibility and inhibition, greater in the PG group
Kalechstein et al. 2007	10PG; 25M; 19C	90% M; 53.7 (9.6)	No current psychiatric disorders	No therapy; Gamblers Anonymous allowed	Frontal lobe functioning including Stoop Color-Word Test, Trail-Making Test, and Ruff Figural Fluency Test	PG subjects performed significantly worse on all measures and significantly worse than Methamphetamine group on Trail-Making Test
Marazziti et al. 2008	20PG; 20C	75% M; 26 (4)	$n = 7$ bipolar II; $n = 5$ OCD; $n = 5$ cocaine and cannabis abuse; $n = 3$ alcohol abuse	No current psychotropic medications	Wisconsin Card Sorting Test (WCST), Wechsler Memory Scale Revised, Verbal Associative Fluency Test	PG subjects had perseverative thinking and deficits in finding different problem-solving methods; failed to learn from mistakes compared controls

AA = abstinent alcohol dependent, C = healthy controls, CPG = pathological gamblers with psychiatric comorbidity, M = Methamphetamine dependent, NCPG = pathological gamblers without psychiatric comorbidity, O = OCD cases, PG = pathological gamblers, SD = substance dependent, SDPG = substance-abuse/dependent pathological gamblers, T = Tourette's.

Fuentes et al. (2006) compared 214 pathological gamblers with 82 control subjects using the Go/No-Go Reaction Test in both an auditory and visual reaction format. Pathological gambling subjects made significantly more errors on both the auditory and visual components of the Go/No-Go Test but did not differ on reaction time. This suggests that pathological gamblers do not have a problem with time integration; rather, they have problems with information processing (Fuentes et al. 2006).

The reverse Stroop Color Word Test measures interference susceptibility by presenting a subject with four color words displayed on a computer screen in a color not matching the word itself. Pathological gambling subjects are consistently significantly slower and less accurate in picking the color word than control subjects, suggesting both automatic and controlled processing impairment (Kertzman et al. 2006; Regard et al. 2003; Rugle and Melamed 1993).

Kalechstein et al. (2007) compared the performance of 10 substance-free pathological gamblers, 25 methamphetamine-dependent subjects, and 19 control subjects on a battery of tests, including the Stroop Color-Word Test, Ruff Figural Fluency Test, and the Trail-Making Test, Part B, all three of which measure frontal lobe impairment. Both the pathological gamblers and methamphetamine-dependent subjects performed significantly worse on all three measures. In addition, the gamblers performed significantly worse than the methamphetamine group on the Trail-Making Test, Part B, suggesting abnormal function in the frontal-subcortical pathways that are implicated in these tasks (Cummings 1993).

Treatment

Psychotherapy

To date, 15 randomized clinical trials using various modifications of cognitive-behavioral therapy (CBT) have been conducted (Table 5.3). Cognitive strategies have included cognitive restructuring, psychoeducation, and "irrational cognition" awareness training. Behavioral approaches have focused on developing alternative activities to compete with reinforcers specific to PG as well as identifying gambling triggers. Although a rich literature of case reports regarding psychodynamic psychotherapy exists and this form of psychotherapy is often incorporated into multimodal, eclectic, and integrated approaches to PG, there are no randomized controlled trials to support its use (Rosenthal 2008). Similarly, although some evidence suggests a beneficial effect of participation in Gamblers Anonymous (GA) (Hodgins, Peden, and Cassidy 2005; Petry et al. 2006; Stewart and Brown 1988; Taber, McCormick, and Ramirez 1987) and in self-exclusion contracts (Ladouceur et al. 2000), we are unaware of any controlled studies of these interventions.

Cognitive Therapy

Three controlled studies have examined the effect of cognitive restructuring in PG. One study ($n = 40$) used a combination of individual cognitive therapy and relapse prevention strategies (Sylvain, Ladouceur, and Boisvert 1997). At 12 months, the treatment group showed significant reductions in gambling frequency and an increase in self-perceived control over their gambling behavior. The same cognitive therapy techniques combined with relapse prevention were compared with a 3-month wait-list control in a group of 88 PG subjects. The treatment group experienced gambling symptom improvement at three months and maintained it at the 12-month follow-up (Ladouceur et al. 2001).

Group cognitive therapy has also been tested in 71 subjects with PG against a wait-list control condition (Ladouceur et al. 2003). Groups met for 2 hours weekly for 10 weeks. After ten sessions, 88% of those in group CBT no longer met PG criteria, compared with 20% in the wait-list condition. At the 24-month follow-up, 68% of the original group's CBT subjects still did not meet the criteria.

Table 5.3 Controlled psychological treatment trials for pathological gambling

Reference	Design/Duration	Subjects	Outcome
Cognitive Therapy Sylvain et al. 1997	Cognitive therapy (CT) + relapse prevention vs. wait list; 30 sessions with 6 month follow-up	40 enrolled, 14 completed treatment, 15 completed wait list	CT: 57% of completers improved on five variables vs. 6% on wait list
Ladouceur et al. 2001	Cognitive therapy + relapse prevention vs. wait list; 20 sessions with 12-month follow-up	88 enrolled, 35 completed teatment, 29 completed wait list	CT: 54% of completers improved on four variables vs. 7% on wait list
Ladouceur et al. 2003	Group cognitive therapy (GCT) + relapse prevention vs. wait list; 10 weeks with 2-year follow-up	71 enrolled, 34 completed teatment, 25 completed wait list	GCT: 88% of completers no longer met PG criteria vs. 20% on wait list at 10 weeks
Behavior Therapy McConaghy et al. 1983	Aversion therapy vs. imaginal desensitization	20 enrolled, 20 completed	Improvement in both treatment groups over 12 months
McConaghy et al. 1988	Imaginal desensitization (ID) vs. imaginal relaxation (IR); 14 sessions in a 1-week period (inpatient sample)	20 enrolled, 20 completed (95% male)	Both ID and IR groups improved at posttreatment, but improvement lessened by 12-month follow-up
McConaghy et al. 1991	Aversion therapy vs. imaginal desensitization vs. in vivo desensitization vs. imaginal relaxation	120 enrolled, 63 available 2 and 9 years later	Imaginal desensitization improved at 1 month and 9 years
Cognitive Behavioral Therapy Echeburua et al. 1996	Stimulus control, in vivo exposure, relapse prevention (SCERP) vs. cognitive restructuring vs. combined treatment vs. wait list; 6 weeks with 12-month follow-up	64 enrolled, 50 completed	At 12 months, abstinence or much reduced gambling present in 69% of SCERP group vs. 38% of cognitive restructuring or combined treatment groups
Milton et al. 2002	Individual CBT vs. CBT + interventions to improve treatment compliance; 8 sessions with a 9-month follow-up	47 enrolled, 40 assigned to treatment (20 in CBT, 20 in CBT + compliance interventions), 20 completed (72.5% male)	65% of CBT + compliance interventions group completed vs. 35% of CBT-only group

(continued)

Table 5.3 (*cont.*)

Reference	Design/Duration	Subjects	Outcome
Melville et al. 2004	Group CBT, group + interactive written assignments (mapping) vs. wait-list control; 290-minute sessions each week for 8 weeks	Exp. #1: 20 enrolled, 13 treated Exp. #2: 28 enrolled, 19 treated (84.2% female)	CBT with mapping group decreased PG symptoms compared with control group. Exp. #2 added depression and anxiety comorbidity, which decreased compliance; maintained at 6-month follow-up
Petry et al. 2006	Manualized CBT in individual counseling vs. CBT workbook vs. Gamblers Anonymous referral; 8 sessions with 1-year follow-up	231 enrolled, 181 completed	CBT was more effective than Gamblers Anonymous and individual counseling more effective than workbook; at 12 months, groups did not differ in abstinence rates
Wulfert et al. 2006	Cognitive-Motivational Behavior Therapy (CMBT) vs. treatment as usual (TAU); mean of 16 sessions with 3-, 6-, and 12-month follow-up	9 of 9 completed CMBT group, 8 of 12 completed TAU group (100% male)	Significant PG symptom improvement was maintained at 12-month follow-up for CMBT group
Grant et al. in press	Manualized CBT treatment using imaginal desensitization and motivational interviewing vs. referral to Gamblers Anonymous	68 enrolled, 55 completed the acute trial	CBT was more effective than Gamblers Anonymous; significant gains maintained at 6-month follow-up
Brief Interventions and Motivational Interviewing			
Dickerson et al. 1990	CBT workbook vs. workbook + a single in-depth interview	29 enrolled	Both groups improved at 6 months
Hodgins et al. 2001	CBT workbook vs. workbook + motivational enhancement intervention via telephone vs. wait list	102 enrolled, 85 available at 12 months	74% with motivational enhancement improved (Clinical Global Impression) vs. 61% with workbook and 44% on wait list
Hodgins & Holub 2007	Single-session motivational interview (MI) with self-help workbook vs. workbook alone. Single session with 12-month follow-up	Unclear	The MI group gambled less often and spent less money at 12-month follow-up vs. the workbook-alone group
Hodgins et al. 2007	Relapse-prevention bibliotherapy – single mailing vs. repeated mailings over a 12-month period Mailings done once for first group ($n = 85$) vs. 7 mailings for second group ($n = 84$), with 12-month follow-up	169 enrolled, 142 available at 12-month follow-up (58% male)	The repeated-mailing group improved more than the single-mailing group but not significantly. However, 70% of the sample still met SOGS criteria for PG at 12-month follow-up

Although both individual and group cognitive therapies have shown promise in treating PG, rates of treatment discontinuation are high (up to 47%). In addition, the cognitive therapy studies have not yet determined the optimal number of sessions needed to reduce gambling symptoms and maintain improvement.

Behavioral Therapy

Behavioral approaches have been examined in three controlled studies. The first compared imaginal desensitization (i.e., subjects were taught relaxation and then instructed to imagine experiencing and resisting triggers to gambling) with traditional aversion therapy (McConaghy et al. 1983). Both therapies had positive effects, but the imaginal desensitization group was more successful in reducing gambling urges and behavior.

In a second study, 20 inpatient subjects were randomized to receive either imaginal desensitization or imaginal relaxation in 14 sessions over a 1-week period. Both groups improved posttreatment, but the therapeutic gains were not maintained by either group at a 12-month follow-up (McConaghy et al. 1988).

In a larger study, 120 subjects were randomly assigned to aversion therapy, imaginal desensitization, in vivo desensitization, or imaginal relaxation. Subjects assigned to imaginal desensitization reported better outcomes at 1 month and up to 9 years later (McConaghy, Blaszczynski, and Frankova 1991).

Although imaginal desensitization has yielded promising results in treating PG, the outcome data are limited. In addition, the studies have not been replicated by an independent investigator, and there are no data indicating how many sessions are needed to achieve the greatest benefit.

Cognitive-Behavioral Therapy

A randomized study of cognitive-behavioral therapy (CBT) in slot-machine–playing pathological gamblers assigned subjects to one of four groups: (1) individual stimulus control and in vivo exposure with response prevention, (2) group cognitive restructuring, (3) a combination of (1) and (2), or (4) a wait-list control (Echeburúa, Baez, and Fernández-Montalvo 1996). At 12-month follow-up, rates of abstinence or minimal gambling were higher in the individual treatment subjects (69%) compared with the cognitive restructuring (38%) and combined treatment (38%) groups. The same investigators also assessed individual and group relapse prevention for subjects completing a 6-week individual treatment program. At 12 months, 86% of those receiving individual relapse prevention and 78% of those in group relapse prevention had not relapsed, compared with 52% of those who received no follow-up treatment (Echeburúa, Fernández-Montalvo, and Baez 2001).

Milton et al. (2002) compared CBT with CBT combined with interventions designed to improve treatment compliance (the interventions included positive reinforcement, identifying barriers to change, and applying problem-solving skills) in 40 subjects receiving eight sessions of manualized individual therapy. Only 35% of the CBT-alone group completed treatment compared with 65% of the CBT-plus-interventions group. At 9-month follow-up, there was no difference in outcomes between treatments, although both produced clinically significant change (Milton et al. 2002).

Melville et al. (2004) described two studies that used a system targeting three topics (understanding randomness, problem solving, and relapse prevention) to improve outcome. In the first study, 13 subjects were assigned to either 8 weeks of group CBT, group CBT with the topic-enhanced treatment, or a wait list. In the second study, 19 subjects were assigned to a topic-enhanced group or a wait-list group for 8 weeks. For those subjects who were in the topic-targeting CBT group, significant improvement was maintained both posttreatment and at a 6-month follow-up (Melville et al. 2004).

Petry et al. (2006) examined an eight-session manualized form of CBT, randomizing 231 subjects to weekly sessions with an individual counselor, therapy in the form of a workbook, or referral to Gamblers Anonymous. Although all groups reduced their gambling, subjects assigned to individual therapy or to the self-help workbook reduced gambling behaviors more than those referred to Gamblers Anonymous (Petry et al. 2006).

In a study examining cognitive-motivational behavior therapy (CMBT), a method that combines gambling-specific CBT with motivational interviewing techniques to aid in resolving treatment ambivalence and improve retention rates, 9 subjects received manualized treatment and were compared with a control group of 12 who received treatment as usual (TAU). All nine subjects (100%) in the CMBT group completed treatment versus only eight (66.7%) in the TAU group. Significant improvements were observed at the 12-month follow-up of the CMBT group (Wulfert, Blanchard, and Freidenberg 2006).

Grant et al. (2009) recently completed a study of 6 sessions of manualized CBT using imaginal desensitization and motivational interviewing compared with Gamblers Anonymous referral in 68 subjects with PG. Of those subjects assigned to the manualized therapy, 66.7% achieved treatment response compared with only 20.0% assigned to Gamblers Anonymous referral. Treatment response was largely sustained at 6-month follow-up (Grant et al. 2009).

Brief Interventions and Motivational Interviewing

Brief treatments are designed to use less professional resources or time than face-to-face interventions. Brief interventions may include single-session interventions, workbooks, or bibliotherapy. Motivational interviewing is often used. The approach is empathic and uses the client's strengths to enhance self-efficacy regarding changes in behavior.

In one study of brief interventions, Dickerson, Hinchy, and England (1990) randomly assigned 29 subjects to either a workbook or to a workbook plus a single in-depth interview. The workbook included CBT and motivational-enhancement techniques. Both groups reported significant reductions in gambling at a 6-month follow-up.

Hodgins et al. (2004) assigned 102 gamblers to a CBT workbook, a workbook plus a telephone motivational-enhancement intervention, or a wait list. Rates of abstinence at 6-month follow-up did not differ between the groups, although the frequency of gambling and amount of money lost gambling were lower in the motivational-intervention group. Compared with the workbook alone, the motivational intervention and workbook together reduced gambling throughout a 2-year follow-up period; notably, 77% of the entire follow-up sample was rated as improved at the 2-year assessment.

A doctoral dissertation study compared a single-session motivational-interviewing (MI) module plus a self-help workbook with the workbook and speaking with an interviewer about gambling for 30 minutes. Half of the sample were randomized to each intervention. At 12-month follow-up, those who received the MI plus the workbook gambled less and spent less money than the workbook-alone group (Hodgins and Holub 2007).

A study using a relapse-prevention bibliotherapy randomized 169 subjects who had recently quit gambling to receive either a summary booklet that detailed all available relapse prevention information (single mailing group) ($n = 85$) or to the same booklet plus seven additional informational booklets mailed over the next 12 months (repeated mailing group) ($n = 84$) (Hodgins et al. 2007). At the 12-month assessment, 24% of the repeated mailing group reported using the strategies regularly to prevent relapse compared with 13% of the single mailing group. However, only 44% of the overall sample reported having not gambled over the 3 months prior to the 12-month assessment.

Pharmacotherapy

No medication is approved by the U.S. Food and Drug Administration (FDA) for treating PG. However, 15 randomized, placebo-controlled pharmacotherapy trials have been conducted in PG (Table 5.4) and suggest that medication may be beneficial for some individuals with this disorder.

Opioid Antagonists

In view of their ability to modulate dopaminergic transmission in the mesolimbic pathway, opioid receptor antagonists have been investigated in the treatment of pathological gambling. An initial double-blind study suggested efficacy for naltrexone, an FDA-approved treatment for alcohol dependence, in reducing the intensity of urges to gamble, gambling thoughts, and gambling behavior (Kim et al. 2001). In an 11-week, double-blind, placebo-controlled study of 45 PG subjects, naltrexone was begun at 25 mg/day and titrated upward to 250 mg/day or maximum symptom relief. Significant improvement was seen in 75% of naltrexone subjects (mean dose 188 mg/day) compared with 24% of placebo subjects. In particular, individuals reporting a higher intensity of gambling urges responded preferentially to treatment (Kim et al. 2001).

The findings of this initial naltrexone study were replicated in a larger, longer study of 77 subjects randomized to either naltrexone 50 mg, 100 mg, or 150 mg/day or a placebo over an 18-week period (Grant et al. 2008). Subjects assigned to naltrexone had significantly greater reductions in gambling urges and gambling behavior than subjects assigned the placebo. The 50 mg/day dose was as effective as the higher doses, but all were well tolerated. Naltrexone subjects also had greater improvement in psychosocial functioning. By the study's endpoint, 39.7% of naltrexone subjects had abstained from all gambling for at least 1 month versus only 10.5% of placebo subjects.

Another opioid antagonist, nalmefene, has shown promise in treating PG. In a large, multicenter trial using a double-blind, placebo-controlled, flexible dose design, 207 subjects were assigned to receive either nalmefene at varying doses or a placebo. At the end of the 16-week study, 59% of those assigned to nalmefene 25 mg/day showed significant reductions in gambling urges, thoughts, and behavior compared with only 34% of the placebo subjects. Higher doses of 50 mg and 75 mg/day were not well tolerated (Grant et al. 2006).

Antidepressants

In a single-subject study, clomipramine 125 mg/day was administered in a double-blind, placebo-controlled trial to a female subject, who reported a 90% improvement in gambling symptoms (Hollander et al. 1992). Gambling behavior remitted at week 3, and improvement was maintained for the next 7 weeks.

Two paroxetine studies have produced mixed results. The first 8-week study, in which paroxetine was titrated from 20 mg/day to 60 mg/day depending on clinical response, demonstrated a significantly greater rate of improvement for pathological gamblers assigned to paroxetine (61%) compared with a placebo (23%) (Kim et al. 2002). A 16-week, multicenter study of paroxetine flexibly dosed from 10 to 60 mg/day, however, failed to find a statistically significant difference between the active drug and the placebo, perhaps in part because of the high placebo response rate (48% vs. 59% for the active drug) (Grant et al. 2003).

Results for fluvoxamine have also been mixed in two placebo-controlled, double-blind studies, with one 16-week crossover study supporting its efficacy at an average dose of 207 mg/day (Hollander et al. 2000) and a 6-month parallel-groups study with high dropout rates finding no significant difference between active drug 2000 mg/day and placebo (Blanco et al. 2002).

A double-blind, 6-month, placebo-controlled trial of sertraline (mean dose 95 mg/day) in 60 pathological gamblers found no statistical advantage over a placebo (Sáiz-Ruiz et al. 2005).

A 12-week, open-label trial followed by an 8-week, double-blind, randomized discontinuation phase for responders used escitalopram in 13 subjects with high levels of anxiety

Table 5.4 Double-blind, placebo-controlled pharmacotherapy trials for pathological gambling

Reference	Medication	Design/Duration	Subjects	Mean Daily Dose (±SD)	Outcome
Antidepressants					
Hollander et al. 1992	Clomipramine	Single subject, 10 weeks	1 enrolled, 1 completed	125 mg	90% improvement in gambling symptoms on medication
Hollander et al. 2000	Fluvoxamine	Crossover, 16 weeks with a 1-week placebo lead-in	15 enrolled, 10 completed (67%)	195 mg (± 50)	Fluvoxamine superior to placebo
Blanco et al. 2002	Fluvoxamine	Parallel design, 6 months	32 enrolled, 13 completed (41%)	200 mg	Fluvoxamine not statistically significant vs. placebo
Kim et al. 2002	Paroxetine	Parallel design, 8 weeks with 1-week placebo lead-in	53 enrolled, 41 completed (77%)	51.7 mg (± 13.1)	Paroxetine group significantly improved vs. placebo
Grant et al. 2003	Paroxetine	Parallel design, 16 weeks	76 enrolled, 45 completed (59%)	50 mg (± 8.3)	Paroxetine and placebo groups had comparable improvements
Saiz-Ruiz et al. 2005	Sertraline	Parallel design, 6 months	60 enrolled, 44 completed (73%)	95 mg	Similar improvements in both groups
Grant and Potenza 2006	Escitalopram	12-week open label followed by 8-week double-blind discontinuation	13 pathological gamblers with anxiety; 4 completed double-blind phase (31%)	25.4 mg	Of the 4 completers randomized, 3 randomized to escitalopram maintained improvement; 1 randomized to placebo lost improvement
Black et al. 2007	Bupropion	Parallel design, 12 weeks	39 enrolled, 22 completed (56%)	324 mg	No difference between groups on any measure
Mood Stabilizers					
Hollander et al. 2005b	Lithium carbonate SR	Parallel design, 10 weeks	40 bipolar-spectrum patients enrolled, 29 completed (73%)	1170 (± 221) mg	Lithium group significantly improved compared with placebo

Table 5.4 (*cont.*)

	Drug	Design	Enrollment/completion	Dose	Results
Atypical Antipsychotics					
Fong et al. 2008	Olanzapine	Parallel design, 7 weeks	23 enrolled, 21 completed (91%)	2.5 mg–10 mg	No differences between groups on any measure
McElroy et al. 2008	Olanzapine	Parallel design, 12 weeks	42 enrolled, 25 completed (60%)	8.9 ± 5.2 mg	No differences between groups on any measure
Opioid Antagonists					
Kim et al. 2001	Naltrexone	Parallel design, 12 weeks with 1-week placebo lead-in	89 enrolled, 45 completed (51%)	188 ± 96 mg	Naltrexone group significantly improved vs. placebo group
Grant et al. 2006	Nalmefene	Parallel design, 16 weeks	207 enrolled, 73 completed (35%)	Fixed dose study (25 mg, 50 mg, 100 mg)	Nalmefene 25 mg and 50 mg significantly improved vs. placebo group
Grant et al. 2008	Naltrexone	Parallel design, 18 weeks	77 enrolled, 49 completed (64%)	Fixed dose (50 mg, 100 mg, 150 mg)	Naltrexone group significantly improved vs. placebo group
Glutamatergic Agents					
Grant et al. 2007	N-Acetylcysteine	8-week open label followed by 6-week double-blind discontinuation	27 enrolled in open label; 13 randomized to double-blind; 13 completed double-blind phase (48%)	1476.9 ± 311.3 mg	83.3% of N-acetyl cysteine group were responders at end of double-blind phase vs. 28.6% of placebo group

and PG (Grant and Potenza 2006). At the end of the open-label phase (escitalopram mean dose 25.4 mg/day), six subjects were responders. Gambling and anxiety improvement were maintained for those continuing escitalopram, but not for those assigned the placebo. A recent study examined flexibly dosed bupropion beginning at 75 mg/day and increasing weekly to 375 mg/day as indicated in a 12-week, double-blind, placebo-controlled design in 39 PG subjects (Black et al. 2007). When subjects with at least one postrandomization visit were assessed, nearly 36% of bupropion subjects and 47% of placebo subjects were rated as much or very much improved. Bupropion was not significantly superior to the placebo on any outcome measures. However, the high treatment discontinuation rate of nearly 44% in this study (placebo 33%, bupropion 55%) make definitive statements regarding the efficacy of bupropion in PG difficult (Black et al. 2007).

Atypical Antipsychotics

Two studies examining olanzapine treatment for PG have not found it effective. In a 12-week, double-blind, placebo-controlled trial of 42 subjects with PG, 66.7% of both the olanzapine group (mean dose 8.9 mg/day) and the placebo group exhibited a 35% or greater reduction in PG-Y-BOCS scores. Thus, no statistically significant treatment effect was noted for olanzapine (McElroy et al. 2008).

Fong et al. (2008) tested olanzapine in 21 PG subjects using a 7-week, double-blind, placebo-controlled design. All subjects reported video poker as their primary form of gambling. Olanzapine was begun at 2.5 mg/day and increased weekly to 10 mg/day. Reductions in gambling cravings and gambling behavior occurred in both the olanzapine and placebo groups, but no statistically significant differences between groups were observed.

Mood Stabilizers

Sustained-release lithium carbonate was studied in a 10-week, double-blind, placebo-controlled trial enrolling 40 subjects with bipolar spectrum disorders and PG. Lithium at a mean dose of 1150 mg/day (mean plasma level 0.87 meq/liter) reduced the thoughts and urges associated with PG. Despite significantly greater improvement recorded by raters using the Y-BOCS PG scale and the Clinical Global Impression-Improvement Scale, no significant differences between groups were found in gambling episodes per week, time spent per gambling episode, or the amount of money lost (Hollander et al. 2005b).

Glutamatergic Agents

Because improving glutamatergic tone in the nucleus accumbens has been implicated in reducing the reward-seeking behavior in addictions (Kalivas et al. 2006), N-acetyl cysteine (NAC), a glutamate-modulating agent, was administered to 27 PG subjects over an 8-week period, with responders randomized to receive an additional 6-week, double-blind trial of NAC or a placebo (Grant et al. 2007). NAC was begun at 600 mg/day for 2 weeks and increased by 600 mg/day every 2 weeks to 1800 mg/day as needed for clinical response. In the open-label phase, 59% of subjects experienced a significant reduction in PG symptoms and were classified as responders. At the end of the double-blind phase, 83% of those assigned to NAC were still responders, compared with only 28.6% of those assigned the placebo (Grant et al. 2007).

Although CBT, opioid antagonists, and lithium appear promising for the treatment of PG, several limitations affect the current body of knowledge. First, the studies have generally lacked a sample large enough for adequate statistical power. Two exceptions are one CBT study (Petry et al. 2006) and the nalmefene study (Grant et al. 2006). Second, no manualized CBT treatment has been examined in a confirmatory study by an independent investigator, and most published studies have relatively small sample sizes. Third, although these treatments appear effective for PG, few studies have systematically compared interventions or examined whether combined treatments are more effective. Fourth, no study has examined whether specific medications or CBT treatments are more likely to benefit PG sufferers who have particular characteristics. Fifth, no study has examined the optimal duration of treatment. Finally, data are limited concerning the effectiveness of treatments for PG subjects with co-occurring psychiatric conditions. One study found that comorbid problem drinking, drug use, and duration of gambling disorder predicted poor treatment compliance (Milton et al. 2002). Evidence also suggests that substance use can adversely affect cognitive processes, leading to poor judgment and increased risk-taking (Baron and Dickerson 1999).

Self-Help Materials

Studies that examined the utility of referral to Gamblers Anonymous were described earlier. Other self-help materials and organizations have not been studied in controlled trials, but clinicians may wish to provide them to patients nonetheless. Contact information for Gamblers Anonymous is:

> P.O. Box 17173
> Los Angeles, CA 90017
> Tel: 213-386-8789
> www.gamblersanonymous.org

Articles written for the public, a directory of state Councils on Compulsive Gambling, and links to related Web sites can be obtained from the Council on Compulsive Gambling of New Jersey, which may be contacted at:

> 3635 Quakerbridge Road
> Suite 7
> Hamilton, NJ 08619
> Tel: 1-800-GAMBLER, or 609-588-5515
> www.800gambler.org

Self-help books written by experts that may be helpful for patients and families include Blaszczynski (1998), Grant and Kim (2003), and National Council on Problem Gambling and National Endowment for Financial Education (2000).

Conclusions

Pathological gambling is a common disabling psychiatric disorder associated with high rates of co-occurring disorders, particularly substance use disorders, and high rates of social and occupational dysfunction. Although psychotherapies and pharmacotherapies have shown promise, the limited data preclude making treatment recommendations with a substantial degree of confidence. Nonetheless, cognitive-behavioral therapy, imaginal desensitization, opioid antagonists, and lithium have all demonstrated benefits.

Clinicians should keep in mind, however, the limitations of our knowledge about treatment described here. In addition, issues such as the duration of treatment are not addressed by the available data. Further research regarding factors related to treatment response will ultimately advance treatment strategies for PG.

References

American Psychiatric Association. *Diagnostic and Statistical Manual of Mental Disorders*, 3rd edition. Washington, DC: American Psychiatric Association, 1980.

American Psychiatric Association. *Diagnostic and Statistical Manual of Mental Disorders*, 4th edition, text revision. Washington, DC: American Psychiatric Association, 2000.

Baron E, Dickerson M. Alcohol consumption and self-control of gambling behaviour. *J Gambl Stud* 15:3–15, 1999.

Bechara A, Damasio AR, Damasio H et al. Insensitivity to future consequences following damage to human prefrontal cortex. *Cognition* 50:7–15, 1994.

Black DW, Arndt S, Coryell WH et al. Bupropion in the treatment of pathological gambling: A randomized, double-blind, placebo-controlled, flexible-dose study. *J Clin Psychopharmacol* 27:143–150, 2007.

Black DW, Monahan PO, Temkit M et al. A family study of pathologic gambling. *Psychiatry Res* 141:295–303, 2006.

Black DW, Moyer T. Clinical features and psychiatric comorbidity of subjects with pathological gambling behavior. *Psychiatr Serv* 49:1434–1439, 1998.

Black DW, Moyer T, Schlosser S. Quality of life and family history in pathological gambling. *J Nerv Ment Dis* 191:124–126, 2003.

Blanco C, Petkova E, Ibáñez A et al. A pilot placebo-controlled study of fluvoxamine for pathological gambling. *Ann Clin Psychiatry* 14:9–15, 2002.

Bland RC, Newman SC, Orn H et al. Epidemiology of pathological gambling in Edmonton. *Can J Psychiatry* 38:108–112, 1993.

Blaszczynski A. *Overcoming Compulsive Gambling: A Self-Help Guide Using Cognitive Behavioral Techniques.* London: Robinson, 1998.

Blaszczynski A, McConaghy N. Anxiety and/or depression in the pathogenesis of addictive gambling. *Int J Addict* 24:337–350, 1989.

Blaszczynski A, Silove D. Pathological gambling: Forensic issues. *Aust NZ J Psychiatry* 30:358–369, 1996.

Blaszczynski A, Steel Z. Personality disorders among pathological gamblers. *J Gambl Stud* 14:51–71, 1998.

Brand M, Kalbe E, Labudda K et al. Decision-making impairments in patients with pathological gambling. *Psychiatry Res* 30(133): 91–99, 2005.

Cavedini P, Riboldi G, Keller R et al. Frontal lobe dysfunction in pathological gambling patients. *Biol Psychiatry* 51:334–341, 2002.

Crisp BR, Thomas SA, Jackson AC et al. Not the same: A comparison of female and male clients seeking treatment from problem gambling counseling services. *J Gambl Stud* 20:283–299, 2004.

Crockford DN, el-Guebaly N. Psychiatric comorbidity in pathological gambling: A critical review. *Can J Psychiatry* 43:43–50, 1998.

Crockford DN, Goodyear B, Edwards J et al. Cue-induced brain activity in pathological gamblers. *Biol Psychiatry* 58:787–795, 2005.

Cummings DL. Frontal-subcortical circuits and human behavior. *Arch Neurol* 50:873–880, 1993.

Cunningham-Williams RM, Cottler LB, Compton WM 3rd et al. Taking chances: Problem gamblers and mental health disorders – results from the St. Louis Epidemiologic Catchment Area Study. *Am J Pub Health* 88:1093–1096, 1998.

Custer RL. Profile of the pathological gambler. *J Clin Psychiatry* 45:35–38, 1984.

Dickerson M, Hinchy J, England SL. Minimal treatments and problem gamblers: A preliminary investigation. *J Gambl Stud* 6:87–102, 1990.

Echeburúa E, Baez C, Fernández-Montalvo J. Comparative effectiveness of three therapeutic modalities in psychological treatment of pathological gambling: Long term outcome. *Behav Cognit Psychother* 24:51–72, 1996.

Echeburúa E, Fernández-Montalvo J, Baez C. Predictors of therapeutic failure in slot-machine pathological gamblers following behavioural treatment. *Behav Cognit Psychother* 29:379–383, 2001.

Eisen SA, Lin N, Lyons MJ et al. Familial influences on gambling behavior: An analysis of 3359 twin pairs. *Addiction* 93:1375–1384, 1998.

Fagan P, Augustson E, Backinger CL et al. Quit attempts and intention to quit cigarette smoking among young adults in the United States. *Am J Public Health* 97:1412–1420, 2007.

Falk DE, Yi HY, Hiller-Sturmhöfel S. An epidemiologic analysis of co-occurring alcohol and tobacco use and disorders: Findings from the National Epidemiologic Survey on Alcohol and Related Conditions. *Alcohol Res Health* 29:162–171, 2006.

Fong T, Kalechstein A, Bernhard B et al. A double-blind, placebo-controlled trial of olanzapine for the treatment of video poker pathological gamblers. *Pharmacol Biochem Behav* 89:298–303, 2008, Epub January 7, 2008.

Fuentes D, Tavares H, Artes R et al. Self-reported and neuropsychological measures of impulsivity in pathological gambling. *J Int Neuropsychol Soc* 12:907–912, 2006.

Gambino B, Fitzgerald R, Shaffer HJ et al. Perceived family history of problem gambling and scores on the SOGS. *J Gambl Stud* 9:169–184, 1993.

Gerstein D, Murphy S, Toce M et al. *Gambling Impact and Behavior Study: Final Report to the National Gambling Impact Study Commission.* Chicago: National Opinion Research Center (NORC), 1999.

Goudriaan AE, Oosterlaan J, de Beurs E et al. Neurocognitive functions in pathological gambling: A comparison with alcohol dependence, Tourette syndrome and normal controls. *Addiction* 101:534–547, 2006.

Grant JE, Donahue CJ, Odlaug BL et al. Imaginal desensitization plus motivational interviewing in the treatment of pathological gambling: A randomized controlled trial. *Br J Psychiatry* 195:226–267, 2009.

Grant JE, Kim SW. Demographic and clinical characteristics of 131 adult pathological gamblers. *J Clin Psychiatry* 62:957–962, 2001.

Grant JE, Kim SW. Parental bonding in pathological gambling disorder. *Psychiatr Q* 73:239–247, 2002.

Grant JE, Kim SW. *Stop Me Because I Can't Stop Myself: Taking Control of Impulsive Behavior.* New York: McGraw-Hill, 2003.

Grant JE, Kim SW. Quality of life in kleptomania and pathological gambling. *Compr Psychiatry* 46:34–37, 2005.

Grant JE, Kim SW, Hartman BK. A double-blind, placebo-controlled study of the opiate antagonist, naltrexone, in the treatment of pathological gambling urges. *J Clin Psychiatry* 69:783–789, 2008.

Grant JE, Kim SW, Odlaug BL. N-acetyl cysteine, a glutamate-modulating agent, in the treatment of pathological gambling: A pilot study. *Biol Psychiatry* 62:652–657, 2007.

Grant JE, Kim SW, Potenza MN et al. Paroxetine treatment of pathological gambling: A multi-centre randomized controlled trial. *Int Clin Psychopharmacol* 18:243–249, 2003.

Grant JE, Potenza MN. Impulse control disorders: Clinical characteristics and pharmacological management. *Ann Clin Psychiatry* 16:27–34, 2004.

Grant JE, Potenza MN. Tobacco use and pathological gambling. *Ann Clin Psychiatry* 17:237–241, 2005.

Grant JE, Potenza MN. Escitalopram treatment of pathological gambling with co-occurring anxiety: An open-label pilot study with double-blind discontinuation. *Int Clin Psychopharmacol* 21:203–209, 2006.

Grant JE, Potenza MN. Commentary: Illegal behavior and pathological gambling. *J Am Acad Psychiatry Law* 35:302–305, 2007.

Grant JE, Potenza MN, Hollander E et al. Multicenter investigation of the opioid antagonist nalmefene in the treatment of pathological gambling. *Am J Psychiatry* 163:303–312, 2006.

Hodgins DC, Currie S, el-Guebaly N. Motivational enhancement and self-help treatments for problem gambling. *J Consult Clin Psychol* 69:50–57, 2001.

Hodgins DC, Currie S, el-Guebaly N et al. Brief motivational treatment for problem gambling: a 24-month follow-up. *Psychol Addict Behav* 18:293–296, 2004.

Hodgins DC, Holub A. Treatment of problem gambling, in *Research and Measurement Issues in Gambling Studies.* Edited by Smith G, Hodgins DC, Williams RJ. Burlington, MA: Elsevier, 2007, pp. 371–397.

Hodgins DC, Peden N, Cassidy E. The association between comorbidity and outcome in pathological gambling: A prospective follow-up of recent quitters. *J Gambl Stud* 21:255–271, 2005.

Hollander E, DeCaria CM, Finkell JN et al. A randomized double-blind fluvoxamine/placebo crossover trial in pathologic gambling. *Biol Psychiatry* 47:813–817, 2000.

Hollander E, Frenkel M, Decaria C et al. Treatment of pathological gambling with clomipramine (letter). *Am J Psychiatry* 149 (5): 710–711, 1992.

Hollander E, Pallanti S, Allen A et al. Does sustained-release lithium reduce impulsive gambling and affective instability versus placebo in pathological gamblers with bipolar spectrum disorders? *Am J Psychiatry* 162:137–145, 2005b.

Hollander E, Pallanti S, Baldini Rossi N et al. Imaging monetary reward in pathological gamblers. *World J Biol Psychiatry* 6:113–120, 2005a.

Ibáñez A, Blanco C, Moreryra P et al. Gender differences in pathological gambling. *J Clin Psychiatry* 64:295–301, 2003.

Ibáñez A, Blanco C, Sáiz-Ruiz J. Neurobiology and genetics of pathological gambling. *Psychiatric Ann* 32:181–185, 2002.

Jacobs J. Examination of sexually abused children. *CMAJ* 141:767, 1989.

Kalechstein AD, Fong T, Rosenthal RJ et al. Pathological gamblers demonstrate frontal lobe impairment consistent with that of methamphetamine-dependent individuals. *J Neuropsychiatry Clin Neurosci* 19:298–303, 2007.

Kalivas PW, Peters J, Knackstedt L. Animal models and brain circuits in drug addiction. *Mol Interv* 6:339–344, 2006.

Kallick MD, Suits T, Deilman T et al. A survey of American gambling attitudes and behavior. Research report series, Survey Research Center, Institute for Social Research. Ann Arbor: University of Michigan Press, 1979.

Kertzman S, Lowengrub K, Aizer A et al. Stroop performance in pathological gamblers. *Psychiatry Res* 142:1–10, 2006.

Kim SW, Grant JE, Adson DE et al. Double-blind naltrexone and placebo comparison study in the treatment of pathological gambling. *Biol Psychiatry* 49:914–921, 2001.

Kim SW, Grant JE, Adson DE et al. A double-blind placebo-controlled study of the efficacy and safety of paroxetine in the treatment of pathological gambling. *J Clin Psychiatry* 63:501–507, 2002.

Ladd GT, Petry NM. Gender differences among pathological gamblers seeking treatment. *Exp Clin Psychopharmacol* 10:302–309, 2002.

Ladouceur R, Jacques C, Giroux I et al. Analysis of a casino's self-exclusion program. *J Gambl Stud* 16:453–460, 2000.

Ladouceur R, Sylvain C, Boutin C et al. Cognitive treatment of pathological gambling. *J Nerv Ment Dis* 189:774–780, 2001.

Ladouceur R, Sylvain C, Boutin C et al. Group therapy for pathological gamblers: A cognitive approach. *Behav Res Ther* 41:587–596, 2003.

Ledgerwood DM, Petry NM. Gambling and suicidality in treatment-seeking pathological gamblers. *J Nerv Ment Dis* 192:711–714, 2004.

Ledgerwood DM, Weinstock J, Morasco BJ et al. Clinical features and treatment prognosis of pathological gamblers with and without recent gambling-related illegal behavior. *J Am Acad Psychiatry Law* 35:294–301, 2007.

Lesieur HR. The compulsive gambler's spiral of options and involvement. *Psychiatry* 2:79–87, 1979.

Lesieur HR, Blume SB. The South Oaks Gambling Screen (SOGS): A new instrument for the identification of pathological gamblers. *Am J Psychiatry* 144:1184–1188, 1987.

Lesieur HR, Rosenthal RJ. Pathological gambling: A review of the literature (prepared for the American Psychiatric Association Task Force of DSM-IV Committee on Disorders of Impulse Control Not Elsewhere Classified). *J Gambl Stud* 7:5–39, 1991.

Linden RD, Pope HG, Jonas JM. Pathological gambling and major affective disorders: Preliminary findings. *J Clin Psychiatry* 47:201–203, 1986.

Marazziti D, Dell'Osso MC, Conversano C et al. Executive function abnormalities in pathological gamblers. *Clin Pract Epidemiol Ment Health* 4:7, 2008.

McConaghy N, Armstrong MS, Blaszczynski A et al. Controlled comparison of aversive therapy and imaginal desensitization in compulsive gambling. *Br J Psychiatry* 142:366–372, 1983.

McConaghy N, Armstrong MS, Blaszczynski A et al. Behavior completion versus stimulus control in compulsive gambling: Implications for behavioral assessment. *Behav Modif* 12:371–384, 1988.

McConaghy N, Blaszczynski A, Frankova A. Comparison of imaginal desensitization with other behavioural treatments of pathological gambling: A two- to nine-year follow-up. *Br J Psychiatry* 159:390–393, 1991.

McCormick RA, Russo AM, Ramirez LF et al. Affective disorders among pathological gamblers seeking treatment. *Am J Psychiatry* 141:215–218, 1984.

McElroy SL, Nelson EB, Welge JA et al. Olanzapine in the treatment of pathological gambling: A negative randomized placebo-controlled trial. *J Clin Psychiatry* 69:433–440, 2008.

Melville CL, Davis CS, Matzenbacher DL et al. Node-link-mapping-enhanced group treatment for pathological gambling. *Addict Behav* 29:73–87, 2004.

Meyer G, Stadler MA. Criminal behavior associated with pathological gambling. *J Gambl Stud* 15:29–43, 1999.

Milton S, Crino R, Hunt C et al. The effect of compliance-improving interventions on the cognitive-behavioural treatment of pathological gambling. *J Gambl Stud* 18:207–229, 2002.

Morasco BJ, Petry NM. Gambling problems and health functioning in individuals receiving disability. *Disabil Rehabil* 28:619–623, 2006.

Morasco BJ, Vom Eigen KA, Petry NM. Severity of gambling is associated with physical and emotional health in urban primary care patients. *Gen Hosp Psychiatry* 28:94–100, 2006.

National Council on Problem Gambling and National Endowment for Financial Education. *Personal Financial Strategies for the Loved Ones of Problem Gamblers.* Greenwood Village, CO: National Endowment for Financial Education, 2000.

National Opinion Research Center. *Gambling Impact and Behavior Study: Report to the National Gambling Impact Study Commission.* Chicago: National Opinion Research Center at the University of Chicago, 1999. Available at http://www.norc.uchicago.edu/new/gamb-fin.htm.

National Research Council. *Understanding Child Abuse Neglect.* Washington, DC: National Academy Press, 1993.

Niederland WG. A contribution to the psychology of gambling. *Psychoanal Forum* 2:175–185, 1967.

Pallanti S, Bernardi S, Quercioli L. The Shorter PROMIS Questionnaire and the Internet Addiction Scale in the assessment of multiple addictions in a high-school population: Prevalence and related disability. *CNS Spectr* 11:966–974, 2006.

Patterson JC 2nd, Holland J, Middleton R. Neuropsychological performance, impulsivity, and comorbid psychiatric illness in patients with pathological gambling undergoing treatment at the CORE Inpatient Treatment Center. *South Med J* 99:36–43, 2006.

Petry NM. Pathological gamblers, with and without substance use disorders, discount delayed rewards at high rates. *J Abnorm Psychol* 110:482–487, 2001.

Petry NM. *Pathological Gambling: Etiology, Comorbidity, and Treatment.* Washington, DC: American Psychological Association, 2005.

Petry NM, Ammerman Y, Bohl J et al. Cognitive-behavioral therapy for pathological gamblers. *J Consult Clin Psychol* 74:555–567, 2006.

Petry NM, Kiluk BD. Suicidal ideation and suicide attempts in treatment-seeking pathological gamblers. *J Nerv Ment Dis* 190:462–469, 2002.

Petry NM, Oncken C. Cigarette smoking is associated with increased severity of gambling problems in treatment-seeking gamblers. *Addiction* 97:745–753, 2002.

Petry NM, Steinberg KL. Childhood maltreatment in male and female treatment-seeking pathological gamblers. *Psychol Addict Behav* 19:226–229, 2005.

Petry NM, Stinson FS, Grant BF. Comorbidity of DSM-IV pathological gambling and other psychiatric disorders: Results from the National Epidemiologic Survey on Alcohol and Related Conditions. *J Clin Psychiatry* 66:564–574, 2005.

Potenza MN, Leung HC, Blumberg HP et al. An FMRI Stroop task study of ventromedial prefrontal cortical function in pathological gamblers. *Am J Psychiatry* 160:1990–1994, 2003b.

Potenza MN, Steinberg MA, McLaughlin SD et al. Illegal behaviors in problem gambling: Analysis of data from a gambling helpline. *J Am Acad Psychiatry Law* 28:389–403, 2000.

Potenza MN, Steinberg MA, McLaughlin SD et al. Gender-related differences in the characteristics of problem gamblers using a gambling helpline. *Am J Psychiatry* 158:1500–1505, 2001.

Potenza MN, Steinberg MA, McLaughlin SD et al. Characteristics of tobacco-smoking problem gamblers calling a gambling helpline. *Am J Addict* 13:471–493, 2004.

Potenza MN, Steinberg MA, Skudlarski P et al. Gambling urges in pathological gambling: A functional magnetic resonance imaging study. *Arch Gen Psychiatry* 60:828–836, 2003a.

Potenza MN, Xian H, Shah K et al. Shared genetic contributions to pathological gambling and major depression in men. *Arch Gen Psychiatry* 62:1015–1021, 2005.

Ramirez LF, McCormack RA, Russo AM et al. Patterns of substance abuse in pathological gamblers undergoing treatment. *Addict Behav* 8:425–428, 1983.

Regard M, Knoch D, Gütling E et al. Brain damage and addictive behavior: A neuropsychological and electroencephalogram investigation with pathologic gamblers. *Cognit Behav Neurol* 16:47–53, 2003.

Reuter J, Raedler T, Rose M et al. Pathological gambling is linked to reduced activation of the mesolimbic reward system. *Nat Neurosci* 8:147–148, 2005.

Rosenthal RJ. Pathological gambling. *Psychiatr Ann* 22:72–78, 1992.

Rosenthal RJ. Psychodynamic psychotherapy and the treatment of pathological gambling. *Rev Bras Psiquiatr* 30 Suppl 1: S41–50, 2008

Rosenthal RJ, Lorenz VC. The pathological gambler as criminal offender: Comments on evaluation and treatment. *Psychiatr Clin North Am* 15:647–660, 1992.

Roy A, Adinoff B, Roehrich L et al. Pathological gambling: A psychobiological study. *Arch Gen Psychiatry* 45:369–373, 1988.

Rugle L, Melamed L. Neuropsychological assessment of attention problems in pathological gamblers. *J Nerv Ment Dis* 181:107–112, 1993.

Sáiz-Ruiz J, Blanco C, Ibáñez A et al. Sertraline treatment of pathological gambling: A pilot study. *J Clin Psychiatry* 66:28–33, 2005.

Shaffer HJ, Hall MN, Vander Bilt J. Estimating the prevalence of disordered gambling behavior in the United States and Canada: A research synthesis. *Am J Pub Health* 89:1369–1376, 1999.

Slutske WS. Natural recovery and treatment-seeking in pathological gambling: Results of two U.S. national surveys. *Am J Psychiatry* 163:297–302, 2006.

Slutske WS, Eisen S, True WR et al. Common genetic vulnerability for pathological gambling and alcohol dependence in men. *Arch Gen Psychiatry* 57:666–673, 2000.

Slutske WS, Eisen S, Xian H et al. A twin study of the association between pathological gambling and antisocial personality disorder. *J Abnorm Psychol* 110:297–308, 2001.

Specker SM, Carlson GA, Christenson GA et al. Impulse control disorders and attention deficit disorder in pathological gamblers. *Ann Clin Psychiatry* 7:175–179, 1995.

Specker S, Carlson G, Edmonson K et al. Psychopathology in pathological gamblers seeking treatment. *J Gambl Stud* 12:67–81, 1996.

Stewart RM, Brown RI. An outcome study of Gamblers Anonymous. *Br J Psychiatry* 152:284–288, 1988.

Sylvain C, Ladouceur R, Boisvert JM. Cognitive and behavioral treatment of pathological gambling: A controlled study. *J Counsel Clin Psychol* 65:727–732, 1997.

Taber JI, McCormick RA, Ramirez LF. The prevalence and impact of major life stressors among pathological gamblers. *Int J Addict* 22:71–79, 1987.

Vitaro F, Arseneault L, Tremblay RE. Dispositional predictors of problem gambling in male adolescents. *Am J Psychiatry* 154:1769–1770, 1997.

Voon V, Potenza MN, Thomsen T. Medication-related impulse control and repetitive behaviors in Parkinson's disease. *Curr Opin Neurol* 20:484–492, 2007.

Welte J, Barnes G, Wieczorek W. Alcohol and gambling pathology among U.S. adults: Prevalence, demographic patterns and comorbidity. *J Stud Alcohol* 62:706–712, 2001.

Westphal JR, Rush J. Pathological gambling in Louisiana: An epidemiological perspective. *J La State Med Soc* 148:353–358, 1996.

Whitman-Raymond RG. Pathological gambling as a defense mechanism against loss. *J Gambl Behav* 4:99–109, 1988.

Wildman RW. Pathological gambling: Marital-familial factors, implications, and treatments. *J Gambl Behav* 5:293–301, 1989.

Winters KC, Rich T. A twin study of adult gambling behavior. *J Gambl Stud* 14:213–225, 1998.

World Health Organization. *International Classification of Diseases, 1975 revision (ICD-9)*. Geneva: World Health Organization, 1977.

World Health Organization. *International Classification of Mental Disorders: The ICD-10 Classification of Mental and Behavioural Disorders – Diagnostic Criteria for Research*. Geneva: World Health Organization, 1992.

Wulfert E, Blanchard EB, Freidenberg BM. Retaining pathological gamblers in cognitive behavior therapy through motivational enhancement. *Behav Modif* 30:315–340, 2006.

6

Pathological Gambling: Promoting Risk, Provoking Ruin

Laura M. Letson, MPA

Introduction

Within the past two decades, gambling in the United States has spread throughout nearly every aspect of the marketplace. Today, Americans spend more money on gambling than on any other form of entertainment (Volberg 2001). From 1995 to 2006, consumer spending on commercial casino gambling almost doubled, from $18 billion to $34 billion. Revenues from casinos, pari-mutuel wagering, lotteries, legal bookmaking, charitable gambling and bingo, Indian reservations, and card rooms experienced similar growth, from $51 billion in 1997 to $94 billion in 2007 (American Gaming Association 2008). These figures do not reveal the amounts actually wagered because gross revenues deduct winnings returned to players. These figures also do not include amounts bet illegally via the Internet or on other unlawful forms of gambling, which total billions each year.

The prevalence of gambling-related difficulties has also increased in recent years. Since 2000, the National Council on Problem Gambling's (NCPG) toll-free and confidential 24-hour helpline has seen its call volume from persons seeking help, information, or resource referrals more than double. Beginning in 2007, calls have consistently surpassed 20,000 per month (National Council on Problem Gambling 2008).

Understanding how gambling impacts our lives, acknowledging who the major stakeholders are, and recognizing associated social impacts are integral components in aiding patients presenting with gambling-related difficulties. Clinicians are in a leading position to assist problem and pathological gamblers, family members, and others adversely affected. To do so effectively, clinicians must be aware of and attentive to social issues so that these may be taken into consideration in the treatment-planning process.

Self-Assessment

It is useful for clinicians to take a quick self-assessment to determine their values and beliefs about legal (e.g., horse racing and lottery games) and unlawful (e.g., sports betting, except in Nevada, and wagering online) forms of gambling, and about money management issues, because personal viewpoints can influence perspectives when treating gamblers. Patients seeking help for a gambling problem will report difficulties with both legal and unlawful forms of gambling and will present with financial challenges requiring immediate attention.

Take a moment to complete the following sentences and consider how your answers may impact your work with patients. Be sure to note any personal differences, depending on whether the gambling form is legal or illegal.

1. The definition of gambling is _____
2. I support, oppose, or take no position on legalized or illegal forms of gambling because _____

3. I do, do not participate in legalized or illegal forms of gambling activities because

_____

4. I do, do not believe that the benefits of legalized gambling outweigh the social costs because _____

5. I do, do not experience difficulties in my financial life because _____

Recognizing Social Impacts of Gambling

One hundred years ago, gambling was essentially outlawed in the United States, and it remained so until 30 years ago, when it was first legalized. By 2007, there were casinos in 32 states, and every state except Hawaii and Utah had some form of legalized gambling (Flynn 2007).

The majority of people who participate in gambling view it as a social activity that does not negatively impact their lives, and, win or lose, they walk away unaffected. When an addicted gambler's life begins to spiral out of control, however, he or she will often engage in desperate acts in attempts to get even or to continue the "action."

Clinicians need to be aware of a multitude of medical, mental health, and related disorders in order to help their diverse patient populations. While screening for alcohol or substance abuse has become fairly commonplace within the medical community, screening for difficulties caused by gambling is rarely done, and many of the presenting symptoms are missed.

Financial Impacts of Problem and Pathological Gambling

Gamblers most often present for treatment after they have depleted their finances and exhausted other options. Several studies have documented a link between the presence of casinos and increased rates of bankruptcy (Barron, Staten, and Wilshusen 2000; Goss and Morse 2004; SMR Research 1997). Credit cards, blank checks issued by credit card companies, and lines of credit provide the gambler with a false sense of security and a loss of a sense of personal responsibility. The level of debt incurred and other financial impacts are typically overwhelming. Unlike alcoholics and drug addicts, pathological gamblers cannot overdose because there is no saturation point, provided they can continue to access money.

The availability of credit prolongs the pathological process and aggravates the associated consequences. Thus, an important treatment element is ensuring that a compulsive gambler cannot gain access to credit or other revenue sources. Given the commonly accrued extent of debt, repayment may take many years and, in some cases, even the course of a patient's lifetime. Frequently, spouses and other loved ones are totally unaware of the amount of gambling debt and only learn specifics when faced with life-altering decisions (e.g., downsizing, filing for bankruptcy, foreclosure). For this reason, bankruptcy may be a reasonable option for gamblers as a means of removing most, if not all, of their debt. In fact, the prevalence of bankruptcy filing of problem and pathological gamblers can be as high as 30% (Gerstein et al. 1999; Lesieur 1998). Nonetheless, it should only be considered as a last resort or when it will considerably aid the welfare of the gambler's family. Casually filed bankruptcy can serve as a bailout for gamblers, whereas part of their treatment should be to accept personal responsibility toward creditors and debt.

Numerous costs of pathological gambling cannot be quantified, such as the emotional pain associated with bankruptcy, divorce, neglect, and related difficulties experienced by gamblers and others in their lives. In the end, society pays the quantifiable costs of these difficulties, which are conservatively estimated at $5 billion annually, with an additional $40 billion in lifetime costs for productivity reductions, social services, and creditor losses (Gerstein et al. 1999). Most research has focused on the societal costs of casino gambling rather than gambling as a whole and therefore understates the scope of overall gambling costs.

For compulsive gamblers and their families, monitoring the patient's progress includes monitoring his or her ability to fulfill financial obligations. Identifying experienced resources that specialize in working with this population and understand the importance of helping patients restore financial health is also critical.

Crime

When problem and pathological gamblers exhaust all legal financial options, they frequently turn to crime to finance the next bet, replace losses, or pay off gambling debts, bookies, or others. Although law enforcement, academic, and other research organizations have attempted to gauge the relationship between crime and certain forms of gambling, these studies have not thoroughly reviewed the types of crimes typically committed by compulsive gamblers (e.g., embezzlement, tax fraud, leaving a minor child unattended in a car parked at a gambling facility).

Arrest and imprisonment histories are, however, common among pathological gamblers (Gerstein et al. 1999; McCorkle 2002). A meta-analysis of studies of prison populations found that 20% of prisoners are probable pathological gamblers (Lesieur 2005). One study noted that criminal behaviors may be more prevalent among adolescent than among adult gamblers (Blaszczynski and Silove 1996). Another analysis uncovered that 17% of incarcerated youths in juvenile residential correctional facilities reported that their imprisonment was gambling related, 46% of whom scored as problem or pathological gamblers (Lieberman and Cuadrado 2002). Studies of gamblers attending Gamblers Anonymous (a self-help support group) or professional treatment revealed crime rates ranging as high as 50%–67% (Lesieur 2005).

Most states do not use a "gambling court" system, analogous to drug and mental health courts, even though evaluations of drug courts confirm that this approach is beneficial (Lesieur 2005). For pathological gamblers, incarceration can worsen their condition because gambling routinely takes place within prisons. Consequently, state and federal correctional oversight bodies need to address gambling within detention centers, jails, and prisons to create a safe space for pathological gamblers and thereby avoid encouraging recidivism. Law enforcement, judicial, and correctional authorities also need to put in place a system that will provide the education, treatment, and support necessary to aid incarcerated gamblers. Furthermore, law students, lawyers, police, probation and parole officers, judges, and others within the criminal justice system need to become better educated about pathological gambling, its relationship to crime, and approaches for best aiding a client while simultaneously assuring justice. These approaches include implementation of screening at intake, intervention during incarceration, and appropriate exit protocols to reduce recidivism (e.g., treatment and related supports, specific probation requirements, community service, etc.).

Clinicians should take into account any legal pressures facing gamblers entering treatment and/or their loved ones. Identifying legal aid resources and using well-established diagnostic assessments that will stand in a court of law (e.g., the South Oaks Gambling Screen [SOGS]) will also be beneficial (see Chapter 5 and Appendix II, this volume). The National Council on Problem Gambling, as well as this organization's affiliate councils, can provide helpful references and background information.

Employment and Productivity Loss

A preoccupation with gambling can result in poor job performance, absenteeism, health problems, job loss, and unemployment. A national study established that problem and pathological gamblers were more than four times as likely as low-risk gamblers to have lost a job and more than three times as likely to have been fired within the past year. They were also six times more likely than their low-risk counterparts to collect unemployment (Gerstein et al. 1999).

Employers of all types would benefit by establishing policies regarding gambling in the workplace, by implementing employee assistance programs to aid personnel struggling with a gambling problem, and by providing health insurance coverage for pathological gambling treatment. (For additional information, see the "Societal Influences on Gambling" section.)

Health and Medical Impacts

Pathological gamblers, and those they adversely affect, frequently experience physical and emotional difficulties, but a patient's symptoms are often not attributed to the underlying gambling problems (Campbell et al. 2008; Gerstein et al. 1999; Mayo Clinic 2007; Pavalko 1999; Petry, Stinson, and Grant 2005; Wiebe 2001). The health effects extend well beyond the gambler to include eight to ten other persons who are negatively impacted. Though these individuals rarely reveal information about the extent of their problems, they, too, experience financial, physical, and psychological symptoms and may suffer abuse (Lorenz and Shuttlesworth 1983; Lorenz and Yaffee 1988). This is also true for children of compulsive gamblers, who have higher levels of risk-taking behaviors and unhappiness (Jacobs et al. 1989).

Simple screening of patients and their family members is an easy and cost-effective approach. For example, one might add a brief inquiry about gambling frequency (e.g., self-rated as never, daily, weekly, monthly, or less than monthly) to patient intake forms that traditionally seek information about alcohol and other substance use. Another option is the two-question Lie-Bet Questionnaire (Johnson et al. 1988), which is highly accurate in identifying pathological gamblers via an affirmative response to one or both of the following questions:

1. Have you ever lied to people important to you about how much you gamble?
2. Have you ever felt the need to bet more and more money?

Including information about gambling pathology, assessment, and treatment in medical school and in training programs for other health care professionals is also vital. Confirming these recommendations, in August 2008, the Florida Medical Association (FMA) approved a resolution that acknowledges problem and pathological gambling as a public health issue, encourages members to become educated about the somatic symptoms and conditions, promotes patient screening and assessment, and advocates referral to the state-recognized 24-hour helpline. The FMA further approved programming for continuing medical education credit (Florida Medical Association 2008). In addition, the American Medical Association has established a policy that encourages physicians to advise their patients of the addictive potential of gambling; prompts states that operate gambling programs to provide a fixed percentage of their revenue for education, prevention, and treatment of compulsive gambling behavior; and requests that states that operate gambling programs affix to all lottery tickets and display at all lottery counters a sign that states that gambling may become a compulsive behavior and that help is available through the local gambling hotline (American Medical Association 2009). (For more information about the health effects of pathological gambling, see Chapter 5 this volume.)

Suicide

When a pathological gambler or loved one becomes hopeless and believes there is no way out, suicide is often considered. According to the National Council on Problem Gambling, approximately 20% of pathological gamblers attempt suicide (National Council on Problem Gambling 1997; Potenza et al. 2002). Pathological gamblers have the highest rate of suicidal ideation and attempts among persons suffering from addictive disorders (National Council on Problem Gambling 1997). A survey of nearly 400 Gamblers Anonymous members revealed that 66% had contemplated suicide, 47% had a definite plan to kill themselves, and 77% stated they wanted to die (Lesieur and Anderson 1995).

Suicide attempts by spouses and partners of pathological gamblers are reported to be three times higher than in the general population (Dickson-Swift, James, and Kippen 2005) and in children occur at twice the rate of their classmates unaffected by familial gambling problems (Jacobs et al. 1989).

Examining suicide rates as they relate to the location of gambling venues is also informative. For example, Nevada's suicide rate is twice the national average. Suicide is the sixth leading cause of death among state residents and the third primary cause of death among youths and young adults ages 10 to 24 years. Nevada senior citizens over 60 years of age have the nation's highest suicide rate, which is more than twice the national average for the same age group (Office of Suicide Prevention 2007).

Suicide prevention personnel, as well as clinicians, need to become well versed about the impacts of pathological gambling on individuals and families to ensure that they are attentive to telltale clues when aiding this population.

Homelessness, Domestic Violence, Neglect, Divorce, and Other Impacts

The number of pathological gamblers and their families that receive services from homeless and domestic violence shelters, rescue missions, food pantries, social service programs, and other organizations servicing the poor or vulnerable is unknown. But social researchers in Australia concluded that gambling addiction is one of the root causes of homelessness and may account for 15%–20% of the homeless population (Hoare 2008). In the United States, nearly 20% of men and women at rescue missions believe that gambling was one cause of their homelessness, and 70% stated that easy access to gambling opportunities inhibited them from bettering their lives (International Union of Gospel Missions 1998).

A national study ascertained that pathological gamblers are three times more likely than nongamblers to have been divorced (Gerstein et al. 1999), and children of pathological gamblers experience almost twice the incidence of broken homes (Jacobs et al. 1989). There further appears to be a relationship between compulsive gambling and intimate partner and spousal violence (Bland et al. 1993; Jejkal 2000; Mullerman et al. 2002; National Research Council 1999). Children of problem gamblers also fall victim to abuse and neglect (*ABC News* 2008; *Associated Press* 1997; Bland et al. 1993; *Chicago Tribune* 1999; Darby 1997; Gerstein et al. 1999; Schneider 2000).

Although many pathological gamblers and their families ultimately present for social service help, gambling behavior is not traditionally evaluated in the application process. Incorporating inquiries about gambling frequency (see the examples given earlier) and asking about activities applicants or patients participate in to relax or for entertainment can reveal an underlying gambling problem (Campbell et al. 2008). Identifying and providing referrals to local resources and programs that provide shelter, food, and other basic necessities to gamblers and their families is also quite helpful.

Societal Influences on Gambling

To understand how problem and pathological gambling affects patients in treatment, clinicians must become acquainted with the multiple ways in which patients are exposed to gambling messages. Whether reading a newspaper, watching television, frequenting a fast food restaurant, shopping at a convenience store, or engaging in some other routine activity, one is reminded that governments, gambling industry operators, academic institutions, houses of worship, employers, retailers, the media, and others promote gambling and encourage participation. Yet, the entities generating these messages typically do not invest time, energy, or money in assuring that there are adequate supports for those negatively affected by gambling.

Federal, State, and Local Governments Encourage Gambling

Federal, state, and local governments promote gambling while simultaneously providing oversight and enforcement responsibilities. Though gambling regulation is usually left to the states, the federal government has the authority to regulate wagering activities that affect interstate commerce, such as online betting, floating casinos, and gambling facilities operated by Native Americans (see Chapter 7 this volume), and monitor certain types of betting businesses, such as those involving wire service (General Accounting Office 2002).

After the introduction of the Internet, millions of individuals were gambling online within a decade's time, spending upward of $10 billion on casinos, sports wagering, cards, and other games. Expenditures are projected to near $20 billion by 2010 (Isidore 2004). Though Internet gambling is not legal within the United States, its sponsoring entities operate offshore and are licensed by foreign governments, making oversight complicated. Federal and state governments have taken steps to prohibit and ban Internet gambling, including civil actions by state prosecutors. This has reduced the number of betting sites, but by the time these measures were undertaken, difficulties had emerged in the marketplace (Stewart 2006). Major credit card companies have similarly attempted to curtail credit card use for such operations. However, despite these efforts, avenues for wagering online continue to exist.

In addition, under federal law, states have little or no authority over Indian reservations, including the ability to tax or regulate gambling (see Chapter 7 this volume). However, while tribal governments have entered into compacts at the state level to permit certain types of gambling, this has been the subject of ongoing controversy. In Florida, for example, following pressure by the federal government, the governor signed a compact in November 2007 allowing the operation of casino card games and slot machines at seven sites. The legislature sued, and less than one year later, in 2008, Florida's Supreme Court ruled that the governor lacked the authority to take such action. Despite the court determination, these tribal casinos are still offering games approved in the compact that are otherwise illegal in Florida, and federal authorities have not required that this be stopped because they feel it is a state issue (Dolinski 2008). Ultimately, to some extent, it is no longer a state's decision as to whether or not it will have gambling or expand gambling because of the pressure from the tribes and the federal government.

Floating casinos, also commonly referred to as cruises to nowhere, are operated in international waters (within just a few miles of state and local jurisdictions), which are regulated by the federal government. These venues present similar challenges to state and local governments because at times these vessels, like tribal compacts, offer gambling options that are otherwise illegal.

An important exception to the federal government's oversight function is the role of the Department of Defense, which has approved the use of slot machines on military bases, which generate significant revenues for military recreational activities. Though slot machines place some military personnel and their families at great risk of becoming problematic or pathological gamblers, these machines remain intact, and assistance to military members experiencing gambling difficulties is inadequate.

Under President Clinton, the federal government in 1996 established the National Gambling Impact Study Commission (NGISC) (National Gambling Impact Study Commission 1999), which was responsible for conducting a nationwide review of the social and economic impacts of gambling. The NGISC recommended a "pause" or moratorium on gambling until certain requirements could be met by all existing and newly licensed gambling operators and tribal–state compacts. The report further outlined steps that state governments should consider in addressing issues related to problem and pathological gambling (National Gambling Impact Study Commission 1999).

To date, the NGISC requirements have been embraced by only some state governments and tribal–state compacts. Most state governments and gambling operators (tribal included) have not adopted mission statements on problem and pathological gambling; initiated thorough public awareness, education, and prevention programs; instituted a "gambling privilege tax" or other assessment; mandated coverage of treatment for problem and pathological gambling in private and public insurance policies; or, within gambling facilities, required the conspicuous posting and dissemination of telephone numbers of state-approved providers of problem gambling information, treatment, and referral support services (National Gambling Impact Study Commission 1999).

State governments promote lotteries as providing support to education and other public programs, while local governments mention lotteries' role in offsetting various program service costs. Despite these contentions, a substantial percentage of the revenues are applied toward marketing, prizes, commissions, and operating expenses (Nixon and Stodghill 2007). Public (Fesling 2008) and private (Dolan and Green 2002) lotteries have also targeted low-income and minority populations (Hill 2002). Gamblers with household incomes of $10,000 or less bet nearly three times as much on lotteries as those with incomes exceeding $50,000 (National Gambling Impact Study Commission 1999). Lower-income individuals also tend to view lottery games as a better way to attain wealth than saving money (Consumer Federation of America and Primerica 1999). Slogans such as "All you need is a dollar and a dream" are advertised by state lotteries and perpetuate a "get rich quick" mentality.

State lotteries have entered into partnerships with outside entities to sell instant tickets featuring sports team logos, popular television shows, and celebrities. And, although lottery games can serve as a gateway to other risk-taking behaviors among adolescents (Volberg 1998), this has not dissuaded some states from using cartoon characters on their instant tickets. In some instances, these marketing efforts have resulted in countervailing legal action (Blumenthal 2003; *New York Times* 2003a, 2003b).

Both state and local legislatures have taken steps to spread gambling options to rejuvenate sectors of the gambling industry. For example, states have secured revenues by transforming some horse-racing pari-mutuel facilities into establishments that function more like casinos (known as "racinos").

State lotteries have instituted new game technology that provides immediate gratification and is increasingly addictive. Video lottery games, referred to by some critics as "video crack," have a high event frequency (i.e., fast outcome and continual staking), involve an element of skill or perceived talent, and create "near misses" that give the illusion of having almost won. The size of the jackpot and stakes, the probability of winning or perception of winning, and the possibility of using credit to play are all associated with higher levels of problematic play (BMA Board of Science 2007; National Research Council 1999).

Governments must be held accountable for promoting gambling and should be required to establish regulatory provisions, mandated insurance coverage, public health educational and research funding, and programs that assure that constituents needing treatment for a gambling problem can gain easy and affordable access to appropriate help. The appointment of one independent and designated regulatory authority within each state is also appropriate in order to eliminate conflicts of interest and ensure that oversight bodies are not functioning as gambling operators and promoters.

In the interim, some patients will require treatment based on an ability to pay (i.e., sliding-scale fees), with a potential for a "zero fee" in some cases. Although imposing a minimal cost for treatment may be therapeutically beneficial, some patients with gambling difficulties will have limited or no available funds. In these instances, clinicians may be able to encourage treatment by identifying local private and government health programs that offer mental health assessment and treatment to the indigent.

The Gambling Industry Promotes Gambling

The gambling industry, which encompasses land-based and riverboat casinos, cruises to nowhere (i.e., floating casinos in international waters), racetracks, card rooms, Internet gambling sites, jai-alai frontons, and other operations, actively markets its games to entice people to play. These entities have modified their venues to be more appealing to women, college students, older adults, and minorities, and have entered into agreements with established institutions that serve these populations. The results of these well-thought-out strategies confirm that such marketing pays off.

The advent of new technology and policies allowing patrons to access money and credit or to play for extended uninterrupted periods have also had negative consequences. Automatic teller machines (ATMs) on or near gambling floors and immediate credit and check-cashing privileges, including paychecks or checks by patrons who have bounced checks, along with incentives for gamblers who reach a certain level of spending, make it increasingly difficult for patrons to take a "break in play" (i.e., step away from the action), which is imperative for those who may lack control. For gamblers who reach a certain level of spending, the industry provides varying inducements, including high credit limits, free alcohol (despite the correlation between gambling addiction and substance abuse), hotel accommodations, and other provisions. Court cases have emerged from such offerings (Schneider 2007).

The gambling industry has partnered with organizations to reach a broader market base and has expanded services to include nongambling amenities and activities (Skolnik 2004). Las Vegas has promoted itself as an "adult playground" (McCarthy 2005), while other locales market their offerings as family vacation destinations because consumers need not leave the premises to shop, eat, exercise, see a movie or a featured performer, or engage in a variety of entertainment and recreational offerings for persons of all ages. Some establishments even encourage patrons to bring children and furnish on-site day care services, which habituate young people to the environment. Such access creates dangerous situations for minors (Evans 2003).

The gambling industry has organized strong groups to represent its interests in political, academic, and other arenas. Several accounts of these relationships have surfaced, bringing the legitimacy of some research and other initiatives into question (Mishra 2004). For example, some industry-subsidized research investigating crime impacts does not examine the types of crime commonly committed by compulsive gamblers and thus underreports gambling-related crime rates.

Efforts to replace words such as "pathological gambling," "compulsive gambling," and "gambling addiction" with the term "disordered" gambling and the like are intended to replace language clinically recognized by the American Psychiatric Association or well established in the literature. Industry also substitutes the word "gaming" for "gambling" in an effort to have the public view their venues purely as entertainment and fun.

Many gambling operators, including tribal casinos, participate in "responsible gaming programs" and/or fund problem gambling initiatives. However, participation and programs vary across states. Programs may include training employees to become educated about problem and pathological gambling, aiding patrons in need of assistance, implementing policies and procedures to curtail addictive behavior, such as restricting credit, ATM access, solicitations, incentives, and patron data compilation, and placing signage featuring the state and/or national toll-free hotline numbers for gambling difficulties in conspicuous locations throughout facilities as well as on advertising and promotional materials.

Some gambling venues offer a self-exclusion option as a protective measure such that patrons can opt in when their gambling is out of control. These programs are often voluntary, and timelines for self-exclusion vary (e.g., 1 year, 3 years, and lifetime), as do restrictions, guidelines, and penalties. Policies even fluctuate within the same corporate structure.

Clinically, self-exclusion is an option that should be seriously considered for any patient with gambling difficulties. Clinicians need to become familiar with facility policies and ensure that patients understand that while establishment personnel may advocate 1-year bans, the minimum period should be no less than 2 years because of the high rate of relapse within the first 12 months of recovery from pathological gambling. Except in very rare instances, gamblers must self-exclude in person, so patients should be accompanied to facilities by trusted friends or family members.

It also appears prudent for gambling regulatory authorities to establish standardized provisions that require gambling operations to implement a "comprehensive" problem gambling awareness program. Requirements should be uniform within a state. Self-exclusion should not necessitate that patrons visit each establishment. Gambling operators must be forbidden to solicit self-excluded patrons to return to facilities. Winnings during an exclusion period should be deposited into a dedicated fund administered by a state regulatory authority for those negatively affected because these gamblers should not be entitled to recover their losses or keep winnings during this time, nor should industry be able to benefit monetarily from such patrons. Industry must also be required to contribute to a dedicated fund for treatment, research, prevention, education, and outreach services; to implement policies that curtail immediate access to credit and paycheck cashing; to prohibit certain types of inducements; and to eliminate practices known to be problematic among this population.

Credit Card and Financial Organizations Facilitate Gambling

Credit card companies, banking and other financial institutions, and ATMs supply the means by which gamblers can wager online or gain access to credit or money to gamble, or to pay back gambling-related debts. Consumers are often targeted with incentives and furnished with credit limits that they lack the ability to repay. Universities and other organizations have entered into agreements with financial institutions that allow promotions on college campuses and office complexes in exchange for monetary benefits based on user spending.

Government must end the practices of financial and other lending institutions that increase consumer debt by providing credit to ineligible persons. Government must further pass laws to prohibit the use of credit in gambling and restrict solicitations and practices that target minors, college students, and other vulnerable populations. Finally, government must hold credit card and financial institutions, as well as partner and sponsoring organizations, accountable when they provide credit to inappropriate populations and/or actively perpetuate consumer debt via gambling.

The Media, Film Industry, and Hollywood Market Gambling

The media and film industry advance legal and illegal forms of gambling through advertising, radio and television programming, and other forums. Even news broadcasts provide information on spreads, favorites, and tips, even though sports betting is illegal everywhere in the United States except within the state of Nevada. Ads for placing wagers online or by phone (800 and 900 numbers) are featured in newspapers, magazines, and elsewhere. The media have aggressively promoted poker and successfully marketed it as an official sporting event. In addition to ESPN, cable television's recognized sports channel, several television shows have been launched based on the popular poker game "Texas Hold 'Em." Reality programs rooted in gambling have also been unveiled in the past decade.

The film industry glamorizes gambling and normalizes gambling behaviors across age groups. Actors in movies with gambling themes often become prominent figures within the gambling industry, as both players and promoters. For a while, some celebrities were promoting online gambling despite its illegal status (Richtel 2005). Here, too, oversight by a government regulatory authority is appropriate to determine the scope of such activities and appropriate courses of action.

Collegiate and Professional Sports May Become Entangled in Gambling

Top collegiate and professional athletes, referees, and other sports figures have become entangled in gambling. At times, their actions have involved illegal bookmakers, affected the outcome of games, and/or resulted in the termination of play and/or prison sentences. Point-shaving scandals have had significant repercussions for individuals, school communities, law enforcement authorities, and others. When the integrity of a sport is placed into question by players or by those responsible for administering the game, the consequences are far-reaching (Ednalino 1998).

Collegiate and professional sports organizations should take steps, alongside government oversight bodies, to curtail illegal sports gambling, including restricting television networks, print media, and others from promoting these activities in areas outside Nevada. These athletic institutions should also implement comprehensive educational programs about gambling, including problem and compulsive gambling, and offer help options for those who experience gambling-related difficulties.

Clinicians need to be aware that athletes who retire or stop playing a sport may seek out action in other areas of their lives, which can mean through gambling. Recovering sports gamblers may need assistance in devising alternatives to watching or listening to sporting events in order to avoid triggering a relapse.

Toy Manufacturers and Retailers Advance Gambling

Toy manufacturers produce simulated gambling games with inappropriate age labels targeting children. Popular retail chains feature poker kits and slot machine handheld games in prominent store placements, clearly aimed at minors, never questioning whether this is appropriate. Fast-food chains, auto dealerships, department stores, and other retailers use scratch-off tickets, raffles, sweepstakes, prizes, and other inducements to entice customers to visit or to purchase certain products. Cell phones even provide features that allow immediate access to placing bets, and wireless companies have faced legal action for enticing customers to engage in illegal gambling by text-messaging wagers on highly viewed television programs (*Business Week* 2008).

Government must devise standards for toy and product manufacturers as well as retail operations and hold companies legally responsible when their actions encourage illegal gambling and/or participation in gambling by underage persons. Such provisions should address product age labels.

Parents, Schools, and Community-Based Organizations May Sponsor Gambling

Parents, schools, and community organizations host gambling parties as social activities or fund-raisers for persons of all ages and view these as safe alternatives to alcohol and drug use among minors. Alarmingly, even substance abuse prevention and rehabilitation programs and other social service organizations have used gambling to raise funds (Booth 2006). Houses of worship are no exception. They, too, sponsor bingo nights and poker tournaments, raffles, and other forms of gambling for recreational purposes and/or to generate funds.

All of these institutions need to assess whether their actions are appropriate. Like gambling operators, they should be required to post a toll-free 24-hour helpline number for gambling difficulties when staging such games and to provide a self-exclusion option when appropriate. Implementing problem gambling prevention and awareness programs within community-based organizations, schools, and houses of worship that sponsor gambling activities would also be reasonable. Academic and parent organizations, law enforcement authorities, and others should apply to gambling activities by minors the same standards they apply to alcohol consumption among underage persons.

Furthermore, public and private funding sources should consider prohibiting alcohol and substance abuse prevention, education, and treatment programs and mental health and social service agencies from engaging in gambling-related activities because these activities can compromise their client populations.

Older Adult Service Organizations May Encourage Gambling Access

Gambling among older adults has become a significant concern in recent years, as prevalence studies have confirmed higher rates of problem gambling among seniors. In addition to gambling establishments heavily targeting seniors and elder service providers, many adult day care centers and older adult programs now offer bingo and other gambling games on-site and/or furnish ready transportation to gambling facilities. At times, these services are also made available to elders who are not mentally equipped to engage in these gambling activities.

While there are very unique issues associated with pathological gamblers who are senior citizens, their caregivers and aides, like family members, often do not pay enough attention to whether gambling is having a negative impact. Elder care organizations need to train staff and clients about adverse impacts of gambling and should monitor how and where their aides spend time with clients, ensuring that neither the client nor the employee is experiencing a gambling problem. These organizations must also explore providing recreational opportunities beyond gambling and should be held to the same standards as gambling facilities when hosting gambling activities (e.g., posting a toll-free 24-hour helpline number and providing for self-exclusion).

Employers and Workplaces May Advocate Gambling

Employers often use gambling incentives and other benefits, including travel to gambling destinations, as a means of rewarding high performance by employees. Businesses use gambling strategies, such as scratch-off tickets or free giveaways, to entice customers to partake in an event or activity without considering whether employees or their patrons may be struggling with, or recovering from, a gambling problem. Most companies do not have gambling-specific policies that address activities such as workplace betting pools or provide supports for persons experiencing a gambling problem. Yet, problem and pathological gamblers frequently turn to the workplace for various forms of bailout (Ashe and Fowler 2006; Maines 2005; O'Malley 2008). These gamblers use company time to gamble, which results in significant costs (Challenger, Gray, and Christmas 2008), and engage in illegal acts, including workplace crimes, to fund their gambling. (See the section on "Employment and Productivity Loss.")

Because gamblers typically spend more awake time on the job than at home, it is important for clinicians to ask patients about their workplace culture to determine whether this environment could be a contributing factor to relapse and compromise recovery efforts. It is also critical for employers to implement programs addressing gambling situations and problem gambling in the workplace, which will help minimize employee impacts and company losses.

Conclusion

In 1999, the National Gambling Impact Study Commission recommended a moratorium on gambling (National Gambling Impact Study Commission 1999). While a decade has since passed and more information is available, a significant gap in research continues. Despite the commission's recommendation, gambling opportunities have exploded, as have the associated social impacts on individuals, families, communities, workplaces, governments, and society as a whole.

Government can no longer afford to delay action. Until government regulatory authorities that are not simultaneously promoting gambling take charge, there will be little hope for change. Fortunately, clinicians will always be a resource to whom pathological gamblers and their families can turn in times of need.

References

ABC News. Kids Left in Car While Mom Allegedly Plays the Slots. May 15, 2008. Available at http://abcnews.go.com/TheLaw/story?id=4853379&page=1. Accessed October 9, 2008.

American Gaming Association. Fact Sheets: Statistics, Gaming Revenue: 10-Year Trends. Available at http://www.americangaming.org/Industry/factsheets/statistics`detail.cfv?id=8, November 2008.

American Medical Association, Health and Ethics Policies of the AMA, H-440.922. Gambling Can Become Compulsive Behavior. Available at http://www.ama-assn.org/ad-com/polfind/Hlth-Ethics.doc, January 7, 2009.

Ashe P, Fowler P. Gambling and problem gambling in the workplace. FOCUS Newsletter, Florida Council on Compulsive Gambling, Fall/Winter 2006.

Associated Press. Police: Baby Died of Dehydration in Car While Mom Gambled in Casino, September 2, 1997.

Barron J, Staten M, Wilshusen S. The impact of casino gambling on personal bankruptcy filing rates, Purdue (West Lafayette, IN) and Georgetown (Washington, DC) Universities, August 18, 2000. Available at http://www.ncalg.org/Library/Studies%20and%20White%20Papers/Bankruptcy/Gambling%20Impact%20on%20Personal%20Filings.pdf. Accessed November 18, 2007.

Bland R, Newman S, Orn, H et al. Epidemiology of pathologic gambling in Edmonton. *Can J Psychiatry* 38:108–112, 1993.

Blaszczynski A, Silove D. Pathological gambling: Forensic issues. *Aust NZ J Psychiatry* 30:338–369, 1996.

Blumenthal R. Attorney General's Opinion, State of Connecticut Attorney General's Office, March 12, 2003. Available at www.ct.gov/AG/cwp/view.asp?A=1770&Q=281962. Accessed March 3, 2008.

BMA Board of Science. *Gambling Addiction and Its Treatment within the NHS: A Guide for Healthcare Professionals.* London: British Medical Association, 2007.

Booth Fr. L. Gambling and fundraising: An issue worthy of question. FOCUS Newsletter, Florida Council on Compulsive Gambling, Fall/Winter 2006.

Business Week. Class-action lawsuits filed against Verizon Wireless, AT&T Mobility Llc, Sprint Nextel Corp., accusing illegal gambling in connection text messaging tied to popular TV shows, March 31, 2008. Available at http://investing.businessweek.com/businessweek/research/stocks/private/snapshot.asp?privcapId=690041.com. Accessed March 31, 2008.

Campbell J, Koshkarova O, Moss A et al, University of Central Florida's Cornerstone Team. *Diagnosis: Pathological Gambling – Medical Providers Guide.* Altamonte Springs: Florida Council on Compulsive Gambling, 2008.

Challenger, Gray, and Christmas. Challenger March Madness Report, Forecast: $1.7 Billion in Lost Productivity. Chicago, IL: Challenger, Gray, and Christmas, 2008.

Chicago Tribune. Mom's Greed, Not SIDS, Killed a Baby, Jurors Told. January 23, 1999. Available at http://wybett.vcn.com/topical/momkills1.htm. Accessed October 9, 2008.

Consumer Federation of America, Primerica. Typical American household has net financial assets of $1,000, related survey shows that most Americans overestimate wealth, underestimate power of saving, October 28, 1999.

Darby J. Sitter Indicted in Toddler's Death. *New Orleans Times-Picayune,* May 23, 1997.

Dickson-Swift V, James E, Kippen S. The experience of living with a problem gambler: Spouses and partners speak out. *J Gambl Issues,* no. 13, March 2005.

Dolan J, Green R. Playing Games: The Poor Play More. *South Florida Sun-Sentinel,* October 7, 2002. Available at http://www.sun-sentinel.com/topic/hc-lotteryday2.artoct07,0,2530772.story?page=1. Accessed February 1, 2008.

Dolinski C. Decision complicates Seminole gaming pact, October 8, 2008. Available at http://www2.tbo.com/content/2008/oct/05/na-decision-complicates-seminole-gaming-pact/imwY./ Accessed October 9, 2008.

Ednalino P. Point Shaving: ASU Officials Take Steps to Head Off Any More Worries about Gambling. *The Bulldog* (Arizona State University), December 11, 1998.

Evans H. Casinos Cash in with Child Care for Players. *Daily News* (New York), February 23, 2003.

Fesling D. Houston's Poor Pay to Play Lottery. Houston Metro, khou.com. February 20, 2008. Available at http://www.khou.com/news/local/houstonmetro/stories/khou080219_ac_lotterystudy.aa83524.html#. Accessed February 28, 2008.

Florida Medical Association, Resolution 08–16, Pathological Gambling – Screening and Referring Patients. Adopted by FMA Association House of Delegates, Annual Meeting, Rosen Shingle Creek Resort, Orlando, FL, July 31–August 3, 2008.

Flynn S. Is Gambling Good for America? *Parade Magazine*, May 8, 2007. Available at http://www.parade.com/articles/editions/2007/edition_05–20-2007/Gambling. Accessed December 27, 2007.

General Accounting Office. Internet Gambling: An Overview of the Issues. Report to Congressional Requesters, United States Government, December 2002.

Gerstein D, Volberg R, Toce M et al. *Gambling Impact and Behavior Study: Report to the National Gambling Impact Study Commission.* Chicago. National Opinion Research Center at the University of Chicago, 1999.

Goss E, Morse E. *The Impact of Casino Gambling on Bankruptcy Rates: A County Level Analysis.* Omaha, NE: Creighton University, 2004.

Hill J. *An Alabama Lottery: A Theft by Consent.* Mountain Brook: Alabama Policy Institute, August 2002.

Hoare D. Problem Gambling a "Root Cause of Homelessness." *ABC News*, January 29, 2008. Available at http://www.abc.net/au/news/stories/2008/02/29/2149351.html. Accessed March 10, 2008.

International Union of Gospel Missions. *1998 Gambling and Homelessness Survey.* Kansas City, MO: International Union of Gospel Missions, Association of Gospel Rescue Missions, 1998.

Isidore C. Don't Bet Against Online Gambling. *CNN*, March 26, 2004. Available at http://money.cnn.com/2004/03/26/commentary/column_sportsbiz/sportsbiz./ . Accessed May 27, 2007.

Jacobs D, Marston A, Singer R et al. Children of problem gamblers. *J Gambl Behav* 5:261–268, 1989.

Jejkal J. University of Nebraska Doctor Contributes to National Domestic Violence Study. *Daily Nebraskan* (University of Nebraska, Lincoln), January 13, 2000.

Johnson E, Harner R, Nora R et al. The lie/bet questionnaire for screening pathological gamblers. *Psychol Rep* 80:83–88, 1988.

Lesieur H. Testimony before the National Gambling Impact Study Commission, January 22, 1998.

Lesieur H. Solutions to the Problem Gambling Crime Connection. Presentation at the Florida Council on Compulsive Gambling and University of Florida Fredric G. Levin College of Law Think Tank on Problem Gambling and Crime: Impacts and Solutions, Orlando, FL, May 2005.

Lesieur H, Anderson C. Results of a 1995 survey of Gamblers Anonymous members in Illinois. Illinois Council on Problem and Compulsive Gambling, June 14, 1995.

Lieberman L, Cuadrado M. Gambling Education and Prevention Needs Assessment for Juveniles in Residential Detention Centers of the Florida Department of Juvenile Justice. Prepared for the Florida Council on Compulsive Gambling, November 2002.

Lorenz V, Shuttlesworth D. The impact of pathological gambling on the spouse of the gambler. *J Community Psychol* 11:67–76, 1983.

Lorenz V, Yaffee R. Pathological gambling: Psychosomatic, emotional and marital difficulties as reported by the spouse. *J Gambl Behav* 4:13–26, 1988.

Maines D. Employee assistance professionals and compulsive gambling. FOCUS Newsletter, Florida Council on Compulsive Gambling, Spring 2005.

Mayo Clinic. Medical Therapy for Restless Leg Syndrome May Trigger Compulsive Gambling, February 8, 2007.

McCarthy M. Vegas Goes Back to Naughty Roots. *USA Today*, April 11, 2005. Available at www.usatoday.com/money/advertising/adtrack/2005–04-11-track-vegas_x.htm. Accessed November 6, 2007.

McCorkle R. Pathological Gambling in Arrestee Populations. Department of Criminal Justice, University of Nevada Las Vegas, Final Report Prepared for the National Institute of Justice, U.S. Department of Justice, August 2002. Available at http://www.ncjrs.gov/pdffiles1/nij/grants/196677.pdf. Accessed December 18, 2007.

Mishra R. Gambling Industry Link to Harvard Draws Questions. *Boston Globe*, November 6, 2004.

Mullerman R, DenOtter T, Wadman M, et al. Problem gambling in the partner of the Emergency Department patient as a risk factor for intimate partner violence. *J Emerg Med* 23:307–312, 2002.

National Council on Problem Gambling. Problem and Pathological Gambling in America: The National Picture, January 1997.

National Council on Problem Gambling. *Helpline Statistics 2000–2008.* Washington, DC: National Council on Problem Gambling, 2008.

National Gambling Impact Study Commission. Final Report, August 31, 1999.

National Research Council. *Pathological Gambling: A Critical Review.* Washington, DC: National Academy Press, 1999.

New York Times. Fears for Children Delay New Lottery Video Game. March 8, 2003a. Available at http://query.nytimes.com/gst/fullpage.html?res=9C05E1D7113FF93BA35750C0A9659C8B63. Accessed December 9, 2008.

New York Times. Computer Lottery Game Canceled. Metro Briefing/Connecticut, Hartford. March 13, 2003b. Retrieved at http://query.nytimes.com/gst/fullpage.html?res=9404EED8133EF930A25750C0A9659C8B63&sec=&spon=.

Nixon R, Stodghill R. For Schools, Lottery Payoffs Fall Short of Promises. *New York Times*, October 7, 2007.

Office of Suicide Prevention. Suicide in Nevada Fact Sheet, 2007. Available at http://www.google.com/search?hl=en&ie=ISO-8859-1&q=nevada+highest+suicide+rate. Accessed June 21, 2008.

O'Malley J. Problem gambling: Addiction or poor choice? Defendants in Northern Nevada courts increasingly are blaming their crimes on gambling addictions. RGJ.com, August 21, 2008. Retrieved at http://www.rgj.com/apps/pbcs.dll/article?AID=/20080821/NEWS/808210352.

Pavalko R. Problem Gambling: The Hidden Addiction, national forum. Available at http:findarticles.com/p/articles/mi_qa3651/is199910/ai_n8875439/print. Accessed March 1, 2008.

Petry N, Stinson F, Grant B. Comorbidity of DSM-IV pathological gambling and other psychiatric disorders: Results from the National Epidemiologic Survey on Alcohol and Related Conditions. *J Clin Psychiatry* 66:564–574, 2005.

Potenza M, Fiellin D, Heninger G et al. Gambling: An addictive behavior with health and primary care implications. *J Gen Intern Med* 17:721–732, 2002.

Richtel M. Celebrities Taking a Gamble. *New York Times*, November 16, 2005.

Schneider G. Children Being Left Alone While Parents Gamble. *Louisville Courier-Journal*, July 18, 2000.

Schneider G. Gambler, Casino Sue Each Other. *Louisville Courier-Journal*, September 3, 2007. Available at http://www.usatoday.com/news/nation/2007–09-03-gambler-N.htm. Accessed November 2, 2007.

Skolnik S. Deck Stacked against Asians; Casinos Play Off Gambling-Intensive Culture. *Seattle Post-Intelligencer*, February 24, 2004.

SMR Research Corporation. *The Personal Bankruptcy Crisis: Demographics, Causes, Implications & Solutions.* Hackettstown, NJ: SMR Research Corporation, 1997, pp. 116–130.

Stewart D. *An Analysis of Internet Gambling and Its Policy Implications.* AGA 10th Anniversary White Paper Series. Washington, DC: American Gaming Association, 2006.

Volberg R. *Gambling and Problem Gambling among Adolescents in New York.* Albany: New York Council on Problem Gambling, March 1998.

Volberg R. *When the Chips Are Down.* Washington, DC: The Century Press Foundation, 2001.

Wiebe J, Single E, Falkowski-Ham A. *Measuring Gambling and Problem Gambling in Ontario.* Toronto: Canadian Centre on Substance Abuse Responsible Gambling Council, 2001.

7

Cash and Casinos: An Indian Perspective

Eileen M. Luna-Firebaugh, JD, MPA

Indian gaming and the development of tribal casinos have a specific purpose: the improvement of conditions that exist in Indian country. Unlike non-Indian casino gambling, the revenue from Indian gaming may be used only for designated purposes. There are no shareholders or corporate interests that control what happens to the profits derived from the gambling activities. Rather, Indian gaming is nonprofit. The distribution of money derived from the gaming enterprise must conform to the law as set forth in the 1999 Indian Gaming Regulatory Act (25 U.S.C. sects. 2701–2721), passed by the 133rd Congress.

Indian country is one of the few land areas in the United States where unemployment, crime rates, and poverty remain largely unaddressed. In 2000, the Associated Press conducted a computer analysis of federal unemployment, poverty, and public assistance records (Pace 2000). Unemployment in Indian country exceeded 50%, attributable largely to factors including geographic isolation, a lack of economic investment, and widespread lack of transportation.

American Indians are disproportionately poor. According to the U.S. Census Bureau, more than one-quarter of all American Indians, and more than 35% of all American Indian children, live below the poverty line, as compared with 12.6% of the total U.S. population. The annual median income of American Indian households in 2005 was $33,627, compared with the national average of $46,037 (Ogunwole 2006).

American Indians often do not have health insurance. The U.S. Census Bureau reports that 29.9% of people who reported American Indian or Alaska Native as their race were without medical coverage, compared with 11.3% of white Americans (Ogunwole 2006).

The American Indian population is both young and undereducated. The median age of American Indians living on tribal lands is 25, compared with the national median age of 35 years. About 33% of the American Indian population is under the age of 18, compared with 26% of the total population (Ogunwole 2006). More than 33% of American Indians living in tribal areas lack a high school education, compared with 20% of the total population (Swisher and Hoisch, 1992). Only about half (51%) of American Indian public high school students finish high school with a regular diploma (Bridgeland et al. 2006).

This comparative youth, lack of education, and lack of economic opportunity combine to create a web of social and psychological problems facing American Indian tribal governments. For example, more than 22% of American Indian juveniles have engaged in illicit drug use, compared with a national average of 10%; 14% have engaged in "binge drinking," compared with a national average of 10%; 22% have gotten into at least one serious fight at school or work, compared with the national average of 20%; 23% have gotten into at least one group-against-group fight, compared with the national average of 16%; and 15% of reservation-based Native American juveniles report some level of gang activity (Clarke et al. 2002–2003).

Yet another critical factor facing Indian country is an Indian youth suicide rate that is three times the national average (Freedenthal and Stiffman 2004). Given the high percentage of American Indian youths, which for many tribes exceeds 60% or more, this problem has reached a crisis level. The crisis is reflected in the 2003 New Mexico Youth Risk and Resiliency Survey, which found that approximately 25% of New Mexico Native American youths in grades 9–12 had attempted suicide (Grisham 2003). Additionally, results from the 2005 Navajo Middle School Youth Risk Behavior Survey indicate that 25% of respondents had seriously thought about killing themselves, 15% reported suicidal thoughts or a plan to kill themselves, and 13% had actually attempted suicide. These statistics make it easy to see why the provision of social and employment services is critical in Indian country (Brener et al. 2004).

Why Indian Gaming?

Economic development, and the resulting enhancement of personal opportunity, is an essential component of social change and community improvement. Indian gaming is one of the few economic development strategies that have worked in Indian country. The possibility of increasing the chances of personal and economic success for tribal members, and particularly for tribal youths, is a prospect that has fueled the development of tribal gaming, whose growth has been explosive. During an 18-year period (1988 to 2006), the revenue from Indian gaming grew from $100 million to $25.7 billion. The industry has created more than 248,000 jobs directly and more than 420,000 jobs indirectly (Taylor and Kalt 2005).

Although the impact of this money has been remarkable, few tribes have received the full benefit. Although there are more than 560 federally recognized tribes in the United States, only 130 have initiated casino gambling. And only a few of these 130 tribes have been highly successful (Luna 2003). Many tribes are located far from populated areas, and thus their opportunities are limited. For others, gaming is not culturally compatible. It may violate traditional values or beliefs, precluding it as a viable approach for enhancing economic opportunity. However, for those tribes where there is a cultural match and a ready market, tribal gaming can be an engine of successful economic development.

Where tribes have been successful, the impact on the lives of reservation Indians has been dramatic. An Associated Press study in 2000 found that, among casino tribes, the use of the U.S. Department of Agriculture's Food Distribution Program rose only 8.2% between 1990 and 1997, compared with an increase of more than 57% among tribes without Las Vegas–style casinos (Associated Press 2000). Between 1990 and 1998, the increase in food stamp use was 5.6% among Indian households in states that allow gambling, compared with 17.7% for analogous households in noncasino states. The county poverty rate where reservations were involved with casino gambling fell more than 2.5% in six years (1989–1995). Median household income rose by more than 30% in these counties during those same six years, and a number of tribes became "welfare-independent" (Luna 2003).

However, even given these results, the idea of Indian gaming as a primary focus of the move to accumulate capital and drive economic development is one about which there is little consensus in Indian country. Many tribes have voted not to proceed with gaming. For some, the cultural adaptation that would have to take place is too problematic. For others, the potential harm to tribal members from the proximity of gaming enterprises outweighs the potential benefits. Depression, alcoholism, and, as noted, suicide are rampant in Indian country (Volberg and Abbott 1997). While the connections with gambling are not clear, these factors, together with the high proportion of adolescents on most reservations, create a situation that could easily induce or exacerbate problematic gaming behaviors among tribal members (Zitzow 1996).

Understanding Tribal Sovereignty

In order to understand the choices faced by American Indian nations and the decisions they make, one must understand tribal sovereignty. The relationship between the Indian nations of the Americas and the colonizing nations began as one of independent sovereign states. The Indian nations had full, independent authority to govern themselves. They did not depend on any other nation to legitimate their acts of government. However, after colonization, the Indian nations accepted specific limitations on their sovereignty, as well as significant losses of land and resources, in exchange for treaty agreements. These treaty agreements and the legal decisions that have been issued subsequently protected the Indian nations' rights of self-government. The powers exercised by tribal governments have been protected by Supreme Court rulings as inherent to sovereigns, not powers granted to Indian nations by the U.S. Constitution.

In the early 1880s, the U.S. Supreme Court decided three cases that remain the basis for the federal–tribal relationship. These three cases (*Johnson v. McIntosh* 21 U.S. (8 Wheat.) 543; *Cherokee Nation v. Georgia* 30 U.S. (5 Pet.) 1; and *Worcester v. Georgia* 31 U.S. (6 Pet.) 515) later came to be known as the Marshall Trilogy. With these cases, Chief Justice John Marshall, writing for the Court, established the fundamental principles for American Indian tribal sovereignty (Luna-Firebaugh 2007):

1. The federal government has "Plenary Power" over Indian matters. State laws may not prevail in Indian country over federal treaties and statutes.
2. Indian nations are recognized as "dependent sovereign nations" to the federal government. Indian nations may not enter into agreements with other countries, nor may they alienate their lands except to the federal government.
3. Treaties between Indian nations and the federal government are legally interpreted to guarantee that Indian nations retain the right to self-government within their territories, without constraint or interference by individuals or state governments.
4. Certain rules of treaty construction govern the interpretation of treaties with Indian nations. These rules include that treaties are to be interpreted as they would have been understood by the Indians when they were negotiated. Any ambiguities within treaties or statutes are to be interpreted in Indians' favor. Treaties and federal Indian laws are to be interpreted liberally and are to favor a retained tribal self-government rather than state or federal authority.
5. The protection of land, guaranteed in the treaties, has been extended to the right to use and develop the resources of the land for the economic self-interest of Indian nations.

Defining "Indian Country"

With regard to tribal gaming, casinos are generally built on Indian trust land, in Indian country, where tribal territorial jurisdiction is complete and unassailable. Some casinos have been built on lands purchased by tribes, where the land has then been put into trust by the federal government. This land-into-trust generally occurs with the concurrence of the state and local governments. The right to conduct casino gaming, whether in Indian country or on land that is purchased and placed into trust, is subject to a tribal–state compact.

In 1948, Congress defined "Indian country" as the land within a reservation and land outside the reservation that is owned by tribal members or by the tribe and is held in trust by the federal government. U.S. federal statutes presently establish both criminal and civil jurisdiction (18 U.S.C.A. sect. 1151). The statutes provide:

[T]he term "Indian country," as used in this chapter, means (a) all land within the limits of any Indian reservation under the jurisdiction of the United States government, notwithstanding the issuance of any patent, and, including rights-of-way running through the reservation, (b) all dependent Indian communities within the borders of the United States whether within the original or subsequently acquired territory thereof, and whether within or without the limits of a state, and (c) all Indian allotments, the Indian titles to which have not been extinguished, including rights-of-way.

Legal and Legislative History of Indian Gaming

The first case to establish the right of tribes to engage in casino-type gaming was *California v. Cabazon Band of Mission Indians* (480 U.S. 202). In this 1987 case, the Supreme Court affirmed that a state could only interfere in Indian gaming if the state law was criminal and prohibitory rather than civil or regulatory. States could not prohibit or regulate gaming on Indian lands if some form of legal gaming occurred elsewhere within the state.

In 1988, subsequent to *Cabazon*, Congress enacted the Indian Gaming Regulatory Act (IGRA) (25 U.S.C. sects. 2701–2721). IGRA established the National Indian Gaming Commission and defined three classes of gaming. The mission of IGRA is to provide a statutory basis for Indian gaming that allows for the promotion of strong tribal governments, tribal economic development, and self-sufficiency. IGRA also created a network of federal regulations and attempted to shield tribal gaming from the possible intrusion of organized crime.

The three classes of Indian gaming set forth in IGRA are regulated differently, depending on their potential social and political impacts:

Class I gaming consists of social games with prizes of minimal value or traditional Indian games of chance held in conjunction with tribal ceremonies or celebrations. Class I gaming is deemed a wholly tribal concern, and thus IGRA does not regulate these activities.

Class II gaming includes bingo, electronic or not, and card games that are either explicitly authorized by state law or not explicitly prohibited by the laws of the state and are played somewhere within the state. Class II gaming is within the jurisdiction of the tribes but subject to the provisions of the Act. Class II gaming requires a tribal ordinance or resolution, and licensing is required. Until February 2008, no tribal–state compact was required.

Class III gaming includes any other form of gaming, including slot machines, banked card games, and other forms of electronic games of chance. The requirements for Class III gaming are similar to those for Class II; however, a tribal–state compact must also be developed and implemented. The net revenues from Class II and Class III gaming may be used only for specific purposes, including:

1. To fund tribal government operations or programs;
2. To provide for the general welfare of the tribe and its members;
3. To promote tribal economic development;
4. To donate to charitable organizations; or
5. To help fund operations of local government agencies.
6. A per capita payment method may only be used if the Secretary of the Interior has approved a plan developed by the tribe and if the interests of minors and other legally incompetent tribal members are protected.

In 2006, the National Indian Gaming Association reported that Indian tribes spent their net revenue as follows: 20% for education, child and elder services, culture, and charity; 19% for economic development; 17% for health care; 17% for police and fire protection; 16% for infrastructure; and 11% for housing. Many gaming tribes provide funding to local and state governments and to local schools, as well as to tribal programs, as part of the state–tribal compact agreements. The money spent on economic development benefits the tribes as well as the local areas, with investments made in diversified enterprises, including agriculture, hotels and conference centers, small businesses, and construction, both on and off reservations. These diversified activities, in addition to casinos, have created an employment base for many rural areas as well as many tribes.

Tribal–State Compacts

The compacting process between the states and the tribes has been difficult at best. States have made expensive financial demands of many tribes, in many instances running to 20%

of net revenues, a factor that has made gaming less lucrative for the tribes. The cost inherent in the development and maintenance of gaming, coupled with the cost of meeting state requirements in the compacting process, has become a significant deterrent to the signing of state–tribal gaming compacts (Worthen and Farnsworth 1996).

The Class III tribal–state compacting process, required by IGRA, gave rise to the 1996 case *Seminole Tribe of Florida v. State of Florida* (517 U.S. 44). *Seminole* significantly altered the effect of IGRA. In this case, the Seminole tribe of Florida sued the state of Florida for refusing to enter into compact negotiations that would have allowed for, and governed, Indian gaming. Florida countersued to dismiss the tribe's action, alleging that it violated the state's sovereign immunity. The U.S. Supreme Court ruled in favor of the state of Florida and against the section of IGRA that allowed the tribe the right to sue a state in federal court. This has now removed that remedy from IGRA and severely limits the ability of tribes to bring states to the bargaining table to negotiate a tribal–state compact.

Nonetheless, this legal obstacle has not stopped many tribes from seeking to implement tribal gaming. Some have attempted to expand tribal gaming through the use of Class II "bingo-type" gaming machines, which until recently did not require a tribal–state compact. However, in October 2007, the National Indian Gaming Commission (NIGC) proposed amendments to the Class II gaming regulations (25 U.S.C. 2071, et seq) that would define "bingo-type" gaming machines (where the players play against each other) as substantially similar to Class III slot machines (where players play against the machine). Thus, the use of these machines would become subject to tribal–state compacting requirements.

Conclusion

The future of American Indian tribal governments and their ability to successfully address the problems existing in Indian country depend on funding, which in turn depends on economic development. Funds can only be accumulated through investment and reinvestment, a process that can be accelerated by Indian gaming. However, questions remain about the long-term benefits of focusing on gaming as the primary tool of Indian economic development. There remain also questions about the feasibility and cultural match of gaming. For many tribes, the risk of gaming exceeds any possible benefit. This risk is often linked in Indian country with the widespread fear that Indian gaming is the "new buffalo"; that is to say, a life-giving resource that could be easily wiped out through actions of the states (Horwit 1996). As a result, for many tribes, the move toward self-determination through economic development does not include a role for Indian gaming. For others, Indian gaming is a valuable, culturally compatible tool that can help break the hold of poverty and despair on many reservations and Indian peoples.

References

Associated Press. Most Indians Haven't Benefited from 1990s Casino Boom, Analysis Shows. August 31, 2008. http://archives.cnn.com/2000/US/08/31/indian.gambling.ap/index.html. Accessed July 25, 2008.

Brener ND, Kann L, Kinchen, Steven A et al. Methodology of the Youth Risk Behavior Surveillance System. 2004. http://www.cdc.gov/MMWR/PDF/rr/rr5312.pdf. Accessed July 24, 2008.

Bridgeland JM, Dijulio JJ, Morison KB. *The Silent Epidemic: Perspectives of High School Dropouts.* Washington, DC: Civic Enterprises for the Bill and Melinda Gates Foundation, 2006.

Clarke AS. Social and emotional distress among American Indian and Alaska Native students. *ERIC Digest*, ED 459988, 2002–2003.

Freedenthal S, Stiffman AR. Suicide behavior in urban American Indian adolescents: A comparison with reservation youth in a southwestern state. *Suicide Life Threat Behav* 34:160–171, 2004.

Grisham ML. New Mexico Risk and Resilience Survey, 2003. Available at: http://www.nmhealth.org/epi/pdf/YRRS2003 FinalReport.pdf. Accessed July 24, 2008.

Horwit W. Note: Scope of gaming under the Indian Gaming Regulatory Act of 1988 after Rumsey v. Wilson: White Buffalo or Brown Cow. Yeshiva Univ Cardozo Arts Entertainment Law J 14:153–212, 1996.

Kennedy PF, Phanjoo AL, Sheki O. Risk-taking in the lives of parasuicides (attempted suicides). *Br J Psychiatry* 119:286, 1971.

Luna-Firebaugh E. *Tribal Policing: Asserting Sovereignty, Seeking Justice.* Tucson: University of Arizona Press, 2007.

National Indian Gaming Association. The Economic Impact of Indian Gaming in 2006. Washington, DC, National Indian Gaming Association.

National Indian Gaming Commission. NIGA Publishes Class II Regulations, Washington DC, October 24, 2007. http://www.nigc.gov/ReadingRoom/PressReleases/PR77102007/tabid/806/Default.aspx. Accessed July 25, 2008.

New York Times. Casino Boom Helps Tribes Reduce Poverty and Unemployment. September 3, 2000, p. 16.

Ogunwole SU. *We the People: American Indians and Alaska Natives in the United States,* Census 2000 Special Reports. Washington, DC: U.S. Census Bureau, 2006.

Pace D. Gaming a Bust for many Indians. *Arizona Daily Star,* September 1, 2000, p. A6.

Perry SW. American Indians and Crime, DOJ/BJS 1992–2002 NCJ 203097.

Swisher K, Hoisch M. Dropping out among American Indians and Alaska Natives. *J Am Indian Educ* 21:2, 1992.

Taylor JB, Kalt JP. Cabazon, American Indians on reservations: A databook of socioeconomic change between the 1990 and 2000 censuses, in *Cabazon, the Indian Gaming Regulatory Act and the Socioeconomic Consequences of American Indian Governmental Gaming: A Ten Year Review.* http://www.indiangaming.org/info/pr/databook/Databook-HPAIED_Gaming_Study.pdf. Accessed July 24, 2008.

Volberg RA, Abbott MW. Gambling and problem gambling among indigenous peoples. *Subst Use Misuse* 32:1525–1538, 1997.

Worthen KJ, Farnsworth WR. Symposium: The dilemma of American federalism: Power to the people, the states, or the federal government? Who will control the future of Indian gaming? A few pages of history are worth a volume of logic. *Brigham Young Univ Law Rev* 1996:407–447.

Zitzow D. Comparative study of problematic gambling behaviors between American Indian and non-Indian adolescents within and near a Northern Plains reservation. *Am Indian Alaska Native Ment Health Res* 7 (2): 14–41, 1996.

Section II

Pellicular Impulses

8

Trichotillomania: Clinical Aspects

Michael R. Walther, BS, Benjamin T. P. Tucker, BA,
and Douglas W. Woods, PhD

History of Psychiatric Attention to the Disorder

Trichotillomania (TTM) is an impulse control disorder characterized by recurrent pulling out of one's hair, resulting in noticeable hair loss (American Psychiatric Association 2000). The first detailed medical account of the disorder appeared in the late nineteenth century, when a French physician, Hallopeau, published case reports (Hallopeau 1889, 1894) of hair pulling, a syndrome he named *trichotillomania* (Christenson and Mansueto 1999).

The *Diagnostic and Statistical Manual of Mental Disorders* (DSM-III-R; American Psychiatric Association 1987) introduced formal diagnostic criteria for TTM, which included, "A) recurrent failure to resist impulses to pull out one's hair, resulting in noticeable hair loss, B) increasing sense of tension immediately before pulling out the hair, C) gratification or a sense of relief when pulling out the hair, and D) no association with a preexisting inflammation of the skin, and not a response to a delusion or hallucination" (p. 328). In DSM-III-R, TTM was classified as an impulse control disorder, but hair pulling was diagnosed as a stereotypy/habit disorder if it was stereotyped, rhythmic, and not preceded by an urge and accompanying gratification.

Current Diagnosis

Several changes to the diagnostic criteria have been made in the DSM-IV-TR (American Psychiatric Association 2000) (Table 8.1). First, hair pulling is an exclusionary criterion in considering a diagnosis of stereotypic movement disorder (formerly stereotypy/habit disorder), and thus hair pulling can only be diagnosed as TTM (Code 312.39). In contrast, the *International Classification of Diseases*, tenth edition (ICD-10; World Health Organization 1992), still allows hair pulling to be diagnosed as either TTM or stereotyped movement disorder with hair plucking. Second, criterion B has expanded to include tension when attempting to resist pulling. Third, patients must report distress or impairment as a result of the disorder. In the current iteration of the DSM, TTM continues to be categorized as an impulse control disorder not elsewhere classified.

Despite these changes, the utility of the current diagnostic criteria for TTM remains controversial. In particular, criteria B and C have been questioned, given that a substantial minority of individuals who chronically pull their hair to the point of significant hair loss do not report either prior tension or gratification when pulling (Christenson, MacKenzie, and Mitchell 1991, 1994; Hanna 1997). In order to inform potential revisions to the diagnostic criteria in DSM-V, studies are needed to examine whether criteria B and C bring incremental validity to characterizing populations and predicting treatment response.

Table 8.1 DSM-IV-TR criteria for trichotillomania (Code 312.39)

A. Recurrent pulling out of one's hair resulting in noticeable hair loss
B. An increasing sense of tension immediately before pulling out the hair or when attempting to resist the behavior
C. Pleasure, gratification, or relief when pulling out the hair
D. The disturbance is not better accounted for by another mental disorder and is not due to a general medical condition (e.g., a dermatological condition)
E. The disturbance causes clinically significant distress or impairment in social, occupational, or other important areas of functioning

Differential Diagnosis

Various conditions can mimic the signs and symptoms of TTM (American Psychiatric Association 2000). If patients presenting with hair loss deny pulling, it is important to consider alternative biological causes of hair loss (e.g., alopecia areata, male-pattern baldness, etc.). Psychiatric disorders can also mimic TTM. First, pulling may occur in response to specific delusions or hallucinations (e.g., pulling in response to auditory hallucinations or the belief that bugs are crawling underneath the scalp). Second, in some cases of obsessive-compulsive disorder (OCD), hair pulling is performed in response to an obsession such as a feared consequence that must be prevented (e.g., death of parents or a natural disaster) or according to rigid rules that elicit anxiety if not followed. In this case, the pulling can be viewed as a compulsion and a symptom of OCD instead of TTM. Third, hair pulling can occur exclusively in response to excessive concern with an imagined defect in one's physical appearance. In this case, the pulling may be a symptom of body dysmorphic disorder.

Clinical Picture

Hair pulling may occur on any area of the body where hair is present. The most common sites include the scalp, eyebrows, and eyelashes, but pulling also occurs frequently on the face, abdomen, legs, arms, armpits, or chest (Christenson, MacKenzie, and Mitchell 1994; Cohen et al. 1995; Woods et al. 2006a). Pulling from the pubic region was once believed to be less common (e.g., approximately 25% of patients reporting pubic pulling; Christenson, MacKenzie, and Mitchell 1994), but larger, more recent studies suggest that approximately half of adults with TTM may pull from this region (Woods et al. 2006a). Individuals typically pull with their fingers, but they may also use instruments such as tweezers, combs, or brushes (Woods et al. 2006b). Pullers commonly manipulate the hair after it has been pulled (e.g., twirling the hair between the fingers, rubbing it on the face or body, chewing or even eating pulled hair; Mansueto et al. 1997).

Trichotillomania patients often pull in response to a variety of cues, both internal and external. In many cases, physical features of the hair (e.g., gray hairs, coarse hairs, etc.) will prompt pulling episodes, with specific cognitions (e.g., "gray hairs are bad" or "my eyebrows should be more symmetrical") playing a role (Christenson and Mansueto 1999; Mansueto et al. 1997; Woods et al. 2006b). Pulling severity has also been associated with appearance-related cognitions such as negative beliefs about appearance and a fear of being negatively evaluated (Norberg et al. 2007). Emotional cues can also prompt the onset of a pulling episode. Negative affective states such as anxiety, tension, loneliness, fatigue, boredom, guilt, sadness, anger, indecision, and frustration may all prompt pulling (Diefenbach, Mouton-Odum, and Stanley 2002; Diefenbach et al. 2008; Mansueto et al. 1997; Woods and Miltenberger 1996). Finally, pulling may occur more often in specific settings or during certain activities (e.g., reading, studying, or watching TV) (Diefenbach, Mouton-Odum, and Stanley 2002; O'Connor et al. 2003; Woods et al. 2006b).

Various reinforcing consequences can maintain pulling. For many, pulling produces pleasurable physical sensations or reduces negative affective states (Diefenbach, Mouton-Odum, and Stanley 2002; Mansueto et al. 1997). Also, postpulling behaviors such as twirling the hair with the fingers, rubbing the hair on the face, or eating the hair can produce reinforcing tactile stimulation (Rapp et al. 1999).

A growing body of phenomenological data suggests that distinct styles of pulling exist. Hair pulling is sometimes performed in an "automatic" fashion, in which the pulling takes place largely out of the individual's awareness while he or she is engaging in another activity (e.g., reading or watching TV). At other times, pulling occurs in a "focused" fashion, in which the individual is intent on pulling and does so in response to bodily urges (e.g., burning or itching), negative affective states, or cognitions. Factor analytic studies support the existence of both styles in children (Flessner et al. 2007) and adults (Flessner et al. 2008b).

Several studies have examined the distribution of focused and automatic pulling in persons with TTM. Percentages have ranged from 5% to 47% for predominantly automatic, 15% to 34% for predominantly focused, and 19% to 80% for mixed pulling (Christenson, MacKenzie, and Mitchell 1994; du Toit et al. 2001). More recent studies have examined the relationship between degrees of focused or automatic pulling and the phenomenology and severity of pulling, depression, anxiety, stress, and disability. Flessner et al. (2008a) found that higher levels of both focused and automatic pulling were associated with greater pulling severity and more symptoms of anxiety and stress. Higher levels of focused but not automatic pulling were associated with increased symptoms of depression and disability. Also, those who were high focused but low automatic pullers were more likely to pull from the eyebrows, eyelashes, and pubic area and less likely to pull from the scalp compared with those who were low in both focused and automatic pulling.

Functional Impairment and Impact on Quality of Life

Trichotillomania can have many negative effects on physical health and psychosocial functioning. Physically, repetitive pulling and associated behaviors lead to hair loss and can cause follicle damage, changes in structure and appearance of regrown hair, scalp irritation, erosion of tooth enamel, gingivitis, and repetitive strain injury (Christenson and Mansueto 1999; O'Sullivan et al. 1996; Woods et al. 2006b). Those who ingest pulled hair are also at risk for developing a trichobezoar (an accumulation of undigested hair in the stomach), which can cause vomiting, anorexia, weight loss, gastric or intestinal bleeding, acute pancreatitis, and rarely death (Bouwer and Stein 1998; Woods et al. 2006b). Trichophagia in children is associated with iron-deficiency anemia (Sullivan 1989); thus, trichophagia is an indication for ordering a complete blood count.

Trichotillomania can also interfere with social, occupational, academic, and psychological functioning. Early studies of functional impairment in TTM patients suggested that concealing the physical effects of pulling from friends and family, avoiding treatment because of embarrassment, low self-esteem, decreased life satisfaction, and a negative impact on day-to-day living were all common (Christenson and Mansueto 1999; Diefenbach et al. 2005; du Toit et al. 2001; Seedat and Stein 1998; Stemberger et al. 2000). In a recent Internet survey of 1,697 adults with chronic hair pulling, the psychosocial impact of pulling was found across several domains (Woods et al. 2006a). Impairment was commonly reported in social functioning (e.g., interference with home management, avoiding social events, and trouble maintaining close relationships), academic and occupational functioning (e.g., difficulty studying, days missed or late to work or school, and interference with job duties). In addition, levels of depression, anxiety, and stress were relatively high and similar to those found in a clinical sample of adults with OCD (Antony et al. 1998). Also, a substantial minority reported using alcohol, tobacco, or illegal drugs to cope with TTM symptoms.

Research on the relationship between cultural or socioeconomic factors and TTM is limited. However, a small body of work has examined unique aspects of hair pulling among African Americans. For example, McCarley et al. (2002) found that African American women were more likely to report hair pulling with noticeable hair loss than individuals of other racial and gender groups. Neal-Barnett et al. (2000) found evidence suggesting that some African American women with TTM symptoms seek cosmetic treatment from their hairdressers. Finally, in a study of hair pulling in over 200 African American college students, none of the 6% who pulled their hair reported distress or impairment from hair pulling (Mansueto, Thomas-McCombs, and Brice 2007). The authors suggested that although both African American and Caucasian hair pullers experience negative emotional impact from pulling, African Americans may be less likely to experience troubling symptoms or seek professional help.

Assessment Instruments

A comprehensive assessment should be multimodal and include diagnostic measures of TTM and other disorders, symptom severity measures, and a functional assessment of pulling. The initial assessment guides treatment development and selection; assessment should continue throughout treatment to measure progress. Although few TTM assessment measures have undergone rigorous psychometric testing, the clinical utility of the best available instruments is discussed here. For more comprehensive reviews of techniques, instruments, and relevant issues in the assessment of TTM, see Carr and Rapp (2001) and Rothbaum, Opdyke, and Keuthen (1999).

The first step in assessing TTM is to determine whether diagnostic criteria for TTM and co-occurring conditions are met. This can be done via a structured diagnostic interview (e.g., the SCID, although this is quite lengthy) (First et al. 2002). The Trichotillomania Diagnostic Interview (Rothbaum and Ninan 1994) is a standardized clinician interview designed to assess DSM-III-R criteria and can be useful. However, further questioning is needed to evaluate the additional criteria described in DSM-IV-TR (e.g., tension when resisting pulling and distress/impairment).

Clinician-rated scales for assessing TTM severity include the Yale-Brown Obsessive Compulsive Scale-Trichotillomania (Y-BOCS-TM) (Stanley et al. 1993), the Psychiatric Institute Trichotillomania Scale (PITS) (Winchell et al. 1992), and the National Institute of Mental Health Trichotillomania Severity and Impairment Scales and Physician Rating of Clinical Progress (NIMH-TSS and TIS) (Swedo et al.1989). Psychometric evaluations of these scales have been mixed. The NIMH scales have demonstrated sensitivity to symptom changes as a result of treatment and acceptable inter-rater reliability (as has the PITS). However, the internal consistencies of the PITS, Y-BOCS-TM, and NIMH-TSS have been below minimal desired levels (Diefenbach et al. 2005; Rothbaum 1992; Stanley et al. 1999; Swedo et al. 1989).

Self-report measures include the Massachusetts General Hospital-Hairpulling Scale (MGH-HPS) (Keuthen et al. 1995) and the Trichotillomania Scale for Children (TSC) (Tolin et al. 2008). The MGH-HPS has acceptable test–retest reliability, convergent and divergent validity, and sensitivity to change (Keuthen et al. 1995; O'Sullivan et al. 1995). A recent factor-analytic study revealed that two factors, "severity" and "resistance and control," are present and may be useful in clinical assessments (Keuthen et al. 2007a). The TSC is the only available paper-and-pencil self-report severity measure for children. It includes separate child- and parent-report versions, each of which contains two components: "severity" and "distress/impairment." Tolin et al. (2008) found that the measure had adequate test–retest reliability, internal consistency, convergent validity, and parent–child agreement. Despite the relative psychometric strength of self-rated scales in measuring TTM severity, such measures are likely to be most useful when administered as part of a comprehensive battery.

Other TTM assessment strategies involve measuring the physical results of pulling. These include collecting and counting pulled hairs or taking photographs of body areas where pulling occurs. Although such techniques are relatively straightforward, one should consider the following before using them: (1) hair loss may be produced by alternative means (e.g., male-pattern baldness); (2) patients may be sensitive to this kind of assessment (e.g., embarrassment over collecting pulled hairs) and may be inaccurate in collecting hairs; and (3) certain measures (e.g., measuring bald spots) may be insensitive to pulling distributed across multiple sites (Carr and Rapp 2001; Rapp et al. 1998).

Direct observation can be used to gather real-time data on pulling as it occurs. Techniques include live observation (e.g., the clinician observes the patient in clinical or natural settings and documents the behavior in real time; Rapp et al. 2001), videotaped observation (e.g., Miltenberger et al. 1999), caregiver observation (e.g., Watson and Sterling 1998), and self-monitoring (e.g., Twohig and Woods 2004). However, hair pulling may be reactive to the observation situation, and patients are less likely to engage in these behaviors when they know they are being watched (Carr and Rapp 2001). Also, the time required to perform direct observation can be considerable. For these reasons, live or videotaped observation is rarely used (Woods et al. 2006b). Caregiver observation or self-monitoring can circumvent these limitations. For a child with TTM, parents, guardians, and teachers can be given a counting device (e.g., hand counter or data sheets) and trained to record pulling as it occurs in the patient's natural environment. Similarly, the patient can be trained and equipped to count instances of hair pulling. However, self-monitoring should be used only with older children and adults who have demonstrated an ability to recognize pulling as it occurs (Carr and Rapp 2001). This is a significant limitation on self-monitoring assessment because pulling often occurs outside the individual's awareness (e.g., automatic pulling).

Gathering functional assessment data is of particular importance in the clinical assessment of TTM. In conducting a functional assessment, clinicians should identify antecedent situations in which pulling is more likely to occur as well as consequences of pulling that may reinforce the behavior. For instance, pulling may be especially likely to occur in certain contexts (e.g., anxiety-producing situations, during particular thoughts, reading, or watching TV). Also, environmental consequences of pulling (e.g., parental attention, tactile stimulation, escape from negative emotions) may serve as reinforcements that maintain pulling. Understanding how environmental factors control pulling can help the clinician formulate treatment strategies incorporating modifications of these antecedents and consequences.

Prevalence

No broad epidemiological studies examining the prevalence of TTM have been published. However, several studies have examined prevalence using samples of convenience, particularly college students. In a sample of 2,579 college students, the lifetime prevalence of TTM was 0.6% (Christenson, Pyle, and Mitchell 1991). However, when the criteria for TTM were modified to include only hair pulling resulting in hair loss, regardless of the presence of tension or relief, the estimate increased to 2.5% (1.5% for males and 3.4% for females). In a study of 794 Israeli adolescents, the prevalence of hair pulling was 1% lifetime and 0.5% for current pulling (King et al. 1995a). Studies have generally reported a much higher proportion of TTM in females than in males (Christenson 1995; Cohen et al. 1995; Swedo and Leonard 1992), but the gender distribution in younger children is believed to be more nearly equal (Chang et al. 1991; Cohen et al. 1995; Muller 1987, 1990).

Age at Onset

Hair pulling may begin as early as the first year of life or well into adulthood (Christenson, Mackenzie, and Mitchell 1991; Cohen et al. 1995). However, a general consensus is that the typical TTM patient experiences onset during early adolescence (i.e., 13 years, SD = 8; Christenson, Mackenzie, and Mitchell 1991). Nonetheless, a subgroup of individuals experience onset in early childhood (2–6 years of age) (Bohne, Keuthen, and Wilhelm 2005), indicating a potential bimodal age of onset.

Natural History and Course of Illness

The severity of TTM waxes and wanes in response to environmental stressors, but given the absence of large longitudinal studies, little is known about its natural course. Moreover, there are few data on how the natural course may differ between treated and untreated cases. Chang et al. (1991) suggested that hair pulling lasting for more than six months is likely to have a more chronic course, but this has not been empirically confirmed. Evidence also suggests that childhood-onset TTM is likely to be relatively benign, transient, and responsive to minimal intervention (Swedo and Leonard 1992; Winchel 1992). However, this hypothesis has yet to be tested using prospective designs (Christenson and Mansueto 1999).

Biological Data

Although there is relatively little research on biological and genetic factors in TTM, several hypotheses and models have been proposed. For instance, family studies suggest that TTM may share a genetic diathesis with OCD and other habit disorders (Bienvenu, Samuels, and Riddle 2000; King et al. 1995b; Lenane et al. 1992). However, as with all family studies, environmental and social learning processes offer alternative explanations. Nonetheless, some studies have found that a small percentage of TTM families have variants of a specific gene, SLITRK1 (Zücher et al. 2006). Mutations in the SLITRK1 gene have also been found in Tourette's syndrome (Abelson et al. 2005), suggesting that rare mutations in this gene may play a role in the development of both disorders.

Other biological models have been built on the observation that TTM patients often do not report pain during hair pulling (Christenson, Mackenzie, and Mitchell 1991) and sometimes report that it feels pleasurable (Stanley et al. 1992). These observations suggest that decreased sensitivity to pain may increase the reinforcing qualities of pulling (Franklin, Tolin, and Diefenbach 2006). This model is consistent with findings that pulling may decrease in response to treatment with opiate receptor antagonists such as naltrexone (Carrion 1995).

A serotonin hypothesis has also been proposed based on studies demonstrating positive effects of selective serotonin reuptake inhibitor treatment for TTM (e.g., Koran, Ringold, and Hewlett 1992). However, placebo-controlled trials have failed to confirm the effectiveness of these medications (see the treatment section of this chapter).

Neuroimaging studies, although quite sparse, have also yielded some interesting findings. Some studies have shown structural abnormalities in TTM patients. For example, O'Sullivan et al. (1997), using magnetic resonance imaging (MRI) to examine ten women with TTM and ten healthy controls, found the TTM group had significantly reduced left putamen volume compared with controls. Keuthen et al. (2007b) found reduced cerebellar volumes in women with TTM compared with controls, which remained significant after correcting for total brain volume and head circumference. Functional neuroimaging studies have also shown increased glucose metabolism in the left and right cerebellum and right superior parietal region in TTM patients compared with controls (Swedo et al. 1991). Finally, although TTM is often conceptualized as an obsessive-compulsive spectrum disorder (Stein et al. 2005), there is growing evidence that TTM and OCD may have distinct brain circuitry profiles. For instance, hyperactivity seen in orbitofrontal-basal ganglia circuits in OCD (Insel 1992) has not been found in TTM (Rauch et al. 2007; Swedo et al. 1991).

Normal and abnormal grooming behaviors in animals have also been examined as potential models of TTM. Psychogenic feather picking in birds, psychogenic alopecia in cats, and acral lick dermatitis in dogs have all been investigated as potential animal analogues to TTM. (For a review of veterinary models of TTM, see Moon-Fanelli, Dodman, and O'Sullivan 1999.)

Comorbid Conditions

Like other psychiatric disorders, TTM is associated with a number of comorbid conditions. However, because TTM has not been extensively studied, psychiatric characterization of TTM samples has been limited.

Available data suggest that mood, anxiety, and substance abuse/dependence disorders are most likely to co-occur with TTM. Christenson (1995), after assessing 186 adults with TTM using a semistructured clinical interview for DSM-III-R disorders, reported the following lifetime diagnosis rates: 51.8% for major depression, 27% for generalized anxiety disorder, 19.4% for alcohol abuse or dependence, 16.1% for other substance abuse or dependence, 18.8% for simple phobia, and 13.4% for OCD. Other studies have reported high rates of personality disorder (e.g., 55%) (Schlosser et al. 1994).

In children with TTM, high rates of depression and anxiety have been reported, but limited sample sizes preclude applying those rates to the general population (Reeve, Bernstein, and Christenson 1992). High comorbidity rates were recently reported in a sample of TTM children, with 30% meeting criteria for at least one other mental disorder (Tolin et al. 2007). Generalized anxiety disorder was the most commonly occurring comorbid diagnosis. Interestingly, OCD was diagnosed in only 6.5% of subjects. In addition, according to parent report, almost two-thirds of first-degree relatives had a history of at least one mental disorder, with depression being the most commonly reported.

Because of the phenomenological similarities and high rates of comorbidity between TTM and OCD, some investigators have suggested that TTM be conceptualized as an obsessive-compulsive spectrum disorder (Stein et al. 2005), while others have countered that it falls within a spectrum of self-injurious behavior disorders (Lochner et al. 2005) or addictive disorders (Grant, Odlaug, and Potenza 2007). Studies of comorbidity rates between TTM and the other impulse control disorders are lacking. However, those with TTM may also frequently engage in other body-focused repetitive behaviors such as chronic skin picking and nail biting (Stein, Chamberlain, and Fineberg 2006).

Treatment

Both psychotherapy and pharmacotherapy are used to treat TTM. Much like treatments for other impulse control disorders, treatments for TTM focus on reducing the hair pulling, managing comorbid conditions that either contribute to or result from TTM, and improving overall well-being and functioning. The mental health care provider treating an individual with TTM should be careful not to convey the idea that therapy will bring a "cure." A more realistic approach to communicate is that treatment is strategy-driven and designed to supply the patient with tools that assist in managing the disorder.

That being said, a number of considerations must be taken into account in treating more severe cases. Individuals with comorbid conditions usually require longer treatment duration. Treatment sequencing must also be considered in such cases. When TTM presents with comorbid mood and/or anxiety disorders, they are usually functionally related to TTM and therefore should be dealt with in the context of TTM treatment (discussed later in this chapter). When co-occurring conditions are relatively independent of or more severe than the TTM, however, these conditions should be treated first.

Treatment compliance is an important predictor of treatment response (Woods, Wetterneck, and Flessner 2006), and a number of strategies can be used to increase it. Behavior reward programs can reward completion of homework and other therapeutic tasks. This strategy is particularly useful and practical in treating children. For adults, a self-imposed reward program may be used in which the patient rewards herself or himself for completing certain therapy tasks. In addition, the therapist should attempt to link the patient's treatment compliance to values the patient holds.

Pharmacotherapy

A recent survey found that pharmacotherapy is the most frequently employed treatment for TTM (Woods et al. 2006b). Medications commonly prescribed include tricyclic antidepressants (e.g., clomipramine) and selective serotonin reuptake inhibitors (SSRIs; e.g., fluoxetine). Both clomipramine and the SSRIs are also used in the treatment of OCD, reflecting the hypothesis that TTM and OCD share some biological features (Stein et al. 2005). Open-label trials have been conducted using other medication classes, including venlafaxine (50–375 mg/day, 12 weeks) (Ninan et al. 2000); lithium (900–1500 mg/day, 1.5–14 months) (Berk et al. 2003; Christenson et al. 1991; Pornnoppadol and Todd 1999); anticonvulsants (topiramate, 25–250 mg/day, 16 weeks) (Lochner et al. 2006); atypical antipsychotics such as olanzapine (2.5–10 mg/day, 12 weeks) (Stewart and Nejtek 2003); risperidone (0.5–3.0 mg/day, 8 months) (Epperson et al. 1999); and naltrexone (50 mg/day, 8 weeks) (Christenson and Crow 1996). These open-label trials and case reports report positive treatment outcomes, but the absence of controlled study designs means that these results must be viewed cautiously.

Swedo et al. (1989) conducted the first randomized, controlled trial (RCT) in individuals with TTM, a double-blind crossover study with 13 females (primarily adults); clomipramine (50–250 mg/day, 5 weeks) was superior to desipramine at posttreatment. Follow-up data 4 years posttreatment indicated that the 40% reduction in symptoms was maintained in the clomipramine group. In another RCT, neither fluoxetine (20–80 mg/day, 6 weeks) nor a placebo improved hair pulling significantly in a double-blind crossover study with 16 adult hair pullers (Christenson et al. 1991). Streichenwein and Thornby (1995) reported similar negative results in a second crossover RCT with fluoxetine (20–80 mg/day, 12 weeks) and a placebo.

Grant et al. (2009) reported efficacy for n-acetylcysteine, a glutamate modulator, in a 12-week RCT involving 50 individuals, 45 women and 5 men, with trichotillomania. N-acetylcysteine at 1200 mg/day was administered for six weeks and then increased as clinically indicated to 2400 mg/day, while matched placebo capsules were identically dosed. Of patients assigned to n-acetylcysteine, 56% were much or very much improved at endpoint, compared with 16% taking placebo; and, similarly statistically significant results were observed using the Massachusetts General Hospital Hair Pulling Scale and the Psychiatric Institute Trichotillomania Scale. No adverse events were reported in patients taking n-acetylcysteine.

Two RCTs have compared medication with cognitive-behavioral therapy (CBT) or behavior therapy. One study randomized 23 TTM patients to 9 weeks of clomipramine, CBT, or placebo and concluded that clomipramine (50–350 mg/day) and the placebo had equal treatment effects. Cognitive-behavioral therapy was superior to both clomipramine and the placebo at posttreatment, but the sample sizes were quite small (Ninan et al. 2000). Similarly, behavior therapy was superior to fluoxetine and a wait-list condition in an RCT conducted with 40 individuals. In this trial, the fluoxetine (20–60 mg/day, 12 weeks) and wait-list groups did not differ in treatment response (van Minnen et al. 2003).

In sum, available research suggests that SSRIs are no more effective than a placebo in the treatment of TTM. However, the studies are limited by small sample sizes, diagnostic variability within the samples, absence of validated assessment instruments, and failure to report intent-to-treat data. In the only two trials comparing CBT and medication, CBT was more effective.

Psychotherapy

Psychotherapy for individuals with TTM typically involves a variety of techniques. At the core are two elements: habit-reversal training (HRT) and stimulus control training. Habit-reversal training involves three main components: awareness training, competing response training, and social support. Additional treatment elements include self-monitoring, motivation enhancement, changing the internal monologue, and teaching coping strategies. Awareness training is designed to enhance a patient's awareness of the behavior they wish to stop. It involves techniques such as describing the pulling and any bodily sensations that precede pulling. The patient may be encouraged to verbalize when these behaviors or sensations occur during the session. In addition, the therapist may try to induce some of these behaviors and instruct the patient to "catch" them each time they happen.

Competing response training involves implementing a behavior or response that is incompatible with hair pulling. For example, the patient may be instructed to place her thumb inside her lightly closed fist each time a preceding bodily sensation (e.g., an urge to pull) occurs, when hair pulling has just begun (e.g., when the hand rises to the head), or when hair pulling is about to begin. Competing responses are: (1) physically incompatible with hair pulling, (2) easily done in multiple contexts, and (3) not noticeable to others. The patient should perform the competing response for 1 minute or until the urge to pull goes away (whichever is longer). The social support component may be particularly useful with children and entails the involvement of one or more support persons (e.g., a parent) who prompts the patient to use strategies learned in therapy and rewards the patient for implementing treatment procedures correctly. (See Chapter 11, this volume, for additional descriptions of HRT interventions.)

Stimulus control involves modifying the antecedent and consequential variables associated with pulling. For example, having a patient remove magnifying mirrors from the bathroom or wear gloves may decrease the probability of pulling by eliminating a trigger (e.g., noticing an "out-of-place" hair) or by changing the tactile sensation from hair manipulation. In addition to HRT and stimulus control procedures, cognitive restructuring is sometimes used to target maladaptive thoughts surrounding pulling (Mansueto et al. 1999). Acceptance-based procedures are included to eliminate the patient's focus on attempting to control unwanted private experiences (e.g., negative thoughts, urges, or emotions).

Two studies already mentioned (Ninan et al. 2000; van Minnen et al. 2003) reported that CBT outperformed a placebo and a wait-list control. In a randomized trial with 34 participants, HRT was also found more effective than negative practice in reducing the number of hair-pulling episodes (Azrin, Nunn, and Frantz 1980). According to the patients' reports, the number of hair-pulling episodes decreased 99% pre- to posttreatment. At follow-up (22 months later), patients reported that they maintained treatment gains, but only about two-thirds participated in the follow-up evaluation.

In another RCT, a combination of HRT and acceptance and commitment therapy (ACT) was compared with a wait list in 25 participants. The active treatment outperformed the wait list on a variety of outcome measures, including hair-pulling severity, impairment, and symptoms of anxiety and depression. Treatment gains were generally maintained at 3-month follow-up (Woods, Wetterneck, and Flessner 2006).

Behavior therapy for TTM has also been conducted in group format. In a study of 24 individuals with TTM, those receiving group behavior therapy reported significantly different improvements in hair-pulling severity and clinician-rated severity than those receiving group supportive therapy, but few participants met criteria for clinically significant change. In addition, 6-month follow-up generally showed symptom relapse (Diefenbach et al. 2006).

A literature search revealed only one controlled trial using combined medication plus psychotherapy treatment approaches. In phase one, adults with TTM were randomized to 12 weeks of the SSRI sertraline or a placebo. In phase two, 11 sertraline nonresponders were treated with HRT. A reduction in hair-pulling severity occurred in both the sertraline ($n = 4$) and combined treatment (sertraline plus HRT) groups, but with better overall gains in the combined treatment group (Dougherty et al. 2006). At this time, strong conclusions cannot be drawn regarding efficacy of combined forms of treatment in TTM, but the aforementioned trial raises the possibility that combined treatments may be more effective than monotherapies.

Hypnosis has also been used as an augmentation to behavior therapy and as a stand-alone treatment in several published case studies and case series (Friman and O'Connor 1984; Galski 1981; Hynes 1982; Kohen 1996; Oakley 1998). Whether adjunctive hypnosis adds any benefit over behavior therapy alone is unknown. In addition, the case study literature is biased in favor of positive reports.

Investigators reporting psychotherapy trial results often fail to utilize a systematic procedure to assess possible adverse events. Nevertheless, because behavior therapy's side effects are believed to be relatively mild, it has been recommended as a first-line treatment for children and adolescents with TTM (Baer, Osgood-Hynes, and Minichiello 1993). Our clinical experience suggests that therapists may wish to convey the message that psychotherapy for TTM may result in minor discomfort and frustration when attempting to alter the habitual pulling pattern and when experiencing the common waxing and waning of symptom intensity.

Summary and Treatment Recommendations

In sum, data regarding treatment response in TTM are not very encouraging. Active medications have generally failed to separate from the placebo, but studies have been small and methodologically limited. In addition, although some forms of psychotherapy have shown promise in small trials, reports on long-term treatment response have been mixed. High rates of relapse suggest the importance of "booster" sessions after the initial psychotherapy phase is complete. The Woods, Wetterneck, and Flessner (2006) protocol of HRT plus ACT calls for the final two treatment sessions to occur every other week (in contrast to the first eight sessions, which occur weekly), in hopes of maintaining treatment gains. Nevertheless, the incremental utility of booster sessions in TTM treatment has not been empirically evaluated.

From available research and our clinical experience, a few suggestions can be made for the clinician. The lack of evidence regarding medication effectiveness for TTM suggests that medication is not an effective stand-alone, first-line treatment for TTM. Thus, we suggest that medication be reserved for severe cases, for individuals who do not wish to or cannot undergo psychotherapy, and for cases in which comorbid conditions (e.g., depression, anxiety) may benefit from pharmacotherapy. Limited evidence supports psychotherapy in the form of HRT, but no treatment can be regarded as well established at this point.

In addition, other mental health professionals may be of help to an individual with TTM. For example, social workers may assist the patient in other domains of functioning, such as job seeking and dealing with family matters. Additionally, support groups for TTM and comorbid conditions may be helpful for both the patient and family members. The Trichotillomania Learning Center (http://www.trich.org) is a national nonprofit organization that provides useful information and support to those affected by trichotillomania and other body-focused repetitive behavior problems.

References

Abelson JF, Kwan KY, O'Roak BJ et al. Sequence variants in SLITRK1 are associated with Tourette's syndrome. *Science* 310:317–320, 2005.

American Psychiatric Association. *Diagnostic and Statistical Manual of Mental Disorders*, 3rd edition, revised. Washington, DC: American Psychiatric Association, 1987.

American Psychiatric Association. *Diagnostic and Statistical Manual of Mental Disorders*, 4th edition, text revision. Washington, DC: American Psychiatric Association, 2000.

Antony MM, Bieling PJ, Cox BJ et al. Psychometric properties of the 42-item and 21-item versions of the depression anxiety stress scales in clinical groups and a community sample. *Psychol Assess* 10:176–181, 1998.

Azrin NH, Nunn RG, Frantz SE. Treatment of hairpulling (trichotillomania): A comparative study of habit reversal and negative practice training. *J Behav Ther Exp Psychiatry* 11:13–20, 1980.

Baer L, Osgood-Hynes D, Minichiello WE. Trichotillomania, in *Handbook of Prescriptive Treatments for Children and Adolescents*. Edited by Ammerman RT, Last CG, Hersen M. Needham Heights, MA: Allyn and Bacon, 1993, pp. 315–331.

Berk M., McKenzie H, Dodd S. Trichotillomania: Response to lithium in a person with comorbid bipolar disorder. *Hum Psychopharmacol* 18:576–577, 2003.

Bienvenu JO, Samuels FJ, Riddle MA et al. The relationship of obsessive-compulsive disorder to possible spectrum disorders: Results from a family study. *Biol Psychiatry* 48:287–293, 2000.

Bohne A, Keuthen N, Wilhelm S. Pathological hairpulling, skin picking, and nail biting. *Ann Clin Psychiatry* 17:227–232, 2005.

Bouwer C, Stein DJ. Trichobezoars in trichotillomania: Case report and literature overview. *Psychosom Med* 60:658–660, 1998.

Carr JE, Rapp JT. Assessment of repetitive behavior disorders, in *Tic Disorders, Trichotillomania, and Other Repetitive Behavior Disorders*. Edited by Woods DW, Miltenberger RG. New York: Springer, 2001, pp. 9–32.

Carrion VG. Naltrexone for the treatment of trichotillomania: A case report. *J Clin Psychopharmacol* 15:444–445, 1995.

Chang CH, Lee MB, Chiang YC et al. Trichotillomania: A clinical study of 36 patients. *J Formos Med Assoc* 90:176–180, 1991.

Christenson GA. Trichotillomania – from prevalence to comorbidity. *Psychiatr Times* 12:44–48, 1995.

Christenson GA, Crow SJ. The characterization and treatment of trichotillomania. *J Clin Psychiatry* 57(suppl 8): 42–49, 1996.

Christenson GA, Mackenzie TB, Mitchell JE. Characteristics of 60 adult chronic hair pullers. *Am J Psychiatry* 148:365–370, 1991.

Christenson GA, Mackenzie TB, Mitchell JE. Adult men and women with trichotillomania: A comparison of male and female characteristics. *Psychosomatics* 35:142–149, 1994.

Christenson GA, Mackenzie TB, Mitchell JE et al. A placebo-controlled, double-blind crossover study of fluoxetine in trichotillomania. *Am J Psychiatry* 148:1566–1571, 1991.

Christenson GA, Mansueto CS. Trichotillomania: Descriptive characteristics and phenomenology, in *Trichotillomania*. Edited by Stein DJ, Christenson GA, Hollander E. Washington, DC: American Psychiatric Press, 1999, pp. 1–41.

Christenson GA, Pyle RL, Mitchell JE. Estimated lifetime prevalence of trichotillomania in college students. *J Clin Psychiatry* 52:415–417, 1991.

Cohen LJ, Stein DJ, Simeon D et al. Clinical profile, comorbidity, and treatment history in 123 hair pullers: A survey study. *J Clin Psychiatry* 56:319–326, 1995.

Diefenbach GJ, Mouton-Odum S, Stanley MA. Affective correlates of trichotillomania. *Behav Res Ther* 40:1305–1315, 2002.

Diefenbach GJ, Tolin DF, Hannan S et al. Trichotillomania: Impact on psychosocial functioning and quality of life. *Behav Res Ther* 43:869–884, 2005.

Diefenbach GJ, Tolin DR, Hannan S et al. Group treatment for trichotillomania: Behavior therapy versus supportive therapy. *Behav Ther* 37:353–363, 2006.

Diefenbach GJ, Tolin DF, Meunier S et al. Emotion regulation and trichotillomania: A comparison of clinical and nonclinical hair pulling. *J Behav Ther Exp Psychiatry* 39:32–41, 2008.

Dougherty DD, Loh R, Jenike MA et al. Single modality versus dual modality treatment for trichotillomania: Sertraline, behavioral therapy, or both? *J Clin Psychiatry* 67:1086–1092, 2006.

du Toit PL, van Kradenburg J, Niehaus DJH et al. Characteristics and phenomenology of hair-pulling: An exploration of subtypes. *Compr Psychiatry* 42:247–256, 2001.

Epperson C, Fasula D, Wasylink S et al. Risperidone addition in serotonin reuptake inhibitor-resistant trichotillomania: Three cases. *J Child Adolesc Psychopharmacol* 9:43–49, 1999.

First MB, Spitzer RL, Gibbon M et al. *Structured Clinical Interview for DSM-IV-TR Axis 1 Disorders – Patient Edition*, SCID-I/P, 11/2002 revision. New York: Biometrics Research Department, 2002.

Flessner CA, Conelea CA, Woods DW et al. Styles of pulling in trichotillomania: Exploring differences in symptom severity, phenomenology, and functional impact. *Behav Res Ther* 46:345–357, 2008a.

Flessner CA, Woods DW, Franklin ME et al. The Milwaukee Inventory for Subtypes of Trichotillomania (MIST-A): Development of an instrument for the assessment of "focused" and "automatic" hair pulling. *J Psychopathol Behav Assess* 30:20–30, 2008b.

Flessner CA, Woods DW, Franklin MF et al. The Milwaukee Inventory for Styles of Trichotillomania – Child Version (MIST-C): Initial development and psychometric properties. *Behav Modif* 31:896–918, 2007.

Franklin ME, Tolin DF, Diefenbach GJ. Trichotillomania, in *Clinical Manual of Impulse Control Disorders*. Edited by Hollander E, Stein DJ. Arlington, VA: American Psychiatric Publishing, 2006, pp. 149–173.

Friman, PC, O'Connor WA. The integration of hypnotic and habit reversal techniques in the treatment of trichotillomania. *Behav Ther* 7:166–167, 1984.

Galski, TJ. The adjunctive use of hypnosis in the treatment of trichotillomania: A case report. *Am J Clin Hypn* 23:198–201, 1981.

Grant JE, Odlaug BL, Kim SW. N-acetylcysteine, a glutamate modulator, in the treatment of trichotillomania. *Arch Gen Psychiatry* 66:756–763, 2009.

Grant JE, Odlaug BL, Potenza MN. Addicted to hair pulling? How an alternate model of trichotillomania may improve treatment outcome. *Harv Rev Psychiatry* 15:80–85, 2007.

Hallopeau H. Alopecie par grattage (tricomanie ou trichotillomanie). *Ann Dermatol Syphil* 10:440–441, 1889.

Hallopeau H. Sur un nouveau cas de trichotillomanie. *Ann Dermatol Syphil* 5:541–543, 1894.

Hanna GL. Trichotillomania and related disorders in children and adolescents. *Child Psychiatry Hum Dev* 27:255–268, 1997.

Hynes JV. Hypnotic treatment of five adult cases of trichotillomania. *Aust J Clin Exp Hypn* 10:109–116, 1982.

Insel TR. Toward a neuroanatomy of obsessive-compulsive disorder. *Arch Gen Psychiatry* 49:739–744, 1992.

Keuthen NJ, Flessner CA, Woods DW et al. Factor analysis of the Massachusetts General Hospital hairpulling scale. *J Psychosom Res* 62:707–709, 2007a.

Keuthen NJ, Makris N, Schlerf JE et al. Evidence for reduced cerebellar volumes in trichotillomania. *Biol Psychiatry* 61:374–381, 2007b.

Keuthen NJ, O'Sullivan RL, Ricciardi JN et al. The Massachusetts General Hospital (MGH) hairpulling scale: 1. Development and factor analysis. *Psychother Psychosom* 64:141–145, 1995.

King RA, Scahill L, Vitulano LA et al. Childhood trichotillomania: Clinical phenomenology, comorbidity, and family genetics. *J Am Acad Child Adolesc Psychiatry* 34:1451–1459, 1995b.

King RA, Zohar AH, Ratzoni G et al. An epidemiological study of trichotillomania in Israeli adolescents. *J Am Acad Child Adolesc Psychiatry* 34:1212–1215, 1995a.

Kohen DP. Hypnotherapeutic management of pediatric and adolescent trichotillomania. *J Dev Behav Pediatr* 17:328–334, 1996.

Koran LM, Ringold A, Hewlett W. Fluoxetine for trichotillomania: An open clinical trial. *Psychopharmacol Bull* 28:145–149, 1992.

Lenane MC, Swedo SE, Rapoport JL et al. Rates of obsessive-compulsive disorder in first degree relatives of patients with trichotillomania. *J Child Psychol Psychiatry* 33:925–933, 1992.

Lochner C, Seedat S, du Toit PL et al. Obsessive-compulsive disorder and trichotillomania: A phenomenological comparison. *BMC Psychiatry* 5:2, 2005.

Lochner C, Seedat S, Niehaus DJH et al. Topiramate in the treatment of trichotillomania: An open-label pilot study. *Int Clin Psychopharmacol* 21:255–259, 2006.

Mansueto CS, Golomb RG, Thomas AM et al. A comprehensive model for behavioral treatment of trichotillomania. *Cognit Behav Pract* 6:23–43, 1999.

Mansueto CS, Stemberger RM, Thomas AM et al. Trichotillomania: A comprehensive behavioral model. *Clin Psychol Rev* 17:567–577, 1997.

Mansueto CS, Thomas-McCombs A, Brice AL. Hair pulling and its affective correlates in an African-American university sample. *J Anxiety Disord* 21:590–599, 2007.

McCarley NG, Spirrison CL, Ceminsky JL. Hair pulling behavior reported by African American and non-African American college students. *J Psychopathol Behav Assess* 24:139–144, 2002.

Miltenberger RG, Rapp JT, Long ES. A low-tech method for conducting real-time recording. *J Appl Behav Anal* 32:119–120, 1999.

Moon-Fanelli AA, Dodman NH, O'Sullivan RL. Veterinary models of compulsive self-grooming: Parallels with trichotillomania, in *Trichotillomania*. Edited by Stein DJ, Christenson GA, Hollander E. Washington, DC: American Psychiatric Press, 1999, pp. 63–92.

Muller SA. Trichotillomania. *Dermatol Clin* 5:595–601, 1987.

Muller SA. Trichotillomania: A histopathologic study in sixty-six patients. *J Am Acad Dermatol* 23:56–62, 1990.

Neal-Barnett AM, Ward-Brown BJ, Mitchell M et al. Hair pulling in African Americans – only your hairdresser knows for sure: An exploratory study. *Cult Divers Ethnic Minor Psychol* 6:352–362, 2000.

Ninan PT, Rothbaum BO, Marsteller FA et al. A placebo-controlled trial of cognitive-behavioral therapy and clomipramine in trichotillomania. *J Clin Psychiatry* 61:47–50, 2000.

Norberg MM, Wetterneck CT, Woods DW et al. Experiential avoidance as a mediator of relationships between cognitions and hair-pulling severity. *Behav Modif* 31:367–381, 2007.

O'Connor K, Brisebois H, Brault M et al. Behavioral activity associated with onset in chronic tic and habit disorder. *Behav Res Ther* 41:241–249, 2003.

O'Sullivan RL, Keuthen NJ, Hayday CF et al. The Massachusetts General Hospital (MGH) hairpulling scale: 2. Reliability and validity. *Psychother Psychosom* 64:146–148, 1995.

O'Sullivan RL, Keuthen NJ, Jenike MA et al. Trichotillomania and carpal tunnel syndrome. *J Clin Psychiatry* 57:174, 1996.

O'Sullivan RL, Rauch SL, Breiter HC et al. Reduced basal ganglia volumes in trichotillomania measured via morphometric magnetic resonance imaging. *Biol Psychiatry* 42:39–45, 1997.

Oakley DA. Emptying the habit: A case of trichotillomania. *Contemp Hypn* 15:109–117, 1998.

Pornnoppadol C, Todd RD. Mania and trichotillomania. *J Am Acad Child Adolesc Psychiatry* 38:1470–1471, 1999.

Rapp JT, Carr JE, Miltenberger RG et al. Using real-time recording to enhance the analysis of within-session functional analysis data. *Behav Modif* 25:79–93, 2001.

Rapp JT, Miltenberger RG, Galensky TL et al. A functional analysis of hair pulling. *J Appl Behav Anal* 32:329–337, 1999.

Rapp JT, Miltenberger RG, Long ES et al. Simplified habit reversal treatment for chronic hair pulling in three adolescents: A clinical replication with direct observation. *J Appl Behav Anal* 31:299–302, 1998.

Rauch SL, Wright CI, Savage CR et al. Brain activation during implicit sequence learning in individuals with trichotillomania. *Psychiatry Res Neuroimaging* 154:233–240, 2007.

Reeve EA, Bernstein GA, Christenson GA. Clinical characteristics and psychiatric comorbidity in children with trichotillomania. *J Am Acad Child Adolesc Psychiatry* 31:132–138, 1992.

Rothbaum BO. The behavioral assessment of trichotillomania. *Behav Psychother* 20:85–90, 1992.

Rothbaum BO, Ninan PT. The assessment of trichotillomania. *Behav Res Ther* 32:651–662, 1994.

Rothbaum BO, Opdyke DC, Keuthen NJ. Asssessment of trichotillomania, in *Trichotillomania*. Edited by Stein DJ, Christenson GA, Hollander E. Washington, DC: American Psychiatric Press, 1999, pp. 285–298.

Schlosser S, Black DW, Blum N et al. The demography, phenomenology, and family history of 22 persons with compulsive hair pulling. *Ann Clin Psychiatry* 6:147–152, 1994.

Seedat S, Stein DJ. Psychosocial and economic implications of trichotillomania: A pilot study in a South African sample. *CNS Spectr* 3:40–43, 1998.

Stanley MA, Breckenridge JK, Snyder AG et al. Clinician-rated measures of hair pulling: A preliminary psychometric evaluation. *J Psychopathol Behav Assess* 21:157–182, 1999.

Stanley MA, Prather RC, Wagner AL et al. Can the Yale-Brown Obsessive Compulsive Scale be used to assess trichotillomania? A preliminary report. *Behav Res Ther* 31:171–177, 1993.

Stanley MA, Swann AC, Bowers TC et al. A comparison of clinical features in trichotillomania and obsessive-compulsive disorder. *Behav Res Ther* 30:39–44, 1992.

Stein DJ, Chamberlain SR, Fineberg N. An A-B-C model of habit disorders: Hair-pulling, skin-picking, and other stereotypic conditions. *CNS Spectr* 11:824–827, 2006.

Stein DJ, Lochner C, Hemmings S et al. Trichotillomania: An obsessive-compulsive spectrum disorder, in *Concepts and Controversies in Obsessive-Compulsive Disorder*. Edited by Abramowitz JS, Houts AC. New York: Springer, 2005, pp. 151–161.

Stemberger RM, Thomas AM, Mansueto CS et al. Personal toll of trichotillomania: Behavioral and interpersonal sequelae. *J Anxiety Disord* 14:97–104, 2000.

Stewart RS, Nejtek VA. An open-label, flexible-dose study of olanzapine in the treatment of trichotillomania. *J Clin Psychiatry* 64:49–52, 2003.

Streichenwein SM, Thornby JL. A long-term, double-blind, placebo-controlled crossover trial of the efficacy of fluoxetine for trichotillomania. *Am J Psychiatry* 152:1192–1196, 1995.

Sullivan C. Trichotillomania (letter). *Br J Psychiatry* 155:869, 1989.

Swedo SE, Leonard HL. Trichotillomania: An obsessive-compulsive spectrum disorder? *Psychiatr Clin North Am* 15:777–790, 1992.

Swedo SE, Leonard HL, Rapoport JL et al. A double-blind comparison of clomipramine and desipramine in the treatment of trichotillomania (hair pulling). *N Engl J Med* 321:497–501, 1989.

Swedo SE, Rapoport JL, Leonard HL et al. Regional cerebral glucose metabolism of women with trichotillomania. *Arch Gen Psychiatry* 48:828–833, 1991.

Tolin DF, Diefenbach GJ, Flessner CA et al. The trichotillomania scale for children: Development and validation. *Child Psychiatry Hum Dev* 39:331–349, 2008.

Tolin DF, Franklin ME, Diefenbach GJ et al. Pediatric trichotillomania: Descriptive psychopathology and an open trial of cognitive behavioral therapy. *Cognit Behav Ther* 36:129–144, 2007.

Twohig MP, Woods DW. A preliminary investigation of acceptance and commitment therapy and habit reversal as a treatment for trichotillomania. *Behav Ther* 35:803–820, 2004.

van Minnen A, Hoogduin KA, Keijsers GP et al. Treatment of trichotillomania with behavioral therapy or fluoxetine: A randomized, waiting-list controlled study. *Arch Gen Psychiatry* 60:517–522, 2003.

Watson TS, Sterling HE. Brief functional analysis and treatment of a vocal tic. *J Appl Behav Anal* 31:471–474, 1998.

Winchell RM. Trichotillomania: Presentation and treatment. *Psychiatr Ann* 22:84–89, 1992.

Winchell RM, Jones JS, Molcho A et al. Rating the severity of trichotillomania: Methods and problems. *Psychopharmacol Bull* 28:457–462, 1992.

Woods DW, Flessner CA, Franklin ME et al. The trichotillomania impact project (TIP): Exploring phenomenology, functional impact, and treatment utilization. *J Clin Psychiatry* 67:1877–1888, 2006a.

Woods DW, Flessner CA, Franklin ME et al. Understanding and treating trichotillomania: What we know and what we don't know. *Psychiatr Clin North Am* 29:487–501, 2006b.

Woods DW, Miltenberger RG. Are persons with nervous habits nervous? A preliminary examination of habit function in a nonreferred population. *J Appl Behav Anal* 29:259–261, 1996.

Woods DW, Wetterneck CT, Flessner CA. A controlled evaluation of acceptance and commitment therapy plus habit reversal for trichotillomania. *Behav Res Ther* 44:639–656, 2006.

World Health Organization. *The ICD-10 Classification of Mental and Behavioural Disorders: Clinical Descriptions and Diagnostic Guidelines*. Geneva: World Health Organization, 1992.

Zücher S, Cuccaro ML, Tran-Viet KN et al. SLITRK1 mutations in trichotillomania. *Mol Psychiatry* 11:888–889, 2006.

9

Trichotillomania: The View from Dermatology

Drew Miller, MD, and Amy McMichael, MD

Introduction

In 1889, Hallopeau, a French dermatologist, reported a self-induced depilation of the scalp and coined the term trichotillomania (Hallopeau 1889). More than 100 years later, the fourth edition of the *Diagnostic and Statistical Manual of Mental Disorders* (DSM-IV) has included trichotillomania (TTM) under the category of impulse control disorders (see Table 8.1). This definition, however, excludes many patients who suffer from a clinically apparent, self-induced hair loss but do not meet full criteria as specified in the DSM-IV guidelines (i.e., tension and release of tension by pulling hair). These patients can be defined more broadly as "hair pullers." The epidemiology of TTM is discussed in Chapter 8 but it should be noted that hair pulling has a higher prevalence than TTM. Large surveys of college students found that while 0.6% met DSM-IV criteria for TTM, 2.5% acknowledged hair pulling that resulted in visible hair loss (Christenson, Pyle, and Mitchell 1991). This chapter extends the discussion of TTM beyond the DSM-IV definition and describes the clinical approach to diagnosis and management of all hair pullers who may present in a dermatology or primary care outpatient setting.

Differences among the patient populations presenting with hair pulling in a dermatologic as compared with a psychiatric setting create unique challenges for diagnosis and management. Patients who seek consultation from a psychiatrist often recognize that they are pulling their hair and are openly seeking help to overcome this tendency. In contrast, many patients who present to a dermatologist or primary care physician lack the insight that they are responsible for their symptoms and instead present with the complaint of general hair loss. This lack of insight, or denial, can create barriers to management that must be addressed in order to achieve a successful outcome.

Patient Presentation

Hair pullers can be divided into two main groups based on the age of presentation: child hair pullers and adult hair pullers. Child hair pulling usually occurs in children age 5 or younger and tends to be both benign and self-limited (Oranje, Peereboom-Wynia, and De Raeymaecker 1986). Some authors suggest that hair pulling in this age group should be considered a separate disorder more analogous to nail biting rather than TTM (Lenane, Swedo, and Rapoport 1992; Mannino and Delgado 1969; Swedo and Rapoport 1991). Studies rarely encompass both age groups, and no longitudinal studies are available to indicate whether patients who develop these symptoms in infancy or childhood are more likely to have TTM later in life (Hautmann, Hercogova, and Lotti 2002). Adult hair pulling has a mean onset of 9–13 years of age and often continues into adulthood (Christensen and Mackenzie 1995); it is associated with more psychopathology and carries a poorer prognosis (Hautmann, Hercogova, and Lotti 2002).

Adult hair pullers can further be subdivided into those with and those without insight. As many as 43% of patients with trichotillomania are estimated to deny that their alopecia

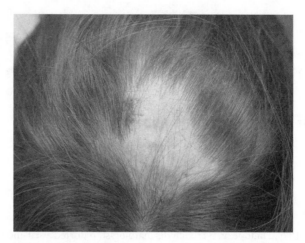

Figure 9.1   Irregular bordered TTM scalp patch with scarring, excoriation, and broken hairs in a teenager.

is self-induced (Christenson, Mackenzie, and Mitchell 1991). In the case of adolescent patients, parents may share in the denial. The approach to diagnosis and treatment must be tailored to the patient's degree of insight.

Patients with hair pulling secondary to another psychiatric disorder, while not included in the DSM-IV TTM category, constitute a significant proportion of patients presenting with alopecia. Common causes may include major depressive disorder, generalized anxiety disorder, or body dysmorphic disorder. It is important to identify any primary disorders and treat appropriately because symptoms may resolve with treatment of the underlying condition.

Clinical Features

In most cases, patients with TTM present with a patchy alopecia of the scalp (Muller 1987). Hair pulling occurs most commonly on the scalp but may also involve the eyebrows, eyelashes, facial hairs, and any other hair-bearing areas. Affected patches vary in size, often have a bizarre pattern with irregular borders, and show a decreased density of hairs that are short but of varying length (Buescher and Resch 2008) (Figures 9.1 and 9.2). Close inspection may reveal perifollicular erythema, hemorrhage, and plucked hairs with a fractured end, as opposed to the finely tapered appearance of a nontraumatized regular hair (Hautmann, Hercogova, and Lotti 2002). This gives rise to a stubbly sensation when gently passing the hand over affected areas. The crown of the scalp is frequently involved, and significant loss in this distribution with maintenance of hair in the occiput is known as the "Friar Tuck sign"

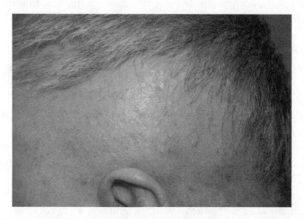

Figure 9.2   Side view. TTM broken hairs in an elderly woman with several other psychiatric diagnoses.

(Dimino-Emme and Camisa 1991). Hair pulling may be biased to the side of handedness, and simultaneous pulling of the ipsilateral eyebrow or eyelashes is common. In severe cases, a full alopecia of the scalp may occur.

Hair pulling can become a ritual that occurs daily and can occupy up to several hours (Soriano, O'Sullivan, and Baer 1996). Such pulling occurs in a particular setting or at a particular time of the day and is often worse in the evening. High-risk settings include watching television, reading, talking on the phone, lying in bed, driving, and writing. Patients may experience feelings of guilt or shame from plucking hair and attempt to conceal the affected areas through creative hairstyling or wearing a wig (Soriano, O'Sullivan, and Baer 1996). There may be periods of exacerbation and remission, but the disorder is generally considered to be chronic (Krishnan, Davidson, and Guarjuardo 1985).

In many cases, biopsy can aid in the diagnosis of TTM. Histology reveals normal growing hairs among empty hair follicles in a noninflammatory dermis. Some follicles show dilated follicular ostia with keratin plugging as well as pigment casts. Hair shafts may be broken or seen as dark bodies.

Differential Diagnosis

Trichotillomania should be distinguished from other causes of patchy alopecia such as alopecia areata, tinea capitis, secondary syphilis, and inflammatory dermatoses (see Table 9.1). Distinguishing alopecia areata (AA) from TTM is often the most challenging. This condition, widely believed to be an autoimmune disorder, leads to rapid and complete hair loss in round or oval patches (James, Berger, and Elston 2006) (Figure 9.3). Patches of complete hair loss give rise to a smooth sensation when passing the hand over the affected area as opposed to the stubbly sensation found in TTM. Just as in TTM, however, AA can occur on the scalp, eyebrows, eyelashes, beard, or any other hair-bearing area. Close examination often reveals "exclamation point" hairs, short hairs composed of a distal end that is broader than the proximal end (Bolognia, Jorizzo, and Rapini 2003). Areas with active borders will display a positive "pull test" performed by pinching approximately 30 hairs between the thumb and index finger and pulling. Loss of three or more hairs with gentle pulling constitutes a positive "pull test." Other diagnostic clues include periodic regrowth

Table 9.1 Primary differential diagnosis of hair pulling

	Hair Pulling	Alopecia Areata	Tinea Capitis
Distribution	Scalp most commonly	Scalp most commonly	Scalp primarily
	May involve any hair-bearing area	May involve any hair-bearing area	
Pattern	Patches vary in size. Bizarre or angular patterns	Patches vary in size Oval-shaped patches	Annular patches most commonly
	"Friar Tuck" sign	Can be diffuse	May involve entire scalp
	May favor the side of handedness		
Patch	Short hairs of varying length (stubbly on exam)	Complete hair loss (smooth on exam)	With or without scaling "Black Dot" tinea
	Decreased hair density	"Exclamation point" hairs	+/− Pustular eruption
	Perifollicular erythema	Short vellus hairs regrowing	
Diagnostic clues	Signs of primary mental disorder	Positive (+) pull test Nail pitting	Posterior cervical lymphadenopathy
	Physical exam generally unremarkable		Spores/hyphae on microscopic examination of hairs

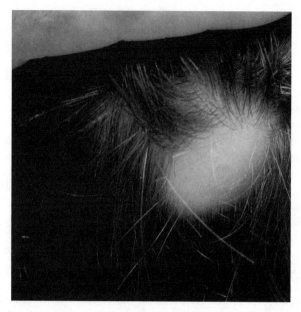

Figure 9.3   Patch of alopecia areata with fine blond hair regrowing.

by history and, on physical examination, visible regrowth of fine, tapered, downy-like hairs and pitting of the nails (Figure 9.4) (James, Berger, and Elston 2006).

Tinea capitis is a fungal infection of the scalp that can mimic TTM. Affecting children with far greater frequency than adults, tinea capitis commonly presents as discrete patches of alopecia with or without scaling. In severe cases, the process may involve the entire scalp. Presentation may vary depending on the causative organism; for instance, infection by the organism *T. tonsurans* can lead to breakage of the hair near the scalp, resulting in a retained hair stuck in the follicular opening, termed "black dot" tinea (Bolognia, Jorizzo, and Rapini 2003). These broken hairs can be confused with the traumatized hairs of TTM (Figure 9.5). Lesions are often annular in tinea as opposed to the bizarre pattern seen in hair pulling. The presence of scaling can be an important diagnostic clue favoring fungal infection. Tinea capitis with more severe inflammation may lead to a pustular eruption, allowing for easy differentiation from TTM. In cases that are difficult to distinguish on inspection alone, the presence of posterior auricular or posterior cervical lymphadenopathy as well as illumination

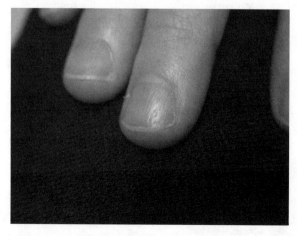

Figure 9.4   Nail pitting that can be seen with alopecia areata.

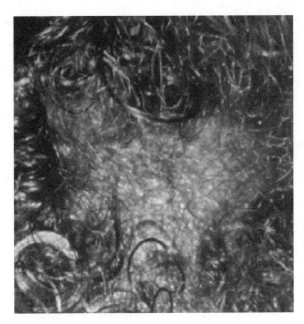

Figure 9.5   Broken hairs of tinea capitis infection mimicking TTM.

by Wood's lamp can aid in the diagnosis of tinea capitis (Hautmann, Hercogova, and Lotti 2002), though most fungal organisms that cause tinea in the United States are not fluorescent. Microscopic examination of affected hairs revealing small round spores or hyphae provides a definitive diagnosis. Fungal culture and skin biopsy are additional means of diagnosing tinea capitis.

Patients with secondary syphilis may experience alopecia syphilitica, composed of small and irregular patches of alopecia that result in a characteristic "moth-eaten" appearance (James, Berger, and Elston 2006). Alopecia syphilitica manifests in less than 10% of individuals with secondary syphilis and is usually reversible with treatment (Bolognia, Jorizzo, and Rapini 2003). The presence of other more prominent signs will aid in diagnosis. More than 80% of patients experience a generalized, nonpruritic eruption of copper-colored lesions that may involve the face, palms, and soles. Systemic manifestations include low-grade fever, malaise, sore throat, lymphadenopathy, weight loss, myalgias/arthralgias, and headache. Condyloma lata are often observed in the anogenital area. Oral involvement may include small, superficial ulcers or mucous patches. Serologic studies during the secondary stage of syphilis provide an easy and reliable means of diagnostic confirmation.

A variety of inflammatory dermatoses can lead to patchy alopecia of the scalp. These can usually be distinguished from TTM on the basis of general signs of inflammation such as erythema and scaling. Inflammatory changes often result in hyper- or hypopigmentation of the scalp that is not expected in TTM.

Treatment

The approach to treating hair pulling will vary among child hair pullers, adult hair pullers with insight, and adult hair pullers without insight (Table 9.2). Hair pulling as a secondary disorder is best managed by identification and treatment of the primary disease process. Basic principles can be applied to each of these groups, and optimal management often relies on successful referral to a psychiatrist. Treatment options include behavioral therapy and pharmacotherapy alone or in combination; a detailed discussion of these modalities can be found in Chapter 8.

Table 9.2 General guidelines to treatment of hair pulling in dermatological practice

Child hair pullers	Support groups (online resources etc.)
	Counseling: cognitive-behavioral modification
Adult with insight	SSRI as first line
	Topical steroids if signs of irritation are present
	If preceding treatments fail, refer to psychiatry for further management (cognitive-behavioral and/or pharmacologic therapy)
Adult without insight	Establish rapport (accusation rarely helpful)
	Biopsy can provide objective evidence if needed
	Treat accompanying symptoms (e.g., itching or unusual sensation of the scalp)
	As physician–patient relationship develops, help the patient to gain insight whenever possible
Hair pulling as a secondary disorder	Treat underlying disorder

Child hair pullers have a better prognosis and generally respond to more conservative measures. Counseling and a supportive family environment should be considered the first line of therapy. Parents are often relieved to hear that other children suffer from the same symptoms, and efforts should focus on guiding parents toward online resources that offer education and support (PsycTech 2002). Patients who do not respond to conservative measures should be referred for psychiatric evaluation.

In adult hair pullers with insight, treatment options include cognitive behavioral therapy, hypnosis, insight-oriented psychotherapy, and pharmacologic therapy. While many reports have demonstrated the efficacy of these various modalities, no treatment approach has been established as effective in a large controlled trial (Hautmann, Hercogova, and Lotti 2002). The combination of cognitive-behavioral therapy and pharmacologic therapy may be better than either alone (Dougherty et al. 2006). In many cases, an initial trial with an SSRI may be warranted as a first line of therapy. Clomipramine has been effective but carries a less favorable side-effect profile than SSRIs (Swedo, Leonard, and Rapoport 1989). Patients who do not respond to an initial trial of medication should be referred to a specialist for further management (see Chapter 8). Trauma to the scalp from hair pulling may manifest as excoriations or thickening of the skin in addition to hair loss. Visible signs of trauma point to local irritation that might trigger further manipulation of the area and lead to increased hair pulling; topical steroids may be a useful adjunct to therapy in this situation.

Adult hair pullers without insight create a unique challenge for the practitioner. Patients who deny or lack the insight that they are responsible for their own hair loss are often unwilling to try psychiatric medications or to be referred to a psychiatrist. In these instances, a strong doctor–patient relationship is crucial to a successful outcome. Accusation or direct confrontation about hair pulling is rarely helpful. Patients who insist their hair loss is due to an alternative process may benefit from a biopsy; providing objective evidence from a pathologist can help the patient come to terms with the diagnosis and open doors for discussion and appropriate management.

In some cases, it may be beneficial to avoid the topic of hair pulling on the initial visit and instead focus on any associated symptoms that are present. For instance, for a patient complaining of an unusual sensation of the scalp in addition to hair loss, it may be necessary to center discussion of treatment recommendations around the unusual sensation rather than addressing the behavior of hair pulling. As the rapport between patient and physician develops over subsequent visits, discussing the issue of hair pulling may become possible. Once the patient gains insight into their behavior, the likelihood of a successful outcome is dramatically increased.

Conclusion

The classification of patients as child hair pullers (age 5 or less) and adult hair pullers (adolescence or adulthood) has significant implications regarding prognosis and approach to management. Whereas the former tend to have a benign and self-limited course, the latter have greater pathology and carry a less favorable prognosis. Diagnosis of children with TTM must exclude common causes of patchy alopecia, notably alopecia areata and tinea capitis. Conservative treatment is usually adequate in this age group; counseling and a supportive family environment often lead to a successful outcome.

In adult hair pullers, the presence or absence of insight into the cause of hair loss dictates the therapeutic approach. Treatment for adult hair pullers includes both cognitive-behavioral and pharmacologic therapy. The addition of topical steroids to treat any visible signs of trauma may be beneficial. Adult hair pullers with insight are often eager to begin therapy and willing to seek psychiatric consultation. In contrast, adult hair pullers without insight will often react negatively to the suggestion of a psychiatric component involving their hair loss. In these challenging situations, the practitioner must work to establish a strong rapport with the patient and slowly bring the patient to terms with the true cause of his or her hair loss whenever possible.

References

Bolognia JL, Jorizzo JL, Rapini RP. Dermatology, vol. 1. London/New York: Mosby/Elsevier, 2003, pp. 1174–1185, 1274–1275.

Buescher L, Resch D. The biophsychosocial aspects of hair disease, in *Hair and Scalp Diseases: Medical, Surgical, and Cosmetic Treatments*. Edited by McMichael A, Hordinsky M. New York: Informa USA, 2008, pp. 267–269.

Christenson GA, Mackenzie TB. Trichotillomania, body dysmorphic disorder, and obsessive-compulsive disorder. *J Clin Psychiatry* 56:211–212, 1995.

Christenson GA, Mackenzie TB, Mitchell JE. Characteristics of 60 adult chronic hair pullers. *Am J Psychiatry* 148:365–370, 1991.

Christenson GA, Pyle RL, Mitchell JE. Estimated lifetime prevalence of trichotillomania in college students. *J Clin Psychiatry* 52:415–417, 1991.

Dimino-Emme L, Camisa C. Trichotillomania associated with the "Friar Tuck sign" and nail biting. *Cutis* 47:107–110, 1991.

Dougherty DD, Loh R, Jenike MA et al. Single modality versus dual modality treatment for trichotillomania: Sertraline, behavioral therapy, or both? *J Clin Psychiatry* 67:1086–1092, 2006.

Hallopeau M. Alopecie par grattage (trichomanie ou trichotillomanie). *Ann Dermatol Syphil* 10:440–441, 1889.

Hautmann G, Hercogova J, Lotti T. Trichotillomania. *J Am Acad Dermatol* 46:807–821, 2002.

James WD, Berger TG, Elston DM. *Andrew's Diseases of the Skin: Clinical Dermatology*, 10th edition. Philadelphia: Saunders Elsevier, 2006, pp. 298–301, 356–359, 749–752.

Krishnan RR, Davidson JR, Guarjuardo C. Trichotillomania: A review. *Compr Psychiatry* 26:123–128, 1985.

Lenane MC, Swedo SE, Rapoport JL. Rates of obsessive compulsive disorder in first degree relatives of patients with trichotillomania: A research note. *J Child Psychol Psychiatry* 33:925–933, 1992.

Mannino FV, Delgado RA. Trichotillomania in children: A review. *Am J Psychiatry* 26:123–128, 1969.

Muller SA. Trichotillomania. *Dermatol Clin* 5:595–601, 1987.

Oranje AP, Peereboom-Wynia JD, De Raeymaecker DM. Trichotillomania in childhood. *J Am Acad Dermatol* 15:614–619, 1986.

PsycTech, Ltd. Stoppicking.*com*. Available at http://www.stoppicking.com/PsycTech/Program/StopPicking/Public/HomePage.aspx. Accessed March 1, 2008.

Soriano JL, O'Sullivan RL, Baer L. Trichotillomania and self-esteem: A survey of 62 female hair-pullers. *J Clin Psychiatry* 57:77–82, 1996.

Swedo SE, Leonard HL, Rapoport JL. A double blind comparison of clomipramine and desipramine in the treatment of trichotillomania (hair pulling). *N Engl J Med* 321:497–501, 1989.

Swedo SE, Rapoport JL. Trichotillomania [annotation]. *J Child Psychol Psychiatry* 32:401–409, 1991.

10

How to Create a National Advocacy Organization

Christina S. Pearson

As a preface to this chapter, let me first review my qualifications. I am not a researcher, clinician, or expert theorist. Instead, I am a woman who grew up suffering from trichotillomania (among other things) and, when I discovered what I had and found that no resources were available, started a national organization to serve those suffering from this little-understood and often misdiagnosed disorder.

I am the Founding Director of the Trichotillomania Learning Center (TLC), an organization I founded in 1990, although we did not receive full nonprofit status until 1991. Today, TLC is flourishing and is considered the leading resource in the world for sufferers of trichotillomania and other related problems, such as skin picking and nail biting.

This chapter is about how to give voice where there is no voice, how to create an oasis of healing in the desert of public denial. It is about developing and cultivating connections, then nurturing them until a solid resource of recovery information is formed that can stand on its own – *and do so effectively*. It is about stepping into the truth of one's experience, breaking the shame barrier (if necessary), and helping others.

I will get to my personal story in just a moment, but first I want to address you, the reader. You are probably reading this book because you are a clinician, researcher, or student, or perhaps you suffer from an impulse control disorder (ICD), or are a parent of an ICD sufferer. Or perhaps you are just interested in the subject matter! This chapter is for all of you, regardless of your reason for reading. If you find yourself indignant and aghast at the dearth of help and are moved by the driving need to help others as a doctor, a sufferer, a mom or dad, or whoever, these disorders all desperately need your help, and this chapter is about how to do just that. In other words, this is a quick "How To" manual if you are interested in developing a successful resource for a disorder that has little or no support for sufferers, coordinated advocacy, or public education.

My own story is rather complicated; it is a book in itself, and I am working on it! Here, I will focus on the impact of trichotillomania on my life and on the resulting decisions that brought me to where I am today. I began hair pulling in earnest in 1970; I was 13 years old, and trichotillomania hit with a vengeance. I had done a little absent-minded pulling prior to this, but never with noticeable damage and not even enough to really become aware of it. Only in hindsight was I able to remember, "Oh yeah, I pulled then, and then.... " So, I guess my pulling behavior started maybe two to three years earlier.

At 13, it was devastating to watch my hands act with what seemed to be a life of their own, fingertips searching, questing, stroking, finding the perfect hair and pulling ever so carefully to preserve the little bulb on the end of the shaft. Then I would touch it to my lip to feel the coolness, the wetness, and pop the bulb between my teeth, then nibble a few centimeters of the hair itself. Obliviously dropping the remainder on the floor, I would immediately begin the search again and again *and again*... for hours at a time.

My pulling created an altered mental state that was unlike anything I had ever experienced, and that is true to this day. It felt, while I was engaged, like this was *exactly* what needed to be happening. It felt like important neurological homework; it just *must* be done. The consequences, however, were disastrous. I remember locking myself in the bathroom, taking off my hat, seeing the mottled pink skin of my bare scalp (I had pulled all the hair from the top of my ears to the crown), and crying in desolation and fear. I thought I must be crazy; yet I didn't *feel* crazy. It was utterly, overwhelmingly excruciating. Thus began a decades-long battle with two body-focused compulsions: to pull my hair and eat it, and to pick at my skin, causing discoloration and damage. I maintain to this day that it is fundamentally easier to kick alcohol, heroin, or cigarettes than to stop pulling and picking (at least with the tools we currently have). If you live in a vulnerable nervous system, beware. For those of us who do, pulling and picking can be more enticing than sleep, more rewarding than chocolate, and more enjoyable than orgasm. They also make many want to die; some do. Believe me – it is a real problem!

OK, I suffered. Let us jump ahead to the reason I wrote this chapter. In 1989, at the age of 33, I learned through a study published in the *New England Journal of Medicine* that there were others with this problem. The article was titled "A double-blind comparison of clomipramine and desipramine in the treatment of trichotillomania (hair pulling)" (Swedo et al. 1989).

As I read, my body shook and would not stop. My world view shattered; fractured pieces of my life went spinning before me. I was not alone, nor had I ever been. *It* had a name. It had been recognized for about 100 years. The journal article gave little good news. Treatment was difficult, with a poor prognosis for chronic sufferers. Most relapsed. I raged for three days. *How could this be?* How could I not have known? I, who was going to be a doctor, go to the moon, be the first female president, all the potential I had hidden, fearful of exposure, suffocating in shame, wanting to die rather than share my awkward truth. *And now they say – no cure?* It was like being kicked in the stomach. Not *only* did it have a poor prognosis, but to add insult to injury, it had an absolutely horrendous name: *trichotillomania*. (Please note that a name change is also on the agenda.)

I begged my way into a trichotillomania (TTM) pilot study on Prozac at Stanford University Medical Center with Lorrin Koran, MD, Director of Stanford's OCD Clinic. I remember interviewing him, while he thought he was interviewing me! (I asked him if he was good at what he did . . . he burst out laughing! At the time, I had *no idea* what a world-respected researcher and clinician he was.) Working with Dr. Koran changed my life. To shorten a long story, about two months into the study, I had the opportunity to do a regional television show (Northwest Afternoon) on TTM in the Seattle area. Dr. Koran graciously agreed to be piped in via telephone as the medical expert for the show.

I came home that night to *hundreds* of calls. People crying, sobbing, begging for help. To discover that there was a possibility of a normal life had literally blown the lid off for them. I had nowhere to send them, no information to give them, no referrals to offer. So I talked. And talked. And talked some more. I spoke to some 600 callers and came to realize that *something* seriously needed to be done. But what? In pondering my own skills as a small businesswoman, I thought that maybe I should go back to school and get a degree to do this work. The problem was that with 17 days of high school under my belt, it would take a long, long time! (Did I mention that I received a psychiatric discharge from high school for pulling out my hair? I did, and I never went back.)

I was propelled from within to serve these sufferers, to reduce the pain, to offer what help I could. But what could I do? By now I was in touch with the Obsessive Compulsive Foundation, but they didn't really address TTM very well. Nor did any other organization that I could find.

I spoke at length about this with Dr. Koran, who gave me absolutely priceless advice and support. When I wavered, fearful of my lack of higher education, he smiled and told me something along the lines of "Christina, you *can* do this. You have the drive, the personal history, and the heart. What I suggest is that to become professional you surround yourself with those who have the degrees, find the very best, let them be the ones who have spent time in academia. Not you. You can coordinate this. People need you to do this."

And I did. Here are the steps I took.

1. Identify the Need

For me, it became crystal clear as I wended my way through all those phone conversations that the need was tremendous. Not only were there no resources, but appropriate treatment was basically nonexistent, and most doctors knew nothing about the disorder. Many of the sufferers I spoke to had been deeply shamed by the very professionals from whom they had sought help.

The big problem had been identified. There was no accessible treatment (in fact, no treatment at all is more like it), uninformed practitioners, overwhelming shame, oceans of denial, and misinformation abounding. Lives were sadly constricted within a behavioral prison, with bars forged of compulsion and no clear way out.

The need I identified was a center, run by an organization, to become a starting point in creating the ability to network, collect data, offer information, and develop recovery tools. I was not sure what the center needed to look like; I just knew it needed to be a public entity, visible and accessible in the real world, and that this in itself would begin the slow and steady process of destigmatizing TTM.

2. Identify the Actions the Organization Will Take to Meet the Need

I made a quick list of the things that would help to meet the need. The list included:

Raise public awareness (destigmatizing was crucial)
Educate treatment professionals (which also meant developing treatment)
Set up regional support networks
Support research
Provide reliable information and resource referrals
Centralize operations and create an ability to communicate (newsletter, Web site, tele-
   phone number)
Act as an archive for relevant data

(I also had things on the list like " cross-cultural genetic studies," but by now you get the idea.)

3. Check Your Degree of Motivation and Commitment

Why is this goal important? What are you willing to do to reach the goal? For me, creating a productive organization was important because I understood the pain from the inside out, and it was appallingly clear that nothing was being done to appropriately serve the TTM community. I also knew that the task was too big for me to complete on my own. I could get things going, but I would need to develop a team consciousness.

Next, I had to ponder what I was truly willing to do. The shame was *so* pervasive and public awareness *so* dismal (in fact, downright demeaning and shaming) that I realized that if I was to do this work, I had better be ready for a *long* haul. I decided that it would take about one human generation to effect significant change. I made an internal commitment to devote 20 years to the project, with the understanding that at that time I would reevaluate and see what the need was and what my role might or might not be. I am now at the 19-year mark, so I am 1 year away from that reevaluation point. And here is the clincher – in some ways we have only just begun! (Hmmmm. . . . I had a hunch it would take a while.)

Now, do not despair! Depending on the need, your time frame may not need to be that long. American society, culture, and communication channels are different now than they were when I started TLC. But, if you do not want to give it 3 to 5 years at least, I would seriously question whether to start on your own. It may be better to get on board with an existing group and help them expand to serve the population to which you want to offer solace.

4. Ask Whether Anyone Is Working to Meet This Need

Look around. What is happening in the arena of service for the people you want to help? Investigate other organizations and the populations they serve. Where does your group of sufferers now turn for help? Is this resource cohesive? Is it useful? Can you coordinate or combine efforts with them? This is important. Clearly, starting a national organization takes a *huge* amount of commitment, motivation, and energy, not to mention money (which I definitely did not have). Most of the time, an attempt to set up a national organization fails. For every national nonprofit that serves a target group, hundreds have failed. You do not want to fail because your target group needs help. So, check out who is doing what, and determine if joining them is the best way to get the need met. If so, work with them to make it happen. Do not reinvent the wheel if there is a good one rolling down the block! Get on the team and make it bigger. There is tremendous power in hooking up with those who have the same or a similar dream, unless, of course, they are doing a poor job. Then, get busy and start on your own!

While I was setting up TLC, I decided to get involved with the Obsessive Compulsive Foundation (OCF). They were doing a fabulous job with OCD and were trying to help hair pullers, but TTM was not their primary focus. *It was mine.* I eventually did serve on the OCF national board of directors for 5 years. I will always be grateful for the tremendous support and advice I received from original founding board members Patti Perkins and Fran Sydney, both of whom had struggled with OCD, and from Jim Broatch, MSW, the executive director during my tenure on the board.

5. Learn All You Can about Your Target Group

Get savvy on current science, demographics (if known), statistics, and treatment options. Identify leading researchers and clinicians. Locate other groups working in your area of interest. Keep notes, so you know who is doing what and where. You will need this information as you begin setting up your team. Use the Internet, and be grateful it exists!

6. Make a List of Resources at Your Disposal

Once I realized that I was going to set up a real entity, I knew that I could not do this alone. I was willing to work hard, but I needed *lots* of advice! My first list of resources looked something like this:

Dr. Koran, Stanford OCD Clinic, my first treatment provider and trusted advisor. He also knew who was working in the field.
Dana Hickerson, my business partner in Quicksilver Voice Mail, our current enterprise.
Quicksilver Voicemail Company, our business. I knew I could set up voicemail for free.
Obsessive Compulsive Foundation, Jim Broatch, MSW, executive director. I had started a telephone dialogue with him about providing services. . . . Just think! Your list can have *me* on it!
Biofeedback Clinic (I was engaging in biofeedback locally.)
Ernie Faitos, our landlord at Quicksilver. I thought he might have an ear open to using some floor space.

Call List (I had six hundred TTM names with phone numbers and addresses from doing the TV show and calling these individuals back.)

Support Group Members (I had just set up a local support group that had seven members.)

7. Define Your Organization's Structure

There is a big difference between a support group and a nonprofit charitable organization. Be clear on how much energy you have and what is manageable for you. Remember that even when you find folks to work with, you may have to be the primary motivator for a long time. You will need to be able to handle what you take on. I started with a local support group and ended up with a national nonprofit. TLC's original board of directors numbered six: three from the support group, one from the Seattle call list, my business partner, and lastly me.

The decision to create a nonprofit entity was based on the fact that a charitable organization can receive tax-deductible contributions, which can and must be used in the service of the target population. Ultimately, this was the only rational choice, but it was painful because I had no clue how to proceed. I paid a CPA who was familiar with nonprofit work to start the process, and I finished it myself with guidance from a Nolo Press book. Doing it this way cost a total of $600, but if you have the money (it can cost a few thousand dollars), pay someone to do it because it can be a real headache! Otherwise, the $30 Nolo Press "How To" book (Pakroo 2007) about starting a legally viable nonprofit is a great help.

8. Set Up the *Very Best* Advisory Board that You Can

This is where the advice of both Dr. Koran and Jim Broatch really paid off. *Work with the best.* I sat down and developed a list of *all* the leading researchers and clinicians I could find, starting with the lead author of the *New England Journal of Medicine* TTM study. I found about ten doctors around the country who had either published research or were doing excellent clinical work on TTM and were familiar with the basics of what effective treatment might look like. I telephoned some of them and tracked others down in person. I told them what I was doing and asked if they would serve on our scientific advisory board. Every single one said yes.

9. Get into Action

This is really where the rubber meets the road. I now had a working executive board, local folks mostly, who could stuff envelopes and help out here and there. I had a list of renowned (and some not-so-renowned) doctors who had agreed to put their stamp of approval on this venture by agreeing to be advisors. I had a telephone number for the organization, and I had arranged with our landlord, Ernie, for a small office space. The first year I could not pay rent, but by the end of the second year, I was paying rent each month and had repaid Ernie in full for the previous year. He was very kind to our cause.

I did not receive a salary for the first 3 years. Originally, every cost came out of my pocket; then, the newsletter I provided to members drew strong interest and the membership grew. By the end of year 2, the organization could pay its bills, but not a salary. When money begins to flow into an organization, formal procedures and clear channels of accountability and decision making become even more important. I eventually resigned from the board to become the organization's executive director and to receive a salary. This meant that the board became my boss. Not everyone can make the transition easily from creator to manager. Pay attention so that you make wise decisions in developing formal policies and structure. I had to make this change because I was devoting full time to the organization at this point and could not do this without a salary.

If you get to this point in your adventure, beware of "Founder's Syndrome." (I started it, I know what is best, I am in charge, no one can do it better than me . . . that kind of stuff.) It can cause great harm (and is often the downfall of a nonprofit with a healthy start). Falling prey to Founder's Syndrome will not support your ultimate goal of being of real service. Keep your ego in check. There is *always* someone who can do things better than you can, so find that person and get him or her on board!

Today, I have a new title, that of founding director. I have once again made a transition, for the good of both myself and the organization as it grows, and we now have a new executive director to oversee operations. In my new role, I focus more on the big picture, working to flesh out programs and spending time fund-raising to put them into action. TLC has grown up. It has been a long time in coming but has been a wonderful and profound journey that I hope you experience for yourself in your own endeavors.

In summary, use other organizations as mentors. There are many incredible people out there who will guide you if you can listen with respect and can honor their wisdom. Pull together the people doing the science. Attract the sufferers and their family members to your cause. Transform your own life while working to help others. Be clear on this if nothing else: the work is not about material gain, it is about love.

May you have the profound and life-altering experience of being an open channel for this process. Do not hesitate for *even a moment* to put me on your list of resources if you choose to walk this path.

In Love and Service, Christina.

For more information on TLC, visit www.trich.org.

References

Pakroo PH. *Starting & Building a Nonprofit: A Practical Guide*. Berkeley: Nolo Press, 2007.

Swedo SE, Leonard HL, Rapoport JL et al. A double-blind comparison of clomipramine and desipramine in the treatment of trichotillomania (hair pulling). *N Engl J Med* 321:497–501, 1989.

11

Skin Picking: Clinical Aspects

Celal Çalıkuşu, MD, and Özlem Tecer, MD

Introduction

Skin picking is a common human behavior and is often performed as part of the daily grooming routine (Bohne et al. 2002a; Keuthen et al. 2000). Some degree of skin picking appears to be normal. Most people pick at their face or hands to a limited extent. Whether the behavior is pathological depends on the duration and extent of the behavior as well as the reasons for picking, the associated emotions, and the resulting problems (Grant and Philips 2003; Keuthen et al. 2000). Individuals with pathologic skin picking report thoughts of picking or impulses to pick that are intrusive and/or senseless and are often described as "irresistible" (Arnold, Auchenbach, and McElroy 2001). Skin-picking disorder (SPD) (also known as psychogenic excoriation, neurotic excoriation, pathological or compulsive skin picking, self-injurious skin picking, self-inflicted dermatosis, acné excoriée, and dermatillomania) has been defined by researchers as recurrent picking accompanied by visible tissue damage resulting in significant distress and/or functional impairment (Bohne et al. 2002a; Keuthen et al., 2000; Simeon et al. 1997; Teng et al. 2002; Wilhelm et al. 1999). The disorder is characterized by excessive scratching, picking, gouging, or squeezing of otherwise healthy skin. The excoriation may also occur in response to an itch or other skin sensation or to remove a lesion on the skin.

History of Psychiatric Attention to SPD

Historically, SPD has received more attention in the dermatologic than in the psychiatric literature. It was first described in 1875 by Erasmus Wilson, who observed self-inflicted excoriations in his neurotic patients and therefore named these behaviors "neurotic excoriations" (Fruensgaard, Hjortshoj, and Nielsen 1978). Since then, skin picking has appeared in the literature under different names and with varying definitions. In 1898, Brocq described excoriations typically occurring in adolescent women as a result of picking acne while in emotional distress and called these lesions "acné excoriée des jeunes filles" (Sneddon and Sneddon 1983). In 1915, Adamson grouped acné excoriée together with acne urticata and neurodermatitis under the concept of "neurotic excoriations" (Fruensgaard, Hjortshoj, and Nielsen 1978). A few years later, McKee defined neurotic excoriations as habitual conditions caused by unconsciously picking small irregularities on the skin, which becomes uncontrollable in severe cases (Fruensgaard, Hjortshoj, and Nielsen 1978). Koo (1989) emphasized that excoriation was a commonly encountered sign in depression marked by psychomotor agitation and irritability. He claimed that excoriations were an expression of agitation in these patients and named these lesions "depressive excoriations."

Diagnosis

Skin-picking disorder is not recognized as a distinct psychiatric disorder in the *Diagnostic and Statistical Manual of Mental Disorders*, 4th edition (DSM-IV) (American Psychiatric

Association 1994) or the *International Classification of Diseases*, 10th revision (ICD-10) (World Health Organization 1992). It has been classified under a number of different diagnostic categories, including impulse control disorders (Arnold et al. 1998; Wilhelm et al. 1999), stereotypic movement disorders (Lochner et al 2002; Wilhelm et al. 1999), obsessive-compulsive disorders (OCDs) (Stein et al. 1993), body dysmorphic disorders (BDDs) (Bohne et al. 2002b; Phillips and Taub1995), and obsessive-compulsive spectrum disorders (Bienvenu et al. 2000; Keuthen et al. 2000). Wilhelm et al. (1999) asserted that skin picking is a heterogeneous behavior and that one cannot include all individuals who engage in this behavior under one diagnosis.

Skin-picking disorder is currently classified in DSM-IV-TR (American Psychiatric Association 2000) as an "impulse control disorder not otherwise specified" (Code 312.30) along with compulsive impulsive (CI) Internet usage disorder, CI sexual behaviors, and CI shopping. This is a residual category for disorders of impulse control that do not meet the criteria for a specific impulse control disorder or for another mental disorder having features involving impulse control (e.g., substance dependence or a paraphilia). Some authors state that most patients with SPD report subjective experiences suggesting an impulse control disorder in that they find themselves acting automatically and experience an increase in tension prior to excoriating and transient relief or pleasure during or immediately after excoriating (Arnold et al. 1998; Simeon et al. 1997; Wilhelm et al. 1999).

Skin-picking disorder is thought to have phenomenological and biological similarities to trichotillomania (TTM) (Christenson, MacKenkie, and Mitchell 1991; Stein and Hollander 1992; Wilhelm et al. 1999). Both conditions are characterized by repetitive unwanted behaviors. In one study (Lochner et al. 2002), TTM and SPD exhibited very similar demographics, psychiatric comorbidity, and personality dimensions. Odlaug and Grant (2008) suggest that there may be a link between SPD, TTM, and compulsive nail biting but not other impulse control disorders such as pathologic gambling or kleptomania.

Skin-picking disorder also manifests similarities to OCD. For example, it is ritualistic, often resisted, and ego dystonic (Stein and Hollander 1992); the patient acknowledges the self-inflicted nature of the disease, has great difficulty controlling the behavior, and fails to do so (Gupta, Gupta, and Haberman 1986). The repetitive, stereotyped nature of skin-picking episodes (Stein et al. 1993) and the tension reduction accompanying the behavior appear similar to compulsions in OCD. Positive treatment response to clomipramine and fluoxetine is another similarity. Some patients excoriate in response to obsessions about an irregularity on the skin or preoccupation with having smooth skin.

A patient's preoccupation with appearance can be severe enough to also meet criteria for BDD, a disorder thought to be related to OCD (Phillips and Taub 1995). Arnold et al. (1998) reported that a minority of their subjects excoriated their skin as part of OCD, and about a third suffered from BDD with a preoccupation about skin appearance. However, some important differences are found between skin picking and OCD or BDD symptoms. Skin picking serves predominantly to regulate emotions, whereas compulsions in OCD serve to neutralize obsessions and repetitive behaviors in BDD serve to check on or improve appearance (Wilhelm et al. 1999). Ferrão et al. (2006), who compared 20 patients with OCD with 20 patients with skin picking and/or TTM, also suggested that OCD and impulse control disorders (ICDs) are qualitatively different.

Wilhelm et al. (1999) noted that their study participants exhibited a high rate of other stereotypic behaviors besides picking their skin and suggested that skin picking can be diagnosed in some cases as a stereotypic movement disorder, because it is a motor behavior that is "repetitive, seemingly driven, and nonfunctional." Both stereotypic movement disorders and skin picking generally have an early age of onset (Odlaug and Grant 2007). On the other hand, while stereotypic movement disorders are usually associated with mental retardation, skin picking is usually seen in individuals with normal intellect (Arnold et al. 1998; Çalıkuşu et al. 2003; Gupta, Gupta, and Haberman 1986).

Table 11.1 Proposed diagnostic criteria for psychogenic excoriation

A. Maladaptive skin excoriation (e.g., scratching, picking, gouging, lancing, digging, rubbing, or squeezing skin) or maladaptive preoccupation with skin excoriation as indicated by at least one of the following:
   1. Preoccupation with skin excoriation and/or recurrent impulses to excoriate the skin that is/are experienced as irresistible, intrusive, and/or senseless.
   2. Recurrent excoriation of the skin resulting in noticeable skin damage.
B. The preoccupation, impulses, or behaviors associated with skin excoriation cause marked distress, are time-consuming, significantly interfere with social or occupational activities, or result in medical problems (e.g., infections).
C. The disturbance is not better accounted for by another mental disorder and is not due to a general medical condition.

Subtypes
Compulsive

1. Skin excoriation is performed to avoid increased anxiety or to prevent a dreaded event or situation and/or is elicited by an obsession (e.g., obsession about contamination of the skin).
2. It is performed in full awareness.
3. It is associated with some resistance to performing the behavior.
4. There is some insight into its senselessness or harmfulness.

Impulsive

1. Skin excoriation is associated with arousal, pleasure, or reduction of tension.
2. It is performed at times with minimal awareness (e.g., automatically).
3. It is associated with little resistance to performing the behavior.
4. There is little insight into its senselessness or harmfulness.

Mixed
Skin excoriation has both compulsive and impulsive features.

(Reprinted with permission from Arnold LM, Auchenbach MB, and McElroy SL. Psychogenic excoriation: Clinical features, proposed diagnostic criteria, epidemiology, and approaches to treatment. *CNS Drugs* 15:351–359, 2001.)

In the early 1990s, an ongoing discussion began about conceptualizing impulse control disorders as part of an obsessive-compulsive spectrum in view of their clinical characteristics, familial transmission, and response to both pharmacological and psychosocial treatment interventions (Hollander et al. 1992; McElroy et al. 1994; Wilhelm et al. 1999). Arnold et al. (1998) noted that the behavior associated with skin picking spans a compulsivity-impulsivity continuum from OCD to impulse control disorders. The DSM-V task force is considering recognizing new disorders, including CI skin picking. These are called compulsive impulsive disorders in view of the impulsive features that initiate the behavior and the compulsive drive that causes the behavior to persist (Dell'Osso et al. 2006).

Arnold, Auchenbach, and McElroy (2001) proposed diagnostic criteria for psychogenic excoriation and suggested a categorization of the disorder into compulsive, impulsive, and mixed subtypes, which they believed would better reflect the heterogeneity of the behavior and would have important treatment implications (Table 11.1).

Differential Diagnosis

The differential diagnosis of SPD includes medical and psychiatric conditions that cause skin picking directly or that create the sensations, such as pruritus, that lead to skin picking. Common dermatologic disorders that need to be ruled out are prurigo nodularis, lichen simplex chronicus, psoriasis, eczematous dermatoses, infestation, and xerosis (Fruensgaard, Hjortshoj, and Nielsen 1978; Koblenzer 1987). Pruritus is a symptom of several systemic diseases, including lymphoma and leukemias, diabetes mellitus, thyrotox-icosis, polycythemia vera, renal and hepatic diseases, infections, allergic reactions, drug toxicity, and neurologic syndromes such as multiple sclerosis (Fruensgaard, Hjortshoj, and Nielsen 1978). Self-mutilation that includes skin picking may be seen in syndromes such as Lesch Nyhan syndrome and Prader Willi syndrome (Dykens and Shah 2003) and in mental retardation. Anticholinergic drugs, amphetamines, methylphenidate, phenelzine, and cocaine may produce tactile sensations that precipitate skin picking (Neziroğlu and Mancebo 2001). Flessner and Woods (2006) reported that picking began after the use of a substance in 3.0% of the participants in their study and as a result of a medical condition in 5.4%.

If skin picking occurs only in response to sensations such as pruritus that cannot be explained by, or are in excess of, what would be expected from a specific medical condition, an undifferentiated somatoform disorder may be diagnosed (Arnold et al. 1998). Alternatively, delusional disorder somatic type, in which patients have a fixed false belief that they are infested with living organisms, may drive skin-picking behavior (Bishop 1983). Factitious dermatitis (dermatitis artefacta) patients intentionally produce skin lesions in order to assume the sick role. Unlike patients with SPD, these patients typically deny the self-inflicted nature of the lesions (Koblenzer 1992).

Clinical Picture

Skin picking is characterized by excessive repetitive scratching, picking, squeezing, digging, or rubbing of normal skin or skin with minor surface irregularities, thus creating and perpetuating lesions (Simeon et al. 1997). Skin lesions such as acne, papules, scabs, scars, and insect bites are sometimes picked; most commonly picked are pimples and scabs (Arnold et al. 1998; Bohne et al. 2002a; Keuthen et al. 2000; Simeon et al. 1997; Wilhelm et al. 1999). Picking may occur in response to skin sensations, most commonly pruritus, but also including burning, warmth, prickling, dryness, and pain (Arnold et al. 1998; Simeon et al. 1997). Subjects who describe primary excoriation may develop secondary disturbing skin sensations that lead to more excoriation. Most patients pick with full awareness of their behavior, and triggers such as the sight or feel of the skin usually precipitate the picking (Odlaug and Grant 2008; Wilhelm et al., 1999). Perfectionism and the desire to improve appearance seem to be common motives as well (Koblenzer 1983; Stein et al. 1993).

Excoriations are typically found in areas that the patient can easily reach, such as the face, scalp, upper back, abdomen, and the extremities. Usually, more than one body area is picked, but the face is the most common site (Arnold et al. 1998; Flessner and Woods 2006; Keuthen et al. 2000; Odlaug and Grant 2008; Simeon et al. 1997; Wilhelm et al. 1999). Excoriations are typically a few millimeters in diameter and weeping, crusted, or scarred with occasional postinflammatory hypopigmentation or hyperpigmentation (Koblenzer 1987; Wilhelm et al. 1999). Clean erosions and dry, adherent scabs may be seen. On physical examina-tion, excoriations, ulcers, and a range of early and late scars are often present, providing a visual time line of the disorder (Bowes and Alster 2004). Facial excoriations in a patient with SPD are shown in Figure 11.1.

Most patients excoriate skin with their fingernails and fingers, but the teeth or instruments (e.g., tweezers, pins, or knives) may also be used (Arnold et al. 1998; Keuthen et al. 2000; Odlaug and Grant 2008; Simeon et al. 1997; Wilhelm et al. 1999). After a skin-picking episode, some subjects roll the picked skin in their fingers before dropping it to the floor, some wipe it in a towel or dispose of it in the trash, and some eat it (Bohne et al. 2002a; Wilhelm et al. 1999). The duration of skin-picking episodes ranges from less than 5 minutes to 12 hours a day (Arnold et al. 1998; Flessner and Woods 2006; Odlaug and Grant 2008; Phillips and Taub 1995; Wilhelm et al. 1999). Skin picking is usually reported to occur in sedentary situations, such as watching television, talking on the phone, or reading

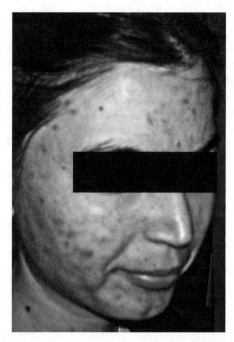

Figure 11.1   Excoriations on the face of a woman with skin-picking disorder (Çalıkuşu, 2008).

(Arnold et al. 1998; Koblenzer 1987). Most subjects pick their skin while they are alone at home, between 8 PM and midnight (Wilhelm et al. 1999).

Patients experience an increasing tension before picking and gratification and mild mesmerization or dissociation during the episode (Wilhelm et al. 1999). Flessner and Woods (2006) reported that 78% of their study subjects reported experiencing urges, feelings, or sensations prior to a picking episode, and 87% reported experiencing pleasure or gratification afterward. Over the course of the skin-picking episode, feelings of shame, guilt, and pain increase (Wilhelm et al. 1999), but most individuals report that they are unable to stop picking until their skin is bleeding (Koblenzer 1992). Skin picking can be an intentionally executed behavior used to regulate feelings of tension, nervousness, and frustration (Arnold et al. 1998; Deckersbach et al. 2002; Stein et al. 1993; Twohig and Woods 2001; Wilhelm et al. 1999). It can also occur as a habitual behavior largely outside an individual's awareness (Simeon et al. 1997). Many skin pickers report that feelings of stress, tension, anger, boredom, sadness, or anxiety precipitate their skin-picking episodes (Arnold et al. 1998; Fruensgaard 1984; Keuthen et al. 2000; Koblenzer 1987; Wilhelm et al. 1999).

Assessment Instruments

Self-monitoring techniques can be used to assess the frequency of skin-picking behavior (Twohig and Woods 2004). Several self-report and clinician-rated scales have also been developed to assess the severity of skin picking and its psychosocial consequences.

The Yale-Brown Obsessive Compulsive Scale (Y-BOCS) (Goodman et al. 1989) modified for psychogenic excoriation is a ten-question, semistructured, clinician-administered scale that assesses the severity of skin picking in the previous week. It measures time occupied, distress, interference with functioning, resistance to and control over preoccupation and behaviors, tension with urge to perform behaviors, release of tension with completion of behaviors, and feelings of comfort or pleasure with behaviors. Scores can range from 0 to 40.

The Skin Picking Scale (Keuthen et al. 2001a) is a self-report instrument consisting of six items: frequency of urges to pick the skin, intensity of urges, time spent, interference with functioning, distress, and avoidance associated with skin picking. Each item is rated on a 5-point severity scale ranging from 0 to 4. It is modeled after the Y-BOCS. Its reliability is satisfactory, with a Cronbach's alpha of 0.8.

The Skin Picking Impact Scale (Keuthen et al. 2001b) is a ten-item self-report scale. It assesses avoidance behaviors, feelings of embarrassment and unattractiveness, and the behavioral sequelae of skin picking. Each question is rated on a 0–5 point scale; the total score cutoff point is 7. It has good internal consistency ($\alpha = 0.88$–0.93), high reliability, and acceptable validity.

The Skin Picking Treatment Scale is a five-item clinician-rated scale modeled after the Y-BOCS. The items assess the intensity of urges to pick, skin-picking frequency, duration of skin picking, control over the behavior, and interference with functioning. Each item is rated on a 0–4 point scale. Its psychometric features have not been investigated (Simeon et al. 1997).

Prevalence

Skin-picking disorder appears to be moderately prevalent, although the exact prevalence in the general population is unknown. In 2004, Keuthen et al. (2009) conducted a random-sample, national telephone survey of 2,513 adults in the United States, using 13 questions to assess skin picking that resulted in noticeable skin damage at some point in life. Skin picking with damage had been experienced by 16.6% of the respondents. Only 0.2% of the sample met strict criteria for SPD, which required noticeable skin damage from picking not attributable to a medical condition or hearing voices, together with related distress and either school or work absences or interference with social functioning. Less strict diagnostic criteria, which required either distress or interference but not both, produced a prevalence estimate of 1.4%.

Skin-picking disorder is seen in approximately 3.8% to 4.6% of college students (Bohne et al. 2002a; Keuthen et al. 2000) and 2% of dermatology clinic patients (Griesemer 1978). Of adolescents hospitalized in a psychiatric facility, 11.8% suffered from SPD (Grant, Williams, and Potenza 2007). Skin picking was reported by 20% of a sample of young women aged 18–25 years, but the behavior was severe enough to cause pain and recurrent bleeding or inflammation in only 8% (Favaro, Ferrara, and Santonastaso 2007). Odlaug and Grant (2008) reported that 28.3% of the skin pickers reported having at least one first-degree relative with picking behavior. Skin-picking disorder is more common in females, and pooled results from large case series of patients with SPD (Arnold et al. 1998; Flessner and Woods 2006; Fruensgaard 1984; Odlaug and Grant 2008; Wilhelm et al. 1999) show a female-to-male ratio of about 7:1.

Age at Onset

The onset of SPD ranges between 3 and 82 years (Arnold et al. 1998). While some studies have reported the age of onset between 30 and 40 years (Arnold et al. 1998; Çalıkuşu et al. 2003; Gupta, Gupta, and Haberman 1986), others have reported that it often begins in adolescence when the subjects develop facial acne (Wilhelm et al. 1999). Simeon et al. (1997) and Lochner et al. (2002) reported an age of onset around 16 years. Recent studies report a mean age of onset of around 12 years (Flessner and Woods 2006; Keuthen et al. 2000; Odlaug and Grant 2008). Odlaug and Grant (2007) found that nearly half of their 40 subjects had onset before 10 years of age. Although childhood- and later-onset skin picking are reported to have similar general sociodemographic and clinical characteristics, patients with childhood onset seem less likely to pick with full conscious awareness of their behavior, more likely to wait a considerable time before seeking treatment, and less likely to seek medication treatment (Odlaug and Grant 2007).

Natural History and Course of Illness

The onset of skin-picking behavior is usually gradual, and its course tends to be chronic (Arnold et al. 1998). The intensity waxes and wanes over time, with rare periods of complete symptom remission (Wilhelm et al. 1999). The mean duration of symptoms has a wide range – between 3 months and 33 years (Arnold et al. 1998; Çalıkuşu et al. 2003; Gupta, Gupta, and Haberman 1986; Simeon et al. 1997; Wilhelm et al. 1999). Most patients engage in the behavior continuously without notable prolonged remissions, but some do it intermittently, with periods of months to years free of the behavior (Koblenzer 1983; Simeon et al. 1997). Skin-picking disorder usually begins after facing stressors. Limitation of physical activity was reported to initiate skin picking in the elderly (Gupta, Gupta, and Haberman 1986). Wilhelm et al. (1999) noted that most women experience a higher frequency of picking during menstruation or shortly before. In one study, the prognosis for patients who had SPD for less than 1 year before presenting to a dermatologist appeared to be better than for those with a longer duration of illness and was worse when concomitant physical complaints such as tension headaches were present (Fruensgaard 1984).

Skin-picking disorder often leads to serious medical complications (Odlaug and Grant 2008). Most subjects with skin picking have noticeable excoriations; some have ulcerations, deep craters, scarring, and recurrent infections that require antibiotics (Odlaug and Grant 2008; Wilhelm et al. 1999). Some individuals experience visible disfigurement as a result of tissue damage (Flessner and Woods 2006; Keuthen et al. 2000; Stout 1990). Odlaug and Grant (2008) reported two subjects who required multiple skin grafts because of picking the area of the graft. Skin picking has caused medical conditions severe enough to warrant hospitalization (Wilhelm et al. 1999) or surgery. For example, a patient tore the dorsum of her hands so severely that her doctors considered amputation (Arnold et al. 1998). Skin-picking disorder may even cause life-threatening conditions. For example, a woman picked her neck with a tweezer and exposed her carotid artery (O'Sullivan et al. 1999).

Effects of Skin Picking on the Patient's Quality of Life

Individuals with skin picking experience social, occupational, and academic impairment, medical and mental health concerns, and financial burdens (Flessner and Woods 2006). Wilhelm et al. (1999) reported that 87% of skin-picking patients felt socially embarrassed, 58% avoided social situations, and more than 80% used clothing or cosmetics to camouflage the damage. Similar findings have been noted in other studies (Arnold et al. 1998; Bloch et al. 2001; Flessner and Woods 2006; Keuthen et al. 2000; Simeon et al. 1997). Arnold et al. (1998) reported that 44% of their subjects withdrew socially and 18% confined themselves to their homes for most of the time. Avoidance of activities that might expose skin lesions to others contributes to restriction in clothing, haircuts, sexual activity, and leisure or sports activities (Simeon et al. 1997).

Comorbid Conditions

Current comorbid Axis I psychiatric conditions were found in 38.3% and at least one lifetime Axis I disorder in 56.7% of the individuals with SPD in one study (Odlaug and Grant 2008). Wilhelm et al. (1999) and Arnold et al. (1998) reported that all subjects in their samples met DSM-IV criteria for at least one current or past Axis I disorder. Keuthen et al. (2007) noted that 13.8% of participants had one additional comorbid psychiatric disorder and 13.8% had two additional comorbid diagnoses.

A high rate of mood disorders has been reported in patients with SPD (Arnold et al. 1998; Çalıkuşu et al. 2003; Simeon et al. 1997; Wilhelm et al. 1999). Current mood disorders, including major depression, bipolar disorder, and dysthymia, were reported in 48%–68% of patients with skin picking, and lifetime mood disorder prevalance was reported as 79% (Arnold et al. 1998). Whether skin picking precipitates or is secondary to the onset of mood disorders is unclear. Lifetime major depression is reported in 16.7% to 47.6% of skin-picking patients (Çalıkuşu et al. 2003; Lochner et al. 2002; Odlaug and Grant 2008; Simeon et al. 1997). Arnold et al. (1998) detected current bipolar disorder in 35%, major depression in 24%, and dysthymia in 12% of 34 patients with SPD. Arnold et al. (1998) noted that 12% of patients reported suicidal ideation because of problems related to skin picking.

Individuals with skin-picking disorder have a high incidence of mild to moderate levels of comorbid anxiety disorders (Arnold, Auchenbach, and McElroy 2001; Çalıkuşu et al. 2003; Keuthen et al. 2000; Wilhelm et al. 1999). Anxiety disorders, including panic disorder, agoraphobia, social phobia, specific phobia, posttraumatic stress disorder, and generalized anxiety disorder, are reported in 41%–65% of patients (Arnold et al. 1998; Wilhelm et al. 1999).

Comorbid lifetime OCD ranges between 6% and 26.7% and current OCD between 6% and 52% (Arnold et al. 1998; Bienvenu et al. 2000; Çalıkuşu et al. 2003; Odlaug and Grant 2008; Simeon et al. 1997; Wilhelm et al. 1999).

About one-third of SPD patients had comorbid BDD in two studies (Arnold et al. 1998; Wilhelm et al. 1999). But BDD was uncommon (5% current and 5% lifetime) in another sample (Odlaug and Grant 2008). Skin picking was reported in 27% and 33% of patients with BDD (Neziroğlu and Mancebo, 2001; Phillips and Taub 1995). In a study of 176 individuals with BDD, 44.9% reported lifetime and 36.9% current skin picking secondary to BDD. Body dysmorphic disorder subjects with skin picking were more likely to be female and to have skin preoccupations and comorbid personality disorders (Grant, Menard, and Phillips 2006).

A high rate of substance or alcohol use has been reported in SPD (Arnold et al. 1998; Favaro, Ferrara, and Santonastaso 2007; Wilhelm et al. 1999). The rates of alcohol and illicit drug abuse/dependence were 39% and 26%, respectively, in one study (Wilhelm et al. (1999). In a Web-based survey, many respondents with skin picking reported drinking alcohol, smoking tobacco, or using illegal drugs to relieve the negative feelings (e.g., anxiety, depression, guilt, worry, and shame) associated with skin picking (Flessner and Woods 2006).

Trichotillomania (TTM) is the most common comorbid impulse control disorder in patients with SPD (Odlaug and Grant 2008). Current comorbidity of TTM ranges between 6% to 36.7%, and lifetime comorbidity ranges between 9% and 38.3% (Arnold et al. 1998; Ferrão et al. 2006; Odlaug and Grant 2008; Simeon et al. 1997; Wilhelm et al. 1999).

Odlaug and Grant (2008) reported a current comorbidity of impulse control disorders other than TTM of 1.6% and a lifetime comorbidity of 3.3%; in addition, the lifetime rate of nail biting was 31.7%. Wilhelm et al. (1999) reported a 16% rate of comorbid kleptomania and a 19% rate of bulimia nervosa. Repetitive behaviors such as body rocking, thumb sucking, knuckle cracking, cheek chewing, head banging, lip biting, and food binges occur in many patients with SPD (Wilhelm et al. 1999). Nail biting during early childhood is also more prevalent in patients with SPD (Çalıkuşu et al., 2002).

Dermatological patients with SPD were reported to have high levels of anxiety and perceived stress and poor sleep quality (Singareddy et al. 2003).

The most common comorbid Axis II disorders are obsessive-compulsive (48%), borderline (26%), and avoidant personality disorders (23%) (Wilhelm et al. 1999). Among first-degree relatives, 20%–45% have been found to have a history of psychiatric disorders, of which mood disorders and psychoactive substance use disorders were the most common (Arnold et al. 1998; Odlaug and Grant 2008; Wilhelm et al. 1999).

Treatment

Individuals with SPD rarely seek psychiatric treatment (Odlaug and Grant 2008; Wilhelm et al. 1999). Many patients first present for treatment to a primary care physician, dermatologist, or surgeon (O'Sullivan et al. 1999). Patients often seek dermatological treatments, such as antihistamines, steroid creams, abrasions, and chemical peels (Simeon et al. 1997), which are ineffective when used alone (Gupta, Gupta, and Haberman 1986).

Few studies have examined the response to psychiatric treatments. The selective serotonin reuptake inhibitors (SSRIs) are the best-studied agents (Arnold et al. 1999; Biondi, Arcangeli, and Petrucci 2000; Bloch et al. 2001; Gupta and Gupta 1993; Kalivas et al. 1996; Keuthen et al. 2007; Simeon et al. 1997).

There are two randomized trials of fluoxetine in SPD. In a placebo-controlled, double-blind, parallel trial (Simeon et al. 1997), fluoxetine, at a mean dose of 55 mg/day for 10 weeks, was significantly superior to a placebo in reducing skin-picking behavior. Baseline level and change in depression, anxiety, or obsessive-compulsive symptoms were not significantly related to change in skin picking. In a 6-week open-label study using a mean fluoxetine dose of 41 mg/day followed by a double-blind, placebo-controlled continuation trial (Bloch et al. 2001), half of 15 women with SPD, whose symptoms had a mean duration of approximately 25 years, responded favorably. Double-blind placebo substitution was associated with relapse within 6 weeks, but the patients who continued double-blind fluoxetine maintained significant improvement (Bloch et al. 2001). Case reports have reported fluoxetine doses of 20 mg/day (Gupta and Gupta 1993; Stein et al.1993) and 40 mg/day (Stout 1990) to be effective. A fluoxetine dose of 80 mg/day was associated with near remission of skin picking secondary to BDD in a patient who had not responded to trials of cognitive behavioral therapy, imipramine, amitriptyline, and benzopdiazepines (Phillips and Taub 1995).

Five patients with acné excoriée improved after 4 weeks of treatment in a double-blind study combining fluvoxamine with supportive psychotherapy (Hendrickx et al. 1991). In a 12-week open trial with 14 subjects, fluvoxamine at a mean dose of 112.5 mg/day was effective in reducing skin picking (Arnold et al. 1999). The reduction in skin-picking–related behaviors was independent of changes in mood, which is consistent with the results of the double-blind fluoxetine study. In a case report, 300 mg/day of fluvoxamine decreased both skin-picking episodes and preoccupation with skin appearance in a woman with delusional BDD (O'Sullivan et al. 1999).

In an open trial of sertraline at a mean dose of 95 mg/day, 19 of 28 patients with skin picking showed significant improvement (Kalivas et al. 1996).

Significant improvement on measures of skin-picking severity and impact, quality of life, and self-rated anxiety and depression were reported in an 18-week, open-label trial of escitalopram up to 30 mg/day in 29 individuals with SPD. Approximately half the sample were full responders and one-quarter were partial responders (Keuthen et al. 2007).

A patient with idiopathic pruritus and skin picking that had not responded to conventional antipruritic drugs had a noteworthy reduction in itching and scratching and total disappearance of excoriation with paroxetine at 30 mg/day and remained improved at 9-month follow-up (Biondi, Arcangeli, and Petrucci 2000). Another patient with pruritus and skin picking experienced improvement on paroxetine 40 mg/day, after failing trials of topical preparations, psychotherapy, and treatment with lorazepam and trazodone (50 mg/day). Improvement was maintained at 1-year follow-up (Ravindran, Lapierre, and Anisman 1999).

In a retrospective treatment review, approximately half of 33 subjects with skin picking secondary to BDD reported significant improvement with SRI treatment (Phillips and Taub 1995).

Although tricyclic antidepressants (TCAs) are frequently used to treat pruritus associated with several dermatologic disorders, evidence of their efficacy in SPD is limited. One patient experienced decreased pruritus and skin picking after 3 weeks of doxepin at 30 mg/day and psychotherapy (Harris, Sheretz, and Flowers 1987). Treatment with clomipramine at 50 mg/day provided marked improvement of both pruritus and excoriation in a patient whose symptoms had not responded to antihistamines and topical corticosteroids (Gupta, Gupta, and Haberman 1987). Tricyclic medications should be used with caution because their side-effect profile includes anticholinergic, sedative, and hypotensive effects, as well as potential cardiac toxicity.

There are only case reports of the use of antipsychotic medications in the treatment of SPD. Gupta and Gupta (2000) reported a patient whose skin picking of 16 years decreased significantly after 4 weeks of treatment with olanzapine at 2.5 mg/day and did not recur after discontinuing the drug. Olanzapine at doses between 2.5 and 7.5 mg/day, either alone or as an adjunctive treatment, was effective in two case series totaling five patients without psychosis (Garnis-Jones, Collins, and Rosenthal 2000; Gupta and Gupta 2000). Christensen (2004) described the case of a 64-year-old woman who had comorbid generalized anxiety disorder and dysthymia, whose SPD did not respond to adequate trials of amitriptyline, sertraline, and behavioral strategies of self-monitoring and habit reversal but resolved with the addition of olanzapine at 5 mg/day to her maintenance dose (40 mg) of fluoxetine. Pimozide at 4 mg/day resolved skin picking in two patients after 1 month of treatment (Duke 1983). Trifluoperazine at 2 mg/day effectively reduced skin picking in two patients (Sneddon and Sneddon 1983). Carter and Shillcutt (2006) reported a woman with comorbid major depressive disorder and generalized anxiety disorder who presented with a 20-year history of SPD with associated alopecia. Her skin picking, which was unresponsive to venlafaxine at 375 mg/day, decreased approximately 50% when risperidone at 1 mg/day was added. However, risperidone had to be discontinued due to the development of edema. The woman's symptoms improved markedly after switching to aripiprazole at 10 mg/day, and the benefit was maintained at the 6-month follow-up.

Lamotrigine, an antiepileptic drug with glutamate-regulating properties, may have efficacy in treating skin picking in patients with no underlying psychopathology. In a 12-week open-label trial, 66.7% of 24 subjects were either very much improved or much improved. Response was achieved after 8 weeks, when the patients were receiving lamotrigine at 200 mg/day. In addition to time spent picking, urges and thoughts about picking also decreased significantly. Patients with a shorter duration of illness and a slightly less severe form of illness tended to respond better to treatment (Grant, Odlaug, and Kim 2007).

An orally active opiate antagonist, naltrexone (50 mg/day), was effective in a patient with skin picking and pruritus whose symptoms had not responded to dermatological treatments (Lienemann and Walker 1989). *[In the editors' experience, doses of up to 250 mg/day may be required. The effect of any given dose is apparent within 2 weeks. At doses above 50 mg/day, one must monitor liver function tests every 3 to 4 weeks for several months because these doses are rarely associated with hepatocellular damage (reversible).]* Naltrexone at 50 mg/day has also been reported to be rapidly effective in other forms of self-injurious behavior (Bystritsky and Strausser 1996; Griengl, Sendera, and Dantendorfer 2001; Roth, Ostroff, and Hoffman 1996).

In one case, skin-picking behavior decreased 4 weeks after inositol at 18 g/day was added to citalopram at 40 mg/day (Seedat, Stein, and Harvey 2001).

Studies of psychotherapeutic treatments of SPD are few. Habit reversal (HR) therapy, a behavioral treatment for modifying habitual behaviors, is the most studied among these and has been examined in controlled trials. It consists of multiple components, including (1) awareness training about habitual behaviors, (2) relaxation training to help reduce tension, (3) competing response training in which patients learn to perform movements that are incompatible with habitual behaviors, (4) rewarding oneself for successfully resisting picking, and, (5) generalization training to learn to control habitual behaviors in different everyday situations (Azrin and Nunn 1973). Awareness training can be complemented by having the patient keep a daily log of picking episodes, including precipitants, time spent, and emotions present before and after picking. Competing response training should be particularized to situations associated with the picking (e.g., watching TV or being in the bathroom). Bathroom picking behavior may be diminished by asking the patient to reduce the intensity of bathroom lighting, discard magnifying mirrors, and set an egg timer running that signals time to exit after a few minutes. (See Chapter 8 for additional descriptions of HR interventions.)

One trial evaluated the effectiveness of simplified habit reversal (SHR) therapy in a multiple-baseline design in two brothers without comorbid psychiatric conditions (Twohig and Woods 2001). Their skin-picking behavior, which had existed since childhood, decreased, but only one brother maintained gains at 3-month follow-up. In a second study, 19 participants were randomized to SHR or a wait-list control group. Simplified habit reversal was more effective, and treatment gains, although not complete, were maintained at 3-month follow-up (Teng, Woods, and Twohig 2006). A third study used an acceptance and commitment therapy (ACT) protocol that specifically avoided components of SHR. Acceptance and commitment therapy decreased anxiety and depression as well as skin picking in four of the five participants, but these gains were not fully maintained for three of the four at follow-up (Twohig, Hayes, and Masuda 2006).

Case reports/series suggest that skin picking can be successfully treated with habit reversal. Rosenbaum and Ayllon (1981) reported on four patients who scratched their skins. Scratching was eliminated in one patient and remained at low levels for the three other patients at 6-month follow-up. Kent and Drummond (1989) found habit reversal successful in a patient with acné excoriée. The improvement was maintained at the 4-month follow-up. Deckersbach et al. (2002) described three patients with skin picking, two of whom had psychiatric comorbidity. Their skin picking decreased following a course of cognitive-behavioral therapy (CBT) that included selected habit-reversal techniques. It is noteworthy that these patients responded to CBT despite the chronicity of the skin-picking behavior and psychiatric comorbidity.

A Web site providing information regarding skin picking is http://www.jfponlive.com. A self-help treatment that incorporates principles of habit reversal and stimulus control is available at www.stoppicking.com. The program involves self-monitoring and a behavior change module designed to be completed in daily sessions over 7–10 weeks, followed by a maintenance model. Although created by experts in cognitive-behavioral therapy and skin picking, the program has not been subjected to evaluation in a controlled trial.

In summary, as a first step, underlying medical or psychiatric conditions should be ruled out before starting the treatment of SPD. SSRIs, which are the best-studied medications for the treatment of SPD, can be recommended as a first-line therapy because of their proven efficacy and safety. It should be kept in mind that treatment of SPD may require high doses of SSRIs for a long duration, like the treatment of OCD. Arnold et al. (1998) suggested that SSRIs may be particularly effective in patients with prominent compulsive features, comorbid mood and anxiety disorders, or BDD. TCAs can also be used with caution because of their side effects. Patients who do not improve with antidepressants may benefit from an augmentation with atypical antipsychotics or from a trial of a medication reported effective in open trials or case reports (i.e., lamotrigine or naltrexone). Patients with impulsive features or comorbid bipolar disorder may benefit from the use of mood stabilizers or atypical antipsychotics (Arnold, Starck, and McElroy 2002). Cognitive-behavioral therapy, especially in the form of habit reversal, may be helpful as an adjunctive treatment in patients who do not respond to medication alone.

References

American Psychiatric Association. *Diagnostic and Statistical Manual of Mental Disorders*, 4th edition. Washington, DC: American Psychiatric Association, 1994.

American Psychiatric Association. *Diagnostic and Statistical Manual of Mental Disorders*, 4th edition, text revision. Washington, DC: American Psychiatric Association, 2000.

Arnold LM, Auchenbach MB, McElroy SL. Psychogenic excoriation: Clinical features, proposed diagnostic criteria, epidemiology, and approaches to treatment. *CNS Drugs* 15(5): 351–359, 2001.

Arnold LM, McElroy SL. The nosology of compulsive skin picking [reply letter]. *J Clin Psychiatry* 60:618–619, 1999.

Arnold LM, McElroy SL, Mutasim DF et al. Characteristics of 34 adults with psychogenic excoriation. *J Clin Psychiatry* 59:509–514, 1998.

Arnold LM, Mutasim DF, Dwight MM et al. An open clinical trial of fluvoxamine treatment of psychogenic excoriation. *J Clin Psychopharmacol* 19(1): 15–18, 1999.

Arnold LM, Starck LO, McElroy SL. Treatment of psychogenic excoriation in the elderly patient. *Clin Geriatr* 10(12): 36–46, 2002.

Azrin NH, Nunn RG. Habit-reversal: A method of eliminating nervous habits and tics. *Behav Res Ther* 11:619–628, 1973.

Bienvenu OJ, Samuels JF, Riddle MA et al. The relationship of obsessive–compulsive disorder to possible spectrum disorders: Results from a family study. *Biol Psychiatry* 48:287–293, 2000.

Biondi M, Arcangeli T, Petrucci RM. Paroxetine in a case of psychogenic pruritus and neurotic excoriations. *Psychother Psychosom* 69(3): 165–166, 2000.

Bishop ER. Monosymptomatic hypochondriacal syndromes in dermatology. *J Am Acad Dermatol* 9:152–158, 1983.

Bloch MR, Elliott M, Thompson H et al. Fluoxetine in pathologic skin-picking: Open-label and double-blind results. *Psychosomatics* 42(4): 314–319, 2001.

Bohne A, Wilhelm S, Keuthen NJ et al. Skin picking in German students: Prevalence, phenomenology, and associated characteristics. *Behav Modif* 26(3): 320–338, 2002a.

Bohne A, Keuthen NJ, Wilhelm S et al. Prevalence of symptoms of body dysmorphic disorder and its correlates: A cross-cultural comparison. *Psychosomatics* 43(6): 486–490, 2002b.

Bowes LE, Alster TS. Treatment of facial scarring and ulceration resulting from acne excoriée with 585-nm pulsed dye laser irradiation and cognitive psychotherapy. *Dermatol Surg* 30(6): 934–938, 2004.

Bystritsky A, Strausser BP. Treatment of obsessive-compulsive cutting behavior with naltrexone (letter). *J Clin Psychiatry* 57:423–3, 1996.

Çalıkuşu C, Yücel B, Polat A et al. Expression of anger and alexithymia in patients with psychogenic excoriation: A preliminary report. *Int J Psychiatry Med* 32(4): 345–352, 2002.

Çalıkuşu C, Yücel B, Polat A et al. The relation of psychogenic excoriation with psychiatric disorders: A comparative study. *Comp Psychiatry* 44(3): 256–261, 2003.

Carter WG, Shillcutt SD. Aripiprazole augmentation of venlafaxine in the treatment of psychogenic excoriation (letter). *J Clin Psychiatry* 67(8): 1311, 2006.

Christensen RC. Olanzapine augmentation of fluoxetine in the treatment of pathological skin picking (letter). *Can J Psychiatry* 49(11): 788–789, 2004.

Christenson GA, Mackenzie TB, Mitchell JE. Characteristics of 60 adult chronic hair pullers. *Am J Psychiatry* 148:365–370, 1991.

Deckersbach T, Wilhelm S, Keuthen NJ et al. Cognitive-behavior therapy for self-injurious skin picking: A case series. *Behav Modif* 26(3): 361–377, 2002.

Dell'Osso B, Altamura AC, Allen A et al. Epidemiologic and clinical updates on impulse control disorders: A critical review. *Eur Arch Psychiatry Clin Neurosci* 256:464–475, 2006.

Duke EE. Clinical experience with pimozide: Emphasis on its use in postherpetic neuralgia. *J AM Acad Dermatol* 8(6): 845–850, 1983.

Dykens EM, Shah B. Psychiatric disorders in Prader-Willi syndrome: Epidemiology and treatment. *CNS Drugs* 17:167–178, 2003.

Favaro A, Ferrara S, Santonastaso P. Self-injurious behavior in a community sample of young women: Relationship with childhood abuse and other types of self-damaging behaviors. *J Clin Psychiatry* 68(1): 122–131, 2007.

Ferrão YA, Almeida VP, Bedin NR et al. Impulsivity and compulsivity in patients with trichotillomania or skin picking compared with patients with obsessive-compulsive disorder. *Compr Psychiatry* 47:282–288, 2006.

Flessner CA, Woods DW. Phenomenological characteristics, social problems, and the economic impact associated with chronic skin picking. *Behav Modif* 30(6): 944–963, 2006.

Fruensgaard K. Neurotic excoriations: A controlled psychiatric examination. *Acta Psychiatr Scand Suppl.* 69:1–52, 1984.

Fruensgaard K, Hjortshoj A, Nielsen H. Neurotic excoriations. *Int J Dermatol* 17:761–767, 1978.

Garnis-Jones S, Collins S, Rosenthal D. Treatment of self-mutilation with olanzapine. *J Cutan Med Surg* 4(3): 161–163, 2000.

Goodman WK, Price LH, Rasmussen SA et al. The Yale-Brown Obsessive Compulsive Scale: Development, use and reliability. *Arch Gen Psychiatry* 46:1006–1011, 1989.

Grant JE, Menard W, Phillips KA. Pathological skin picking in individuals with body dysmorphic disorder. *Gen Hosp Psychiatry* 28(6): 487–493, 2006.

Grant JE, Odlaug BL, Kim SW. Lamotrigine treatment of pathologic skin picking: An open-label study. *J Clin Psychiatry* 68(9): 1384–1391, 2007.

Grant JE, Phillips KA. Captive of the mirror: I pick at my face all day, every day. *Curr Psych* 2:45–52, 2003.

Grant JE, Williams KA, Potenza MN. Impulse control disorders in adolescent psychiatric inpatients: Co-occurring disorders and sex differences. *J Clin Psychiary* 68(10): 1584–1592, 2007.

Griengl H, Sendera A, Dantendorfer K. Naltrexone as a treatment of self-injurious behavior: A case report. *Acta Psychiatrica Scand* 103:234–236, 2001.

Griesemer RD. Emotionally triggered disease in a dermatologic practice. *Psychiatr Ann* 8:407–412, 1978.

Gupta MA, Gupta AK. Fluoxetine is an effective treatment for neurotic excoriations: Case report. *Cutis* 51:386–387, 1993.

Gupta MA, Gupta AK. Olanzapine is effective in the management of some self-induced dermatoses: Three case reports. *Cutis* 66(2): 143–146, 2000.

Gupta MA, Gupta AK, Haberman HF. Neurotic excoriations: A review and some new perspectives. *Compr Psychiatry* 27:381–386, 1986.

Gupta MA, Gupta AK, Haberman HF. The self-inflicted dermatoses: A critical review. *Gen Hosp Psychiatry* 9(1): 45–52, 1987.

Harris BA, Sheretz EF, Flowers FP. Improvement of chronic neurotic excoriations with oral doxepine therapy. *Int J Dermatol* 26:541–543, 1987.

Hendrickx B, Van Moffaert M, Spiers R et al. The treatment of psychocutaneous disorders: A new approach. *Curr Ther Res Clin Exp* 49:111–119, 1991.

Hollander E, Stein DJ, DeCaria CM et al. Disorders related to OCD-neurobiology. *Clin Neuropharmacol* 15:259–260, 1992.

Kalivas J, Kalivas L, Gilman D et al. Sertraline in the treatment of neurotic excoriations and related disorders. *Arch Dermatol* 132:589–590, 1996.

Kent A, Drummond LM. Acne excoriée: A case report of treatment using habit reversal. *Clin Exp Dermatol* 14(2): 163–164, 1989.

Keuthen NJ, Deckersbach T, Wilhelm S et al. Repetitive skin picking in a student population and comparison with a sample of self-injurious skin pickers. *Psychosomatics* 41(3): 210–215, 2000.

Keuthen NJ, Deckersbach T, Wilhelm S et al. The Skin Picking Impact Scale (SPIS): Scale development and psychometric analyses. *Psychosomatics* 42(5): 397–403, 2001b.

Keuthen NJ, Jameson M, Loh R et al. Open-label escitalopram treatment for pathological skin picking. *Int Clin Psychopharmacol* 22:268–274, 2007.

Keuthen NJ, Koran LM, Aboujaoude E et al. Prevalence of pathological skin picking (PSP) in the general population. *Compr Psychiatry*, in press 2009.

Keuthen NJ, Wilhelm S, Engelhard IM et al. The Skin Picking Scale (SPS): Scale construction and psychometric analyses. *J Psychosom Res* 50:337–341, 2001a.

Koblenzer CS. Psychosomatic concepts in dermatology: A dermatologist-psychoanalyst's viewpoint. *Arch Dermatol* 119:401–512, 1983.

Koblenzer CS. *Psychocutaneous Disease.* New York: Grune and Stratton, 1987.

Koblenzer CS. Cutaneous manifestations of psychiatric disease that commonly present to the dermatologist: Diagnosis and treatment. *Int J Psychiatry Med* 22:47–63, 1992.

Koo JYM. *Psychodermatology: Current Concepts.* Kalamazoo, Mich: Upjohn, 1989, pp. 1–14.

Koo JY. Psychotropic agents in dermatology. *Dermatol Clin* 11:215–224, 1993.

Koo J, Lebwohl A. Psychodermatology: The mind and skin connection. *Am Fam Physician* 64(11): 1873, 2001.

Lienemann J, Walker FD. Reversal of self-abusive behavior with naltrexone. *J Clin Psychopharmacol* 9(6): 448–449, 1989.

Lochner C, Simeon D, Niehaus DJH et al. Trichotillomania and skin picking: A phenomenological comparison. *Depress Anxiety* 15:83–86, 2002.

McElroy SL, Phillips KA, Keck PE et al. Obsessive compulsive spectrum disorder. *J Clin Psychiatry* 55 (10 suppl): 33–53, 1994.

Neziroğlu F, Mancebo M. Skin picking as a form of self-injurious behavior. *Psychiatric Annals* 31:549–555, 2001.

Odlaug BL, Grant JE. Childhood-onset pathologic skin picking: Clinical characteristics and psychiatric comorbidity. *Compr Psychiatry* 48:388–393, 2007.

Odlaug BL, Grant JE. Clinical characteristics and medical complications of pathologic skin picking. *Gen Hosp Psychiatry* 30:61–66, 2008.

O'Sullivan RL, Phillips KA, Keuthen NJ et al. Near-fatal skin picking from delusional body dysmorphic disorder responsive to fluvoxamine. *Psychosomatics* 40(1): 79–81, 1999.

Phillips KA, Taub SL. Skin picking as a symptom of body dysmorphic disorder. *Psychopharmacol Bull* 31:279–288, 1995.

Ravindran AV, Lapierre YD, Anisman H. Obsessive-compulsive spectrum disorders: Effective treatment with paroxetine. *Can J Psychiatry* 44(8): 805–807, 1999.

Roth AS, Ostroff RB, Hoffman RE. Naltrexone as a treatment for repetitive self-injurious behavior: An open-label trial. *J Clin Psychiatry* 57:233–237, 1996.

Rosenbaum MS, Ayllon T. The behavioral treatment of neurodermatitis through habit-reversal. *Behav Res Ther* 19(4): 313–318, 1981.

Seedat S, Stein DJ, Harvey BH. Inositol in the treatment of trichotillomania and compulsive skin picking (letter). *J Clin Psychiatry* 62:60–61, 2001.

Simeon D, Favazza AR. Self-injurious behaviors, phenomenology and assessment, in *Self-Injurious Behaviors, Assessment and Treatment.* Edited by Simeon D, Hollander E. Washington, DC: American Psychiatric Publishing, 1995, pp. 1–28.

Simeon D, Stein DJ, Gross S et al. A double-blind trial of fluoxetine in pathologic skin picking. *J Clin Psychiatry* 58:341–347, 1997.

Singareddy R, Moin A, Spurlock L et al. Skin picking and sleep disturbances: Relationship to anxiety and need for research. *Depress Anxiety* 18:228–232, 2003.

Sneddon J, Sneddon I. Acne excoriée: A protective device. *Clin Exp Dermatol* 8(1): 65–68, 1983.

Stein DJ, Hollander E. Dermatology and conditions related to obsessive-compulsive disorder. *J Am Acad Dermatol* 26:237–242, 1992.

Stein DJ, Hutt CS, Spitz JL et al. Compulsive picking and obsessive compulsive disorder. *Psychosomatics* 34:177–181, 1993.

Stout RJ. Fluoxetine for the treatment of compulsive facial picking [letter]. *Am J Psychiatry* 147:370, 1990.

Teng EJ, Woods DW, Twohig MP. Habit reversal as a treatment for chronic skin picking: A pilot investigation. *Behav Modif* 30(4): 411–422, 2006.

Teng EJ, Woods DW, Twohig MP et al. Body-focused repetitive behavior problems: Prevalence in a nonreferred population and differences in perceived somatic activity. *Behav Modif* 26(3): 340–360, 2002.

Twohig MP, Hayes SC, Masuda A. A preliminary investigation of acceptance and commitment therapy as a treatment for chronic skin picking. *Behav Res Ther* 44:1513–1522, 2006.

Twohig MP, Woods DW. Habit reversal as a treatment for chronic skin picking in typically developing adult male siblings. *Journal of Applied Behavior Analysis* 34:217–220, 2001.

Twohig MP, Woods DW. A preliminary investigation of acceptance and commitment therapy and habit reversal as a treatment for trichotillomania. *Behavior Therapy* 35:803–820, 2004.

Wilhelm S, Keuthen NJ, Deckersbach T et al. Self-injurious skin picking: Clinical characteristics and comorbidity. *J Clin Psychiatry* 60(7): 454–459, 1999.

World Health Organization. *International Classification of Diseases*, 10th revision. Geneva: World Health Organization, 1992.

12

Skin Picking: The View from Dermatology

Rungsima Wanitphakdeedecha, MD, and Tina S. Alster, MD

Introduction

The psychocutaneous disorders span a vast range of entities from primary skin conditions known to have psychologic sequelae (e.g., psoriasis, pemphigus, alopecia, acne vulgaris) to psychological or psychiatric conditions resulting in severe skin morbidity (Folks and Warnock 2001). The psychiatric conditions with skin manifestations are difficult to diagnose and are often misdiagnosed. Commonly, these "psychodermatoses" are grouped into one broad category generally known as "psychogenic excoriation" (O'Sullivan et al. 1999). This designation conflicts with the proper identification of psychiatric disorders from which the patient may suffer and limits the extent and proper selection of required treatment modalities.

Psychogenic excoriation (also referred to as neurotic excoriation, compulsive skin picking, dermatotillomania, and acne excoriée) is characterized by excessive picking and scratching of normal skin or skin with minimal surface texture irregularities (Arnold, Auchenbach, and McElroy 2001). This condition affects up to 2% of patients in dermatology clinics and leads to marked functional disability, further emotional distress, and medical complications (e.g., infections, limb loss, severe bleeding). Individuals suffering from psychogenic excoriation report significant distress and psychosocial impairment, including occupational and marital difficulties (Folks and Warnock 2001). This condition has received special attention from pediatricians and mental health professionals because of the underlying presence of obsessive-compulsive personality and body dysmorphic disorders affecting many patients with severe excoriations (Arnold et al. 1998; Bach and Bach 1993; Deckersbach et al. 2002; Gupta, Gupta, and Schork 1996; Koo and Smith 1991a, 1991b; Wilhelm et al. 1999).

Clinical Characteristics

Prevalence rates of psychogenic excoriation in the general population are unknown, but studies have found that the behavior occurs in 4% of college students (Arnold et al. 1998), 2% of dermatology patients (Gupta, Gupta, and Schork 1996), 11.8% of adolescent psychiatric inpatients (Grant, Odlaug, and Kim 2007), and 44.9% of individuals with body dysmorphic disorder (Grant, Menard, and Phillips 2006). The female-to-male ratio is approximately 8:1; however, this ratio may reflect the differences between the number of men and women seeking treatment (Wilhelm et al. 1999).

Although psychogenic excoriation generally has its onset in adolescence, it may occur at any age (Arnold et al. 1998; Odlaug and Grant 2007). The mean age of onset ranges from 15 to 45 years and the mean duration of symptoms spans 5 to 21 years (Arnold, Auchenbach, and McElroy 2001). The symptoms often begin with dermatological disorders such as acne, eczema, or psoriasis (Wilhelm et al. 1999). The picking behavior may result in significant tissue damage and scarring, sometimes warranting surgery. However, because of embarrassment or the mistaken belief that their condition is untreatable, those afflicted

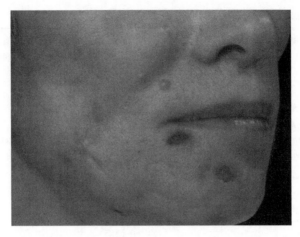

Figure 12.1   Disfiguring ulcers and scars on the face resulting from uncontrollable skin picking.

with skin picking rarely seek dermatological or psychiatric treatment (Grant, Odlaug, and Kim 2007). Patients often develop disfiguring ulcers and scars as a result of uncontrollable skin picking and gouging (Figure 12.1). This further aggravates the situation because much of the skin mutilation stems from the patient's falsely perceived imperfection or ugliness.

Patients with acne excoriée resulting in disfiguring facial ulcers and scars pose a true treatment challenge for the physician. On physical examination, excoriations, ulcers, and a range of early and late scars are often present, providing a visual time line of the disorder. There commonly exists at least one comorbid psychiatric diagnosis, such as obsessive-compulsive personality disorder or body dysmorphic disorder, rendering multimodal (dermatologic and psychiatric) treatment a necessity (Arnold et al. 1998; Wilhelm et al. 1999).

Diagnosis

Psychogenic excoriation is not explicitly classified in the *Diagnostic and Statistical Manual of Mental Disorders*, 4th edition (DSM-IV), but implicitly falls within the category of "impulse control disorders not otherwise specified" (American Psychiatric Association 2000). Arnold, Auchenbach, and McElroy (2001) proposed preliminary operational criteria for its diagnosis and subtypes based on a number of studies of patients with this condition (see Table 11.1 and Table 12.1). These criteria take into account the heterogeneity of behavior associated with psychogenic excoriation and allow for subtyping along a compulsivity-impulsivity spectrum.

Treatment

Treatment of skin picking has proven to be challenging (O'Sullivan et al. 1999). Special emphasis should be placed on interrupting the repetitive cycle of events that perpetuates this psychodermatosis. The psychiatric disorders affecting many of these patients can often be managed with behavior modification or cognitive-behavioral psychotherapies and/or psychiatric medication (Arnold, Auchenbach, and McElroy 2001) (see Chapter 11). Clinicians not only need to recognize the emotional and psychosocial impacts of picking to provide appropriate treatment but also must be aware of possible medical sequelae of picking so that appropriate interventions can be provided.

A detailed account of the psychiatric treatment of patients with skin picking is presented in Chapter 11.

Table 12.1 Psychogenic excoriation subtypes

Compulsive type

Skin excoriation is performed to avoid increased anxiety or to prevent a dreaded event or situation and/or is elicited by an obsession (e.g., obsession about contamination of the skin).
It is performed in full awareness.
It is associated with some resistance to performing the behavior.
There is some insight into its senselessness or harmfulness.

Impulsive type

Skin excoriation is associated with arousal, pleasure, or reduction of tension.
It is performed at times with minimal awareness.
It is associated with little resistance to performing the behavior.
There is little insight into its senselessness or harmfulness.

Mixed type

Skin excoriation has both compulsive and impulsive features.

Dermatological Management: Topical Treatments

From the dermatological point of view, active acne vulgaris lesions, as well as the associated excoriations, ulcers, and scars, should be treated simultaneously. Nonirritating topical antibiotics as well as oral antibiotics should be prescribed for any observable acne and/or secondarily infected excoriations or ulcers. Semiocclusive protective dressings are particularly helpful in preventing further trauma and excoriations of the picked areas. Using isotretinoin, a common treatment for moderate to severe or persistent acne, may not be safe in treating these patients because of the possibility of continued excoriations and the known detrimental effect of isotretinoin on wound healing. Compliance requirements, the risk of inducing depression, and the need for close laboratory monitoring, including pregnancy, lipid, and liver function tests, also argue against using isotretinoin in treating these patients (Barth et al. 1993; Wysowski, Pitts, and Beitz 2001).

Dermatological Management: Pulsed Dye Laser Treatment

A variety of erythematous, atrophic, hypertrophic, and keloid scars respond favorably to 585-nm pulsed dye laser (PDL) irradiation (Alster 1994, 2003; Alster and Greenberg 2005; Alster and Handrick 2000; Alster and McMeekin 1996; Alster and Nanni 1998; Alster and Tanzi 2003; Alster and Williams 1995; Alster and Zaulyanov-Scanlon 2007; Alster et al. 1993; Bowes and Alster 2004; Dierickx, Goldman, and Fitzpatrick 1995; Handrick and Alster 2001; Lupton and Alster 2002; Manuskiatti, Fitzpatrick, and Goldman 2001; Patel and Clement 2002; Rostan et al. 2001). The improvement of hypertrophic scars following treatment with PDL was first demonstrated in argon laser-induced fibrosis in port-wine stains (Alster et al. 1993). Subsequent studies of patients with erythematous facial acne scars who received one or two treatments with a PDL also reported significant improvement in skin texture and erythema (Alster and McMeekin 1996).

The positive effect of PDL irradiation on hypertrophic surgical scars, either alone (Alster 1994; Alster and Williams 1995; Dierickx, Goldman, and Fitzpatrick 1995) or in combination with intralesional corticosteroids as adjunctive therapy (Alster 2003), has also been demonstrated. Scar response depends on the wavelength, fluence (laser beam energy), and number of treatments applied. A 585-nm wavelength, low fluences (3–5 J/cm^2), and repetitive treatments (usually two or more) produce the most favorable clinical outcome (Manuskiatti, Fitzpatrick, and Goldman 2001; Reiken et al. 1997). Even atrophic scars and rhytides (wrinkles) have shown improvement after PDL irradiation (Handrick and Alster 2001; Patel and Clement 2002; Rostan et al. 2001). Microvasculature-specific PDL irradiation has been postulated to lead to release of growth factors (e.g., platelet-derived growth factor) from the blood vessels into the dermal milieu, initiating a cascade of events that culminate in fibroblast activation and enhanced dermal collagen deposition (Alster and

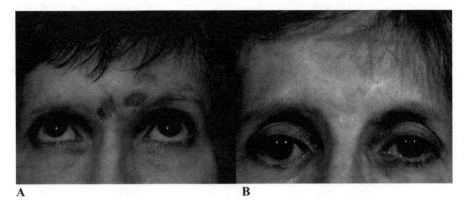

A   B

Figure 12.2   Facial ulcerations and scars before (A) and after (B) 585-nm pulsed dye laser irradiation.

Tanzi 2003). Such events could also explain, at least in part, the reduction in depth and size of atrophic acne scars noted after PDL treatment (Patel and Clement 2002). Therefore, a 585-nm pulsed dye laser may offer advantages in the treatment of facial acne and traumatic scars because the coexistence of the hypertrophic, erythematous, and atrophic components can each be effectively treated with the same laser (Alster and McMeekin 1996; Bowes and Alster 2004) (Figures 12.2A and 12.2B).

Other treatments for facial scars that result from trauma and/or acne are available to resurface skin, including dermabrasion with a rotating wire brush, using various topical acids, chemical peels, and vaporizing lasers (such as CO_2 or erbium) (Tanzi and Alster 2007). Each of these treatments is more aggressive in nature, involving a degree of injury to the epidermis and dermis that may not be suitable for patients with acne excoriée (Alster and Tanzi 2008). The uncontrollable skin-picking habits of acne excoriée patients may severely impair the wound healing process and could lead to further scarring and secondary infection. In view of the possible risks associated with these treatments and the distinct possibility of patient exacerbation of the problem, 585-nm PDL irradiation may be a preferable treatment for scars and ulcers in these cases.

Conclusion

Self-inflicted skin ulcers and scars are often observed in patients with compulsive skin picking. The term "psychogenic excoriation" has been used to describe this condition and may or may not be present in patients with other true skin pathologies, such as acne. Psychogenic excoriation poses a diagnostic and treatment challenge because patients often also have an undiagnosed underlying psychiatric disorder. Thus, when treating a patient with skin picking, it is important to identify any underlying psychiatric disorder that could account for the skin-picking behavior. Early and ongoing psychotherapeutic intervention will increase the likelihood of more effective management of this complex psychodermatosis. Additionally, simultaneous implementation of a skin-treatment regimen will provide faster resolution of lesions, which in turn will improve the patient's self-image, decrease the risk of further skin manipulation, and render behavior modification more effective. Therefore, collaboration between dermatologists and psychiatrists is an essential key for successful treatment of patients whose excoriation has resulted in visible, chronic damage.

References

Alster T. Laser scar revision: Comparison study of 585-nm pulsed dye laser with and without intrale-sional corticosteroids. *Dermatol Surg* 29:25–29, 2003.

Alster TS. Improvement of erythematous and hypertrophic scars by the 585-nm flashlamp-pumped pulsed dye laser. *Ann Plast Surg* 32:186–190, 1994.

Alster TS, Greenberg HL. Laser treatment of scars and striae, in *Principles and Practice in Cutaneous Laser Surgery*. Edited by Kauvar ANB, Hruza G. New York: Taylor & Francis, 2005, pp. 619–635.

Alster TS, Handrick C. Laser treatment of hypertrophic scars, striae, and keloids. *Semin Cutan Med Surg* 19:287–292, 2000.

Alster TS, Kurban AK, Grove GL et al. Alteration of argon laser-induced scars by the pulsed dye laser. *Lasers Surg Med* 13:368–373, 1993.

Alster TS, McMeekin TO. Improvement of facial acne scars by the 585-nm flashlamp-pumped pulsed-dye laser. *J Am Acad Dermatol* 35:79–81, 1996.

Alster TS, Nanni CA. Pulsed dye laser treatment of hypertrophic burn scars. *Plast Reconstr Surg* 102:2190–2195, 1998.

Alster TS, Tanzi EL. Hypertrophic scars and keloids: A review of etiology and management. *Am J Clin Dermatol* 4:235–243, 2003.

Alster TS, Tanzi EL. Complications in laser and light surgery, in *Lasers and Lights*, vol. II. Edited by Goldberg DJ. Philadelphia: Saunders Elsevier, 2008, pp. 99–112.

Alster TS, Williams CM. Treatment of keloid sternotomy scars with the 585 nm flashlamp-pumped pulsed-dye laser. *Lancet* 345:1198–1200, 1995.

Alster TS, Zaulyanov-Scanlon L. Laser scar revision: A review. *Dermatol Surg* 33:131–140, 2007.

American Psychiatric Association. *Diagnostic and Statistical Manual of Mental Disorders*, 4th edition, text revision. Washington, DC: American Psychiatric Association, 2000.

Arnold LM, Auchenbach MB, McElroy SL. Psychogenic excoriation: Clinical features, proposed diagnostic criteria, epidemiology and approaches to treatment. *CNS Drugs* 15:351–359, 2001.

Arnold LM, McElroy SL, Mutassim DF et al. Characteristics of 34 adults with psychogenic excoriation. *J Clin Psychiatry* 59:509–514, 1998.

Bach M, Bach D. Psychiatric and psychometric issues in acne excoriée. *Psychother Psychosom* 60:207–210, 1993.

Barth JH, MacDonald-Hull SP, Mark J et al. Isotretinoin therapy for acne vulgaris: A re-evaluation of the need for measurements of plasma lipids and liver function tests. *Br J Dermatol* 129:704–707, 1993.

Bowes LE, Alster TS. Treatment of facial scarring and ulceration resulting from acne excoriée with 585-nm pulsed dye laser irradiation and cognitive psychotherapy. *Dermatol Surg* 30:934–938, 2004.

Deckersbach T, Wilhelm S, Keuthen NJ et al. Cognitive-behavior therapy for self-injurious skin picking: A case series. *Behav Modif* 26:361–367, 2002.

Dierickx C, Goldman MP, Fitzpatrick RE. Laser treatment of erythematous/hypertrophic and pigmented scars in 26 patients. *Plast Reconstr Surg* 95:84–90, 1995.

Folks DG, Warnock JK. Psychocutaneous disorders. *Curr Psychiatry Rep* 3:219–225, 2001.

Grant JE, Menard W, Phillips KA. Pathological skin picking in individuals with body dysmorphic disorder. *Gen Hosp Psychiatry* 28:487–493, 2006.

Grant JE, Odlaug BL, Kim SW. Lamotrigine treatment of pathologic skin picking: An open-label study. *J Clin Psychiatry* 68:1384–1391, 2007.

Gupta MA, Gupta AK, Schork NJ. Psychological factors affecting self-excoriative behavior in women with mild-to-moderate facial acne vulgaris. *Psychosomatics* 37:127–130, 1996.

Handrick C, Alster TS. Laser treatment of atrophoderma vermiculata. *J Am Acad Dermatol* 44:693–695, 2001.

Koo JY, Smith LL. Obsessive-compulsive disorders in the pediatric dermatology practice. *Pediatr Dermatol* 8:107–113, 1991a.

Koo JY, Smith LL. Psychologic aspects of acne. *Pediatr Dermatol* 8:185–188, 1991b.

Lupton JR, Alster TS. Laser scar revision. *Dermatol Clin* 20:55–65, 2002.

Manuskiatti W, Fitzpatrick RE, Goldman MP. Energy density and number of treatments affect response of keloidal and hypertrophic sternotomy scars to the 585-nm flashlamp-pumped pulsed-dye laser. *J Am Acad Dermatol* 45:557–565, 2001.

Odlaug BL, Grant JE. Childhood-onset pathologic skin picking: Clinical characteristics and psychiatric comorbidity. *Compr Psychiatry* 48:388–393, 2007.

O'Sullivan RL, Phillips KA, Keuthen NJ et al. Near-fatal skin picking from delusional body dysmorphic syndrome responsive to fluvoxamine. *Psychosomatics* 40:79–81, 1999.

Patel N, Clement M. Selective treatment of acne scarring with 585-nm flashlamp pulsed dye laser. *Dermatol Surg* 28:942–945, 2002.

Reiken SR, Wolfort SF, Berthiaume F et al. Control of hypertrophic scar growth using selective photothermolysis. *Lasers Surg Med* 21:7–12, 1997.

Rostan E, Bowes LE, Iyer S et al. A double-blind, side-by-side comparison study of low-fluence long pulse dye laser to coolant treatment for wrinkling of the cheeks. *J Cosmet Laser Ther* 3:129–136, 2001.

Tanzi EL, Alster TS. Skin resurfacing: Ablative lasers, chemical peels, and dermabrasion, in *Fitzpatrick's Dermatology in General Medicine*, 7th edition, vol. 2. Edited by Wolff K, Goldsmith LA, Katz SI et al. New York: McGraw-Hill, 2007, pp. 2364–2371.

Wilhelm S, Keuthen NJ, Deckersbach T et al. Self-injurious skin picking: Clinical characteristics and comorbidity. *J Clin Psychiatry* 60:454–459, 1999.

Wysowski DK, Pitts M, Beitz J. An analysis of reports of depression and suicide in patients treated with isotretinoin. *J Am Acad Dermatol* 45:515–519, 2001.

13

Onychophagia (Nail Biting): Clinical Aspects

Timothy Ivor Williams, MD

History of Psychiatric Attention to the Disorder

Onychophagia (nail biting) is a word of Greek origin (from ονυξ, meaning nail, and φαγειν, meaning to eat). It is unlikely that it was recognized as a problem by the Greeks of classical times because it does not appear in classical literature. There is some evidence, however, that well-kept nails were noticed. Theophrastus (ca. 370 BCE–ca. 285 BCE) describes the appearance of fingernails in the characterization of people. Specifically, he regarded well-manicured fingernails as a sign of the oligarch (Ολιγαρχιας) or authoritarian personality (Jebb 1870). Onygophagist (sic) appears in the Compact Edition of the *Oxford English Dictionary* as a misspelling in Southey's book *The Doctor* (Southey 1836). This chapter uses the phrase "nail biting" rather than onychophagia because "nail biting" is more easily understood.

The earliest reference to nail biting as a nervous habit occurs in a late sixteenth-century French history that describes nail biting as associated with anxiety (de Lisle 1577). The *Oxford English Dictionary* records the admonition "don't bite your nails" in a translation of the works of Quevedo, a sixteenth-century Spanish writer (Stevens 1707). Other European traditions have defined nail biting (mordre les ongles, Nagelkauen, comerse las uñas) as being linked to anxiety or anxious personality types.

Freud is often regarded as having suggested that nail biting represented a return to the oral stage of development. Psychoanalytic tradition identified nail biting as representing a conflict of two drives: the desire for the breast represented by putting things in one's mouth and an aggressive motivation represented by biting (Rosow 1954; Solomon 1955). Although psychoanalytic publications on nail biting continued through the 1950s, related research began to concentrate on measuring aspects of personality (Billig 1941) before the behavioral tradition exemplified by Azrin's work (Azrin and Nunn 1973) appeared. A peak of treatment research activity that focused on behavioral principles in the late 1970s and early 1980s has been followed by a relative dearth of new research on nail biting. However, since the study of other repetitive behavior problems such as trichotillomania and pathologic skin picking has increased, nail biting has been discussed as part of the proposed obsessive-compulsive disorder (OCD) spectrum. For instance, Nestadt et al. (2003) linked nail biting and skin picking in a multivariate cluster of symptoms in a study examining possible OCD subtypes. Thus, the current literature regards nail biting either as a form of obsessive-compulsive spectrum disorder, often with an implied neurological malfunction, or as a maladaptive learned behavior. These two views are not incompatible because behavioral change and neurological change can co-occur.

Diagnosis

Nail biting is not recognized as a disorder in the fourth edition of *Diagnostic and Statistical Manual of Mental Disorders Text Revision* (DSM-IV-TR) (American Psychiatric Association

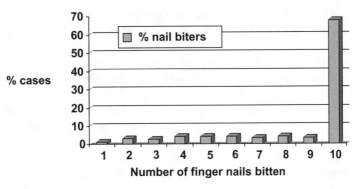

Figure 13.1   Distribution of numbers of fingernails bitten in a large sample (*n* = 4,587) (Malone and Massler 1952).

2000), but the research interest in repetitive behavior disorders suggests that subsequent revisions (DSM-V) may recognize nail biting as a disorder if it affects the person's life or causes damage to health. While DSM-V will probably include a category for repetitive behavior disorders, this author doubts that nail biting can be regarded as a "disorder" in childhood. A second possible placement of nail biting would be within a category of body-focused repetitive behaviors. Again, whether the term "disorder" could be applied to a behavior that has few ill effects and is common among certain age groups is dubious. Finally, DSM-V could include a wide-ranging category of obsessive-compulsive spectrum disorders into which nail biting might be placed.

Clinical Picture

Although most nail biters bite only their fingernails, some people bite their toenails as well (Leung and Robson 1990) or overclip their toenails (Leonard et al. 1991). Malone and Massler (1952) described the distribution of numbers of fingernails bitten by both age (5–18 years) and gender. Their data show that about two-thirds of nail biters bite all ten nails (see Figure 13.1). Both the extent of nail damage and the extent of damage to the cuticle and the skin around the nails vary considerably.

Occasionally people may bite their nails as part of a behavioral disorder occasioned by intense pain. One series (Mailis 1996) describes four individuals with severe pain caused by both central and peripheral nerve malfunctions, of whom two showed severe nail biting that caused loss of the whole nail. In rare cases, nail biting may cause infections that damage the tissues of the digits (Tosti et al. 1994). In a more extreme case, a Brazilian woman removed the upper joint of one finger by biting her nails as well as damaging most of her other fingers (Dalanora et al. 2007).

Nail biters are often ashamed of their habit (Joubert 1993) and view themselves in a more negative way than people who do not bite their nails (Hansen et al. 1990). Nail biters are also perceived more negatively than people who do not bite their nails (Wells, Haines, and Williams 1998), and this perception may lead to fewer opportunities for valued activities such as employment (Long et al. 1999).

Assessment Instruments

Nail biting can be reliably and simply measured by using calipers. The nails are measured from the "base of the nail where it separates from the cuticle to the centre point of the top of the nail" (Allen 1996). Some authors have reported total nail length over all ten fingers (Frankel and Merbaum 1982) or mean nail length (i.e., total nail length divided by the number of fingers; see Davidson, Denney, and Elliott 1980). Either figure will provide a simple and reliable indication of nail growth as long as a baseline (pretreatment) measure is taken.

Ladouceur (1979) has argued, however, that nails may grow even though the person is biting them and that a measure of damage to the nails is to be preferred. He used photographs and an observer to determine whether or not nails had been bitten. Interobserver reliability for this measure was 97.8%. Ratings of appearance have also been used by other investigators (Allen 1996; Davidson, Denney, and Elliott 1980; Frankel and Merbaum 1982; Glasgow, Swaney, and Schafer 1981; Twohig et al. 2003). Davidson, Denney, and Elliott (1980) describe their measure as a Cosmetic Appearance Checklist containing six items related to damage to the cuticles and nails, with an interrater reliability of $r = 0.99$. Frankel and Merbaum (1982) used the same checklist and found an interrater reliability of $r = 0.98$. Glasgow, Swaney, and Schafer (1981) used a specially devised measure of nail appearance, the details of which are contained in an MSc thesis. No interrater reliability data were presented in the published paper. Twohig et al.'s (2003) measure, called the Social Validity Scale, contained three 7-point ratings of nail damage, degree of problem, and need for treatment, all rated by judges from photographs of their participants' hands. No interrater reliability data are presented. The Cosmetic Appearance Checklist used by Davidson, Denney, and Elliott seems preferable in that it measures both nail and cutical appearance and has very good interrater reliability.

Malone and Massler (1952) described a simple 4-point rating scale for each (finger) nail that is bitten. While this has the advantage of simplicity, it is more subjective than measuring the length of the nail. Nevertheless, this measure has been used in a number of studies (e.g., Allen 1996) to compare interventions. There are no data on the measure's reliability or validity.

The number and duration of nail-biting episodes have also been measured in treatment trials. Azrin, Nunn, and Frantz (1980) used the number of nail-biting episodes per day to compare two treatment conditions that included, as part of the habit reversal intervention, instruction in self-monitoring and recording of nail biting. Because this is a self-report measure, the influence of the demand characteristics of the study is uncertain. In Davidson, Denney, and Elliott's (1980) study, the statistical tests showed different effects depending on which measure was being analyzed. It is therefore difficult to recommend a self-report of nail-biting episodes as the sole measure of treatment efficacy.

Leonard et al.'s (1991) study stands out from others in both its use of medication as the intervention and in its choice of measures. The authors used three measures. First was an adaptation of the trichotillomania adaptation of the Yale-Brown Obsessive Compulsive Scale (Y-BOCS –TTM) (Swedo et al. 1989) that contained five items, each rated on a scale of 0–5. The items measured the amount of time spent biting nails, intensity of the nail-biting urge, resistance against the urge, and distress and degree of interference in daily life. The second measure was the Nail Biting Impairment Scale, a single 11-point rating scale of impairment caused by nail biting. Finally, the researchers used clinical progress, rated by the clinician on a 0–20 scale. Interrater reliability was reported as kappa scores between 0.78 and 1.00. These scales have not achieved widespread acceptance.

Prevalence

Although nail biting appears to be a common behavior, there are very few scientifically robust studies of its prevalence. For instance, whereas Wechsler (1931) reported that 44% of children were nail biters at age 13 years, Deardoff, Finch, and Royall (1974) found only 12% were nail biters at a similar age. Figure 13.2 shows the rates of nail biting as reported in studies that surveyed individuals over age ranges varying from 10 to 20 years. Nail biting clearly peaks in childhood and seems to decline over the teenage and early adult period.

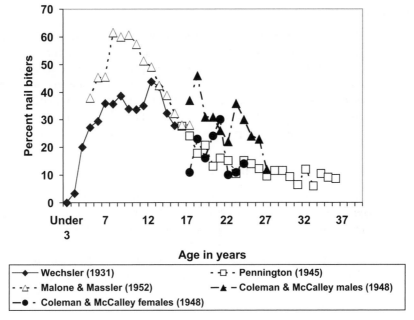

Figure 13.2   Prevalence of nail biting at different ages as reported in four surveys.

Nail biting may be less common in women than in men, but the data are from only one study of subjects in the late teens and early adulthood (Coleman and McCalley 1948). The one study that included people in their thirties and forties suggests a slight ongoing reduction in the proportion of nail biters with increasing age, but the data need replication.

Drawing clear conclusions about the cross-cultural prevalence of nail biting is difficult because the ascertainment methods differ markedly between studies and because the data are not clearly presented. Thus, one study of oral habits in children from Delhi, India, suggested that less than 1% of schoolchildren bit their nails (Kharbanda et al. 2003), whereas another study of Indian children suggested that as many as 13% of schoolchildren did so (Guaba et al. 1998). In a study of minority populations in China (Li et al. 2001), no ethnic differences were reported, although the level of nail biting reported was very low (1.1%). Similarly wide ranges from the studies of developmental patterns discussed earlier imply that the difficulty may lie in defining the behavior sufficiently to allow studies of cross-cultural prevalence to be meaningful.

One review of nail biting (Wells, Haines, and Williams 1998) tabulated several studies that had identified nail biting both in the general population and in psychiatric patients. Like the cross-cultural literature, the variability of the findings means that determining whether nail biting occurs more or less often in conjunction with mental illness is difficult. For instance, one study found that about one-quarter of young people with depression also bit their nails (Calitz et al. 2007).

More recently, a number of studies have been conducted to determine whether nail biting occurs as part of a putative spectrum of obsessive-compulsive behaviors. Initial studies confirmed that "grooming disorders" such as nail biting occurred more frequently among patients with OCD and their relatives (Bienvenu et al. 2000), but statistical modeling suggests that the association is as strong with general anxiety disorder as with OCD (Nestadt et al. 2003). Nestadt et al. (2003) also demonstrated that the association was strongest for those people who suffered from multiple disorders (a mean of 5+ disorders).

Age at Onset

When nail biting starts is unclear. The prevalence figures shown in Figure 13.2 suggest that nail biting is largely a school-age phenomenon, with the highest rates in the age range 5 to 17 years. For older teenagers and adults, the data from Malone and Massler's (1952) study indicate that fewer girls and women than boys and men bite their nails. This could reflect the emphasis young women place on nail treatments such as nail polish and manicures. However, as Friman, Byrd, and Oksol (2001) have observed, the prevalence figures are not robust, and each study appears to produce different results.

Natural History and Course of Illness

Early studies of nail biting concentrated on the natural history of the problem. These studies suggest that the majority of people who bite their nails stop during childhood and adolescence. One might speculate that as children reach their teens they become more self-conscious and aware of the social disapproval associated with nail biting. Beyond adolescence, the surveys suggest that people stop biting their nails over time. Coleman and McCalley's (1948) study advanced a number of reasons: social disapproval, realization of the social value of long, well-kept nails, fear of being infected by germs from the nails, and imitation of parental care for their hands. Our experience with asking people why they have stopped biting their nails has suggested that they made a decision to do so and then were sufficiently determined to carry it out. A less optimistic view was expressed by Mangweth et al. (2005), who suggested that nail biting is one of the behaviors that predisposes people to both eating disorders and "polysubstance abuse," suggesting a common pathway in terms of using physical means to control unpleasant feelings.

Comorbid Conditions

A number of studies have tried to validate the assertion that nail biting is a nervous habit or is characteristic of nervous people. The results have been mixed, with some studies finding associations between anxiety and nail biting (e.g., Billig 1941; Klatte and Deardoff 1981) whereas others did not (Deardoff, Finch, and Royall 1974; Joubert 1993). A wide range of questionnaires have been used, ranging from personality tests (e.g., Bernreuter Personality Inventory – Billig 1941) to specific measures of anxiety (e.g., Manifest Anxiety Scale – Klatte and Deardoff 1981; State Trait Anxiety Inventory – Gilleard, Eskin, and Savasir 1988). Some authors have suggested instead that nail biting, like other repetitive behaviors, serves either a self-stimulatory or an anxiety-reducing function (Wells, Haines, and Williams 1998; Woods and Miltenberger 1996).

Studies of obsessive-compulsive spectrum disorders have often revealed quite high levels of nail biting, among other habits (e.g., Grant et al. 2006). However, many of these studies have not used comparison groups, making it difficult to determine whether the finding applies to all clinical groups, just to groups with OCDs, or to groups with other impulse control disorders.

Treatments

Only one trial of pharmacological agents has been described, in which clomipramine and desimipramine were compared in a double-blind, randomized study (Leonard et al. 1991). Although the results favored clomipramine, the high dropout rate suggests that medication is not an option that nail biters easily adopt. This study also used unique measures, which has rendered comparison of the efficacy of medication with psychological interventions problematic. Pharmacological treatments for other habit disorders have largely used newer

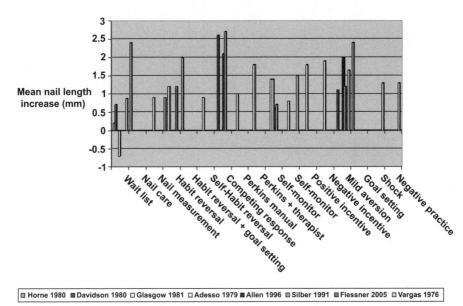

Figure 13.3   Mean nail-length increase for different treatment methods used in controlled studies. Habit reversal is the full habit-reversal intervention as described by Azrin and Nunn (1973). Self-habit reversal is self-administered habit reversal.

selective serotonin uptake inhibitors (SSRIs) such as fluoxetine (e.g., trichotillomania, see van Minnen et al. 2003). Treatment trials using one or more of the SSRIs to determine whether they have better utility than clomipramine seem indicated.

A wide range of psychological treatments for nail biting have been suggested. Those with the most evidence are based on behavioral methods that manipulate the events controlling the occurrence of nail biting. In preparing this chapter, I attempted a systematic review of the treatment literature. The search terms onychophagia and nail biting *and* (treatment *or* intervention) were searched on Google scholar, World of Knowledge, Embase, and Medline. The 15 trials identified are shown in Table 13.1.

Of the 15 trials using group comparison designs (Table 13.1), most failed to provide sufficient details of the baseline, end of treatment, and follow-up data to enable a meta-analysis to be undertaken. In particular, the published trials frequently do not present means for the separate groups and/or measures of the confidence intervals of the means. Figure 13.3 shows the data for the change in nail length from the beginning to the end of treatment as described in published group comparison trials. For several of these trials, data had to be estimated from the published figures. The three left-hand interventions (wait list, nail care, and nail measurement) in Figure 13.3 can be described as control interventions in that they are not designed to change nail length or nail-biting behavior. Two of these interventions (wait list and nail measurement) do not seem to reduce nail biting. However, in one study (Horne and Wilkinson 1980), nail care (not described) had a major beneficial effect compared with habit reversal or goal setting (which included nail care).

Although habit reversal is often recommended in the literature as the treatment of choice, Figure 13.3 does not provide unequivocal support and suggests that simply setting goals for nail-length increase may be sufficient to produce significant increases. One method of determining whether a particular intervention is effective is to conduct a meta-analysis of outcomes across trials. For this chapter, I extracted data from the published literature to find treatment trials that compared active interventions with a waiting list or placebo control. In general, all the treatments showed beneficial effects. However, one treatment, the habit-reversal treatment of Twohig et al. (2003), showed particularly promising results

Table 13.1 Group comparison treatment trials

Reference	Design (n)	Treatments	Significant Results	Notes	Measures
Adesso, Vargas, and Siddall (1979)	Random group comparison (40) (5 groups)	Self-monitoring, positive incentive, negative incentive, nail measurement alone, minimal contact	No significant difference between groups		Nail length, self-monitored nail-biting episodes
Allen (1996)	Group comparison, community volunteers (45)	Competing response, mild aversion (chemical), self-monitoring	Mild aversion > self-monitoring	All groups showed improvements over time	Nail length, Malone and Massler rating, skin damage rating, urges to bite nails
Azrin, Nunn, and Frantz (1980)	Random allocation, group comparison	Habit reversal, negative practice	Habit reversal > negative practice		Nail-biting episodes per day
Davidson, Denney, and Elliott (1980)	Random allocation, group comparison (5 groups)	Combined treatment, positive treatment, negative treatment, placebo treatment, untreated control	Positive component and combined treatment > others		Nail length, cosmetic appearance checklist
Flessner et al. (2005)	Random allocation, group comparison (40) (2 groups)	Awareness training + social support + competing response, awareness training + competing response	No significant group difference		Nail length, frequency of nail biting
Frankel and Merbaum (1982)	Random allocation, group comparison (75)	Habit reversal manual with five regular weekly face-to-face sessions, five telephone contacts, no contact	Contract > no contact	Nail-length data not reported	Nail length, cosmetic appearance, Rosenbaum self-control schedule

Reference	Design	Treatments	Results	Comments	Outcome measures
Glasgow, Swaney, and Schafer (1981)	Group comparison, random assignment (43)		No significant group differences		Appearance ratings, nail length
Horne and Wilkinson (1980)	Group comparison (4 groups)	Simplified habit reversal, simplified habit reversal plus goal setting, nail care and goal setting, wait list	No statistics provided	Habit reversal better for preventing relapse	Nail length, absence of nail biting
Ladouceur (1979)	Group comparison (5 groups)	Habit reversal, habit reversal and self-monitoring, self-monitoring and graph plotting, wait list	No significant group differences, all better than wait list	No data published	Photographs of nails judged for nail biting
Leonard et al. (1991)	Group comparison, blind allocation and assessment (24)	Clomipramine (CMI) Desimpramine (DMI)	CMI > DMI	Substantial dropout rate (46%)	Nail biting severity scale, nail biting impairment scale, clinical progress scale
Miltenberger and Fuqua (1985)	Group comparison (mixed habits – nail biters = 5)	Contingent competing response, habit reversal	?		Number of episodes of nail biting
Silber and Haynes (1992)	Group comparison (21)	Competing response, mild aversion (chemical), self-monitoring	Competing response > mild aversion > self-monitoring		Nail length, skin damage ratings, nail-biting episodes, nail-biting urges
Twohig et al. (2003)	Random group comparison (25)	Habit reversal, talking about nail biting	Habit reversal > talking		Nail length, cosmetic appearance
Twohig and Woods (2001)	Group comparison	5-second competing response (CR), 1-minute CR, 3-minute CR		No statistical tests. Results suggest 3-min CR = 1-min CR > 5-sec CR	Nail length, cosmetic appearance
Vargas and Adesso (1976)	Group comparison, random assignment (61)	Shock, negative practice, bitter substance, attention control split between self-monitoring or no self-monitoring	Self-monitoring > no self-monitoring, no other treatment effects		Nail length, nail-biting episodes

compared with a placebo treatment, in which nail biting was discussed. The habit-reversal treatment of Twohig et al. (2003) incorporated a particularly stringent training criterion for the awareness component, which may explain the treatment's particularly beneficial effects (see Chapters 8 and 11, this volume, for additional descriptions of habit reversal interventions).

If increased awareness of nail biting is sufficient to produce beneficial effects, trials that compared self-monitoring with other interventions should show this. Figure 13.4 shows a forest plot of the outcomes of various interventions compared with self-monitoring in two studies. If any treatment was more effective than self-monitoring, then that treatment's mean effect should differ statistically significantly from the mean effect of self-monitoring. In the forest plot, this would be represented by a horizontal line that did not cross the vertical line of no benefit (i.e., mean difference from self-monitoring (MD) – standard error > 0). Figure 13.4 shows that the overall mean effect of the treatments is less than that of self-monitoring! Furthermore, the therapist-aided use of the Azrin and Nunn (1973) habit reversal manual did not produce beneficial effects when compared with self-monitoring. Ladouceur (1979) had previously reported no difference between habit reversal and self-monitoring, but no data were published so these data are not included in Figure 13.4.

Most treatment trials predate the development of improved analytic techniques to determine the function of a behavior. Meta-analysis has shown that these analytic techniques improve the outcomes of behavioral treatments (Didden, Duker, and Korzilius 1997). At their simplest, behavioral interventions modify either the preceding events or the consequences of a behavior. More complex interventions, such as habit reversal, attempt to modify both simultaneously. The last 25 years have seen a move away from studies of straightforward behavioral interventions toward studies including interventions that concern the cognitive processes associated with behavior.

Stimulus Control

Another means of refining behavioral treatments of nail biting is to define the situations under which nail biting is more and less likely to occur. Behaviorists distinguish between *motivating operations*, which alter the reinforcing or punishing effectiveness of events, and *discriminative stimuli*, which signal the availability of a reinforcer. These distinctions have not yet been applied in studies of nail-biting treatments, although some experiments have demonstrated the importance of the settings in which nail biting occurred (e.g., Williams, Rose, and Chisholm 2007; Woods and Miltenberger 1996). In general, these studies have found that nail biting can be reliably evoked by stressful situations or abated by the presence of another person.

The implications of finding that stress promotes nail biting are clear – stress management interventions should reduce nail biting (e.g., relaxation as suggested by Barrios 1977). How to design interventions that can capitalize on the presence of others to reduce nail biting is less clear. The effects that others have on this behavior have been known since the late nineteenth century.

The research literature has not, however, been able to explain the effect satisfactorily (Aiello and Douthitt 2001). Theories have variously posited effects on arousal, attention, and motivation. Recent research has suggested that the effect may be produced by the knowledge that the person is being evaluated (Feinberg and Aiello 2006). Unfortunately, unpublished research from our lab indicates that high social desirability (the drive to do the right thing, measured by the Marlowe-Crown social desirability scale) does not correlate with suppression of nail biting in the presence of another person (Williams and Zucchelli unpublished), even when more detailed measures of the components of social desirability (i.e., impression management, socially desirable responding) are used (Williams, Smith, and Soorty, unpublished).

Study ID	Year	Exposed n[e]/M[e]/SD[e]	Control n[c]/M[c]/SD[c]	Forest plot - MD (IV)	Weight (%)	Association measure with 95% CI
Glasgow Azrin self	1981	6.3/10.5/1.9	6.3/10.7/2.1		2.56%	-0.2 (-2.4114 to 2.0114)
Glasgow Azrin therapist	1981	6.3/12/1.6	6.3/10.7/2.1		5.38%	1.3 (-0.7616 to 3.3616)
Glasgow Perkins self	1981	6.3/9.6/3.2	6.3/10.7/2.1		2.56%	-1.1 (-4.0888 to 1.8888)
Glasgow Perkins therapist	1981	6.3/10.5/2	6.3/10.7/2.1		4.46%	-0.2 (-2.4645 to 2.0645)
Glasgow self-monitoring therapist	1981	6.3/10.8/1.7	6.3/10.7/2.1		5.13%	0.1 (-2.0098 to 2.2098)
Adesso Positive incentive	1979	8/6.0365/0.8414	8/5.9492/1.2343		21.32%	0.0873 (-0.9478 to 1.1224)
Adesso Negative incentive	1979	8/5.6237/0.9604	8/5.9492/1.2343		19.45%	-0.3254 (-1.4092 to 0.7583)
Adesso Nail measurement	1979	8/5.1633/1.0755	8/5.9492/1.2343		17.75%	-0.7858 (-1.9203 to 0.3486)
Adesso Minimal contact	1979	8/4.2743/0.9723	8/5.9492/1.2343		19.27%	-1.6748 (-2.7636 to -0.586)
META-ANALYSIS:					100%	-0.4784 (-0.9564 to -0.0004)

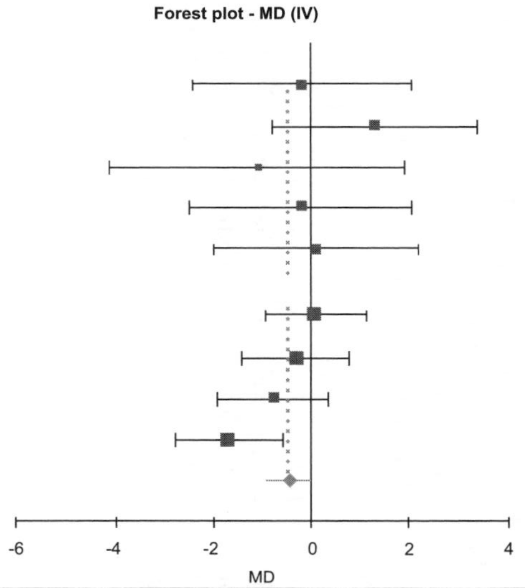

MD axis: -6 -4 -2 0 2 4

Figure 13.4 Forest plot comparing various treatments against self-monitoring of nail biting. It can be seen that most of the lines depicting the confidence intervals of the means cross the line of no effect and that most of the means fall on the negative side of the axis, suggesting that most of the treatments are less effective than self-monitoring. The meta-analytic mean is represented by the diamond on the gray line at the bottom of the figure and demonstrates that the line of no effect (MD = 0) crosses the 95% confidence interval for the overall mean of the treatments.

Interventions Using Consequences

The consequences of behavior may change its subsequent probability through appetitive or aversive reinforcement. An appetitive reinforcer increases the likelihood of a behavior, whereas an aversive reinforcer acts to decrease its likelihood. In the case of nail biting, interventions seek to decrease the likelihood of the behavior.

One of the simplest means of attempting to influence nail biting is to paint unpleasant-tasting substances on the nail. This has become a common commercial remedy for nail biting. A brief Internet search found the following products: THUM (contains Cayenne pepper); Stop'n Grow or Mavala (sucrose octa-acetate and denatonium benzoate); Stop-Bite (ingredients not known); Orly No-Bite (denatonium benzoate); Control-it nail-biting treatment (ingredients unclear). Although these are widely recommended as effective treatments, very few trials have been published that show the claimed benefits. Vargas and Adesso (1976) compared both shock and negative practice with painting an unpleasant tasting substance (believed to be THUM) on the participants' nails. Figure 13.3 shows three group comparison studies that evaluated the potential of aversion to increase nail length. One study (Davidson, Denney, and Elliott 1980) used an imaginal aversion method, whereas the others (Allen 1996; Silber and Haynes 1992) used Stop'n Grow. Allen (1996) concluded that "the results of this study are less encouraging than anticipated." It is therefore difficult to draw firm conclusions about the efficacy of aversive substances. Nevertheless, reputable scientific journals state that mild aversion is the treatment of choice for nail biting that is severe enough to warrant intervention (Jabr 2005).

No studies using appetitive reinforcers have been published. An intervention could be devised that rewarded the absence of nail biting (in technical terms, the intervention would involve a differential reinforcement of other behavior, or DRO, schedule). Naturally occurring rewards for having nails that are not bitten, such as people commenting favorably on well–cared-for nails, could also be studied.

Conclusions

Nail biting is a common repetitive behavior of childhood that tends to decline in prevalence starting in the mid-teens. How it should be classified, and even whether it should be considered a disorder in DSM-V, remains unclear. A number of interventions have been proposed, but none has shown clear superiority in adequately designed trials. Future trials should include measures of nail length, cosmetic appearance of the hands, and the number of episodes of nail biting. Further research is needed to understand the motivation underlying nail biting in order to facilitate the design of interventions targeting the motivation rather than the behavior itself. Drug treatment has not proven acceptable to people who bite their nails, but attempting a trial of one of the newer SSRIs for severe cases of nail biting may be worthwhile.

Resources

The Web site http://www.onychophagia.com/ provides some information about nail biting and remedies that may be available to readers, but does not offer evaluations of evidence.

The Web site http://health.yahoo.com/beauty-overview/nail-biting/healthwise–tw9722 spec.html provides a number of suggestions for helping to overcome nail biting, but without evaluation of their empirical support.

References

Adesso V J, Vargas JM, Siddall JW. Role of awareness in reducing nail-biting behavior. *Behav Ther* 10:148–154, 1979.

Aiello JR, Douthitt EA. Social facilitation from Triplett to electronic performance monitoring. *Group Dynamics Theor Res Pract* 5:163–180, 2001.

Allen KW. Chronic nailbiting: A controlled comparison of competing response and mild aversion treatments. *Behav Res Ther* 34:269–272, 1996.

American Psychiatric Association. *Diagnostic and Statistical Manual of Mental Disorders*, 4th edition, text revision. Washington, DC: American Psychiatric Association, 2000.

Azrin NH, Nunn RG. Habit reversal: A method of eliminating nervous habits and tics. *Behav Res Ther* 11:619–628, 1973.

Azrin NH, Nunn RG, Frantz SE. Habit reversal vs negative practice treatment of nailbiting. *Behav Res Ther* 18:281–285, 1980.

Barrios BA. Cue-controlled relaxation in reduction of chronic nervous habits. *Psychol Rep* 41:703–706, 1977.

Bienvenu OJ, Samuels JF, Riddle MA et al. The relationship of obsessive-compulsive disorder to possible spectrum disorders: Results from a family study. *Biol Psychiatry* 48:287–293, 2000.

Billig AL. Finger nail-biting: Its incipiency, incidence, and amelioration. *Genet Psychol Monogr* 24:13–148, 1941.

Calitz FJW, Veitch M, Verkhovsky A et al. The general profile of children and adolescents with major depression referred to the Free State Psychiatric Complex. *S Afr J Psychiatry* 13:132–136, 2007.

Coleman JC, McCalley JE. Nail biting among college students. *J Abnorm Soc Psychol* 43:517–525, 1948.

Dalanora A, Uyeda H, Empinotti JC et al. Destruição de falanges provocada por onicofagia. *An Dermatol* 82:5, 2007.

Davidson AM, Denney DR, Elliott CH. Suppression and substitution in the treatment of nail-biting. *Behav Res Ther* 18:1–9, 1980.

De Lisle F. A legendarie conteining an ample discourse of the life and behaviour of Charles Cardinal of Lorraine, and the house of Guise, 1577.

Deardoff PA, Finch AJ, Royall LR. Manifest anxiety and nail-biting. *J Clin Psychol* 30:378, 1974.

Didden R, Duker PC, Korzilius H. Meta-analytic study on treatment effectiveness for problem behaviors with individuals who have mental retardation. *Am J Ment Retard* 101:387–399, 1997.

Feinberg JM, Aiello JR. Social facilitation: A test of competing theories. *J Appl Soc Psychol* 36:1087–1109, 2006.

Flessner CA, Miltenberger RG, Egemo K et al. An evaluation of the social support component of simplified habit reversal. *Behav Ther* 36:35–42, 2005.

Frankel MJ, Merbaum M. Effects of therapist contact and a self-control manual on nail-biting reduction. *Behav Ther* 13:125–129, 1982.

Friman PC, Byrd MR, Oksol EM. Characteristics of oral digital habits, in *Tic Disorders, Trichotillomania, and Other Repetitive Behavior Disorders: Behavioral Approaches to Analysis and Treatment*. Edited by Woods DW, Miltenberger RG. Boston: Kluwer, 2001, pp. 197–222.

Gilleard E, Eskin M, Savasir B. Nail-biting and oral aggression in a Turkish student population. *Br J Med Psychol* 61:197–201, 1988.

Glasgow RE, Swaney K, Schafer L. Self-help manuals for the control of nervous habits: A comparative investigation. *Behav Ther* 12:177–184, 1981.

Grant JE, Mancebo MC, Pinto A et al. Impulse control disorders in adults with obsessive compulsive disorder. *J Psychiatr Res* 40:494–501, 2006.

Guaba K, Ashima G, Tewari A et al. Prevalence of malocclusion and abnormal oral habits in North Indian rural children. *J Indian Soc Pedodont Prev Dent* 16:26–30, 1998.

Hansen DJ, Tishelman AC, Hawkins RP et al. Habits with potential as disorders: Prevalence, severity, and other characteristics among college-students. *Behav Modif* 14:66–80, 1990.

Horne DJ de L, Wilkinson J. Habit reversal treatment for fingernail biting. *Behav Res Ther* 18:287–291, 1980.

Jabr FI. Severe nail deformity. *Postgrad Med Online* 118:3, 2005.

Jebb RC. *The Characters of Theophrastus*. London: Macmillan and Company, 1870.

Joubert CE. Relationship of self-esteem, manifest anxiety, and obsessive-compulsiveness to personal habits. *Psychol Rep* 73:579–583, 1993.

Kharbanda OP, Sidhu SS, Sundaram KR et al. Oral habits in school going children of Delhi: A prevalence study. *J Indian Soc Pedodont Prev Dent* 21:120–124, 2003.

Klatte KM, Deardorff PA. Nail-biting and manifest anxiety of adults. *Psychol Rep* 48:82, 1981.

Ladouceur R. Habit reversal treatment: Learning an incompatible response or increasing the subjects awareness. *Behav Res Ther* 17:313–316, 1979.

Leonard HL, Lenane MC, Swedo SE et al. A double-blind comparison of clomipramine and desipramine treatment of severe onychophagia (nail biting). *Arch Gen Psychiatry* 48:821–827, 1991.

Leung AKC, Robson WLM. Nailbiting. *Clin Pediatr* 29:690–692, 1990.

Li Y, Shi A, Wan Y et al. Child behavior problems: Prevalence and correlates in rural minority areas of China. *Pediatr Int* 43:651–661, 2001.

Long ES, Woods DW, Miltenberger RG et al. Examining the social effects of habit behaviors exhibited by individuals with mental retardation. *J Dev Phys Disabil* 11:295–312, 1999.

Mailis A. Compulsive targeted self-injurious behaviour in humans with neuropathic pain: A counterpart of animal autotomy? Four case reports and literature review. *Pain* 64:569–578, 1996.

Malone AJ, Massler M. Index of nail biting in children. *J Abnorm Soc Psychol* 47:193–202, 1952.

Mangweth B, Hausmann A, Danzl C et al. Childhood body-focused behaviors and social behaviors as risk factors of eating disorders. *Psychother Psychosom* 74:247–253, 2005.

Miltenberger RG, Fuqua RW. A comparison of contingent vs. non-contingent competing response practice in the treatment of nervous habits. *J Behav Ther Exp Psychiatry* 16:195–200, 1985.

Nestadt G, Addington A, Samuels J et al. The identification of OCD-related subgroups based on comorbidity. *Biol Psychiatry* 53:914–920, 2003.

Pennington LA. Incidence of nail biting among adults. *Am J Psychiatry* 102:241–244, 1945.

Rosow HM. The analysis of an adult nail biter. *Psychoanal Q* 35:333–345, 1954.

Silber KP, Haynes CE. Treating nailbiting: A comparative analysis of mild aversion and competing response therapies. *Behav Res Ther* 30:15–22, 1992.

Solomon JC. Nail biting and the integrative process. *Psychoanal Q* 36:393–395, 1955.

Southey R. *The Doctor*. New York: Harper and Brothers, 1836.

Stevens J. The comical works of F. de Quevedo. London: John Morphew, 1707.

Swedo SE, Leonard HL, Rapoport JL et al. A double-blind comparison of clomipramine and desipramine in the treatment of trichotillomania (hair pulling). *N Engl J Med* 321:497–501, 1989.

Tosti A, Peluso AM, Bardazzi F et al. Phalangeal osteomyelitis due to nail biting. *Acta Derm Venereol* 74:206–207, 1994.

Twohig MP, Woods DW, Marcks BA et al. Evaluating the efficacy of habit reversal: Comparison with a placebo control. *J Clin Psychiatry* 64:40–48, 2003.

van Minnen A, Hoogduin KAL, Keijsers GPJ et al. Treatment of trichotillomania with behavioral therapy or fluoxetine: A randomized, waiting-list controlled study. *Arch Gen Psychiatry* 60:517–522, 2003.

Vargas JM, Adesso VJ. A comparison of aversion therapies for nailbiting behaviour. *Behav Ther* 7:322–329, 1976.

Wechsler D. The incidence and significance of nail biting in children. *Psychoanal Rev* 18:201–209, 1931.

Wells JH, Haines J, Williams CL. Severe morbid onychophagia: The classification as self-mutilation and a proposed model of maintenance. *Aust NZ J Psychiatry* 32:534–545, 1998.

Williams TI, Rose R, Chisholm S. What is the function of nail biting? An analog assessment study. *Behav Res Ther* 45:989–995, 2007.

Woods DW, Miltenberger RG. Are persons with nervous habits nervous? A preliminary examination of habit function in a nonreferred population. *J Appl Behav Anal* 29:259–261, 1996.

14

Nail Biting and Other Oral Habits: A Dentist's Perspective

Sven E. Widmalm, DDS, Dr Odont, and Duane C. McKay, DDS

From a dentist's perspective, nail biting raises questions about the presence of serious dental problems. Nail biting and its substitutes – biting on a pencil, a pipe stem, or similar hard objects – are termed oral parafunctions (OPFs). Those that do not involve biting include bruxism (tooth gnashing, grinding), teeth clenching, and sucking on a finger. Nail biting is often accompanied by one or more additional OPFs, and isolating the effects of any one OPF can be difficult (Westling 1988; Widmalm, Gunn, and Christiansen 1995). These behaviors may cause not only mechanical wear of the teeth, which dentists are well trained to repair, but also temporomandibular joint disorders (TMDs), for which there is no generally recognized cure or prevention. This chapter will discuss the cumulative effect of OPFs on the health of a patient's natural dentition, dental restorations, oral soft structures, and temporomandibular joints (TMJs).

For many dentists, OPF is synonymous with bruxism and its deleterious effects upon the dentition (Figure 14.1). Other OPF behaviors, however, including thumb and finger sucking, may prevent proper growth of the mouth and can contribute to an anterior open bite (AOB) (Figure 14.2). Advice about the risks and management of such problems has been widely explored in dental journal articles (Ware 1980). Because the role of OPFs in damaging and disrupting a patient's craniomandibular system is unclear and because most dentists are not trained to treat underlying parafunctions, the dentist's role may be to detect the OPF, protect the craniomandibular system, and refer the patient to professionals able to provide treatment.

Pathophysiology, Signs, and Symptoms

The TMJ is a stress-bearing joint. Therefore, too much loading can lead to joint pain and dysfunction. Both nail biting and bruxism cause repetitive loading of the TMJ and may lead to pain and dysfunction by overloading components of the masticatory system (Westling 1988). The TMJ is more heavily loaded during incisor chewing and habitual movements, and thus during nail biting, than during molar (posterior) chewing (Brehnan et al. 1981; Hylander and Bays 1979; Ito et al. 1986; Westling 1988).

The cardinal signs of temporomandibular joint disorder (TMD) are pain, joint sounds, and restrictions in jaw movement: pain in the jaw joint area, the jaw muscles, and during palpation of the jaw muscles and the temporomandibular joint (TMJ); joint sounds such as cracking, popping, and/or clicking sounds from either one or both TMJs during jaw movements; and restricted mandibular movement in one or all directions of motion. These cardinal signs may result from direct injury to the TMJ, which causes these signs via swelling and inflammation, or OPFs. Therefore, patients with temporal muscle pain or neck pain complaints should be questioned about oral habits such as nail biting, in

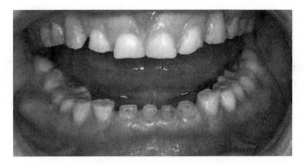

Figure 14.1   Bruxism. Severe wear of all teeth, especially those in the lower jaw.

which the jaw assumes a forward-jutting position (Scott and Lundeen 1980) (Figures 14.3 and 14.4).

A nail-biting habit may be relatively harmless if a patient's dentition is soundly supported with good bone density and alveolar height. Alveolar height is a clinically assessed measure of the degree of bone support between adjacent teeth. This bone height is diminished by gum disease; the greater the reduction, the less support for the remaining dentition. Nail biting and other OPFs may be dangerous when imposed on tooth restorations and/or implants with insufficient bone support. An accurate evaluation of the patient's parafunctional habits is advisable when designing such restorations. Other negative effects of severe nail biting include apical root resorption (the apical root is the root-tip portion of a tooth) (Odenrick and Brattström 1983) and the transfer into the oral cavity of bacteria buried under the surface of the nail (Bayda et al. 2007).

Prevalence of OPFs

In a group of 749 randomly selected children and adolescents ages 7–18, 75% reported OPFs (Nilner 1985). Nail biting was evenly distributed by age, while grinding and clenching decreased with age. Widmalm, Gunn, and Christiansen (1995) examined 540 4- to 6-year-old children and found almost exactly the same prevalence; only 28% of the children had no history of a parafunction. A history of nail biting was common (41%) but was an isolated behavior in only 8.6%. Farsi (2003) examined 1,940 randomly selected schoolchildren and found that nail biting was the most common OPF (27.7%), while bruxism was the least common (8.4%). OPFs in childhood are persistent in many subjects and predict the existence of the same OPFs 20 years later (Egermark, Carlsson, and Magnusson 2001).

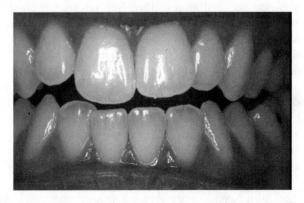

Figure 14.2   Anterior open bite in a teenage girl. Such opening can be caused by thumb or finger sucking, but can also develop because of pathological changes in the TMJs caused by rheumatoid arthritis.

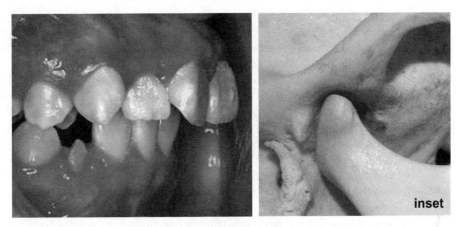

Figure 14.3   The figure shows how upper and lower teeth come together when a young nail-biting patient with a large horizontal overbite achieves maximal intercuspation/centric occlusion (CO). Intercuspation is the fitting together of the cusps of opposing teeth, creating an occlusion (bite) between the upper and lower dentitions. The inset in the lower right corner illustrates normal skeletal relationships between condyle and fossa when biting in CO.

Association between OPFs, Orofacial Pain, and TMDs

Because nail biting commonly occurs with other OPFs and the contribution of each individual OPF to the patient's complaints can be difficult to disentangle, data regarding other OPFs are briefly summarized here. Epidemiologic studies of the etiologic role of OPFs in oral pain, diseases, and dysfunctions have produced varying statistics, mostly because the modes of ascertainment and definition are not standardized. In many studies, patients answered self-administered questionnaires, but the questions varied from study to study. The duration of the parafunction was not always reported, making it difficult to deduce incidence. In addition, the intensity of the OPF behavior was seldom explored.

The reliability of information obtained by interviewing children without their parent(s) present was questioned by Castelo et al. (2005), who did not find any association between parafunctional habits and signs and symptoms of TMD in children aged 3–5 years. In contrast, Widmalm, Gunn, and Christiansen (1995) found significant correlations between

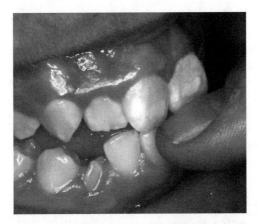

Figure 14.4   The patient in Figure 14.1 now protrudes the lower jaw to bite her fingernail. The upper left corner inset shows the effect on the nail. The lower right corner inset illustrates how the condyle is moved forward during lower jaw protrusion into an unphysiological position where clenching may harm the internal TMJ structures.

observable signs of parafunctions and the answers of children aged 4–6 years and regarded this information as reliable. Widmalm, Gunn, and Christiansen (1995) found that nail biting was significantly associated with two of ten pain variables: chewing pain and palpation pain in the posterior TMJ area. Bruxism was significantly associated with eight of the ten pain variables: recurrent TMJ pain; recurrent neck pain; chewing pain; pain at jaw opening; palpation pain in the lateral and posterior TMJ area; and anterior temporalis and masseter areas. Thumb or finger sucking was significantly associated with three of ten pain variables: palpation pain in the lateral TMJ, posterior TMJ, and masseter areas. The results indicated that TMD signs and symptoms are common in young children and thus that TMD may have an early onset.

A broad consensus exists regarding the importance of parafunctional habits in the etiopathogenesis of TMD (Manfredini et al. 2003). Macfarlane et al. (2003), in a cross-sectional population-based survey involving 2,504 participants, found a significant association between OPFs (chewing pens or biting fingernails, tooth grinding) and TMD signs and symptoms, including orofacial pain, a history of the jaw getting stuck or locked, jaw joint clicking or grating sounds when opening or closing the mouth, and difficulty in opening the mouth wide. Winocur et al. (2006) found that nearly all oral habits were risk factors for TMD. In children aged 7–14 years, correlations have been found between nail biting on one jaw side and recurrent headache and/or pain in the temporal region (Nilner 1985). Some studies, however, have not found an association between OPFs and TMD signs and symptoms (Castelo et al. 2005; Meulen et al. 2006). Also, most studies have been cross-sectional, and although many authors report significant associations between OPFs and TMD signs and symptoms, association does not prove causation.

A majority of studies have found a relationship between bruxism and TMD, but the subject remains complicated by the absence of universally accepted definitions of these two terms. The variables studied – frequency, duration, and intensity of episodes, for example – have not been standardized. The role of bruxism is therefore both controversial and unresolved (Kalamir et al. 2007; Rugh 1991).

The most important conclusions to be drawn from these studies are that examination for OPFs and signs and symptoms of TMD should start in very young children and that prospective longitudinal studies are needed (Farsi 2003; Widmalm, Gunn, and Christiansen 1995).

Diagnosis of OPFs in Dental Practice

Dentists must be aware of the effects of emotional problems on teeth. Patients can be very emotional and at times somewhat irrational concerning the appearance of their teeth. Such reactions are easier to understand if teeth are considered in their (usually symbolic) role as weapons and as significant features for gaining respect, love, and admiration. Because of shame and embarrassment, OPF sufferers often fail to admit the self-inflicted nature of their physical damage (Bohne, Keuthen, and Wilhelm 2005). While this reticence complicates recognition and differential diagnosis, the dentist needs to be particularly attentive to physical signs that indicate these behavior disorders. Because nail biting is socially unacceptable in adults, substitution behaviors often emerge that may cause significant wear of teeth, such as biting on a pipe stem or pencil.

Treatment of the Effects of OPFs in Dental Practice

Occlusal splints, occlusal adjustment, biofeedback and relaxation training, and behavioral treatments have all been recommended as therapies for individuals with OPFs associated with dental problems.

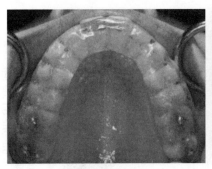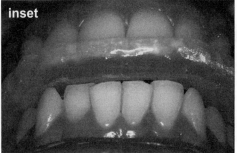

Figure 14.5   A typical occlusal splint made of plastic for covering the upper teeth. The inset shows an anterior view of the splint and the teeth.

Occlusal splints

An occlusal splint (Figure 14.5) is a removable device that is usually made of plastic and placed on the upper or lower teeth, covering all or part of the occlusal surfaces. Its primary purpose in patients with bruxism is to protect teeth from being worn by preventing direct contact between the upper and lower teeth. Westling (1988) describes valuable examples showing how occlusal splints can effectively and safely arrest nail-biting and sucking habits. Most of her patients with signs of extensive wear on frontal teeth, who in questionnaires had reported nail biting, also had other oral habits, especially clenching. Consequently, the factors contributing to cessation of the patient's nail biting were difficult to evaluate.

Occlusal Adjustment (OA)

The once widely accepted theory that occlusal interferences (Figure 14.6) can trigger muscular hyperactivity and OPFs through activating periodontal receptors has lost credibility (Manfredini et al. 2003). Instead, the hypothesis that OPFs stem from a central nervous system etiology has found greater acceptance. Unfortunately, to evaluate fairly the role of OA as a cure for OPFs and therefore the theory regarding removal of triggering occlusal interference is presently impossible. Even skillful clinicians with lifelong training and experience in OA acknowledge that the procedure is often difficult to perform and that many years of practice are needed (Ash 2007). Unless mastered, OA treatment can damage the patient's occlusion and cause irreversible harm. As with evaluations of occlusal splint therapy, OA researchers judge the quality of the adjustments they themselves have performed. The absence of independent evaluation sorely limits the conclusions that can be drawn. At present, concluding that interferences affect condylar position and the loading of internal structures (as illustrated in Figure 14.6) is as reasonable as conclusions regarding periodontal receptor-triggered muscular hyperactivity.

Biofeedback and Relaxation Training

Progressive muscle relaxation is a technique of stress management developed to reduce anxiety by relaxing muscular tension (Jacobson 1948). Biofeedback and relaxation training have been applied with positive results in patients with OPFs (Dahlström 1989; Gramling et al. 1997). In dental practice, biofeedback-supported relaxation has been used on the jaw muscles, although effective relaxation training should commence with arm and leg muscles (Jacobson 1948).

Behavioral Treatment

Most dental textbooks contain brief segments about counseling the patient to avoid stress and to discontinue harmful habits. Dental students, however, are rarely trained to include in

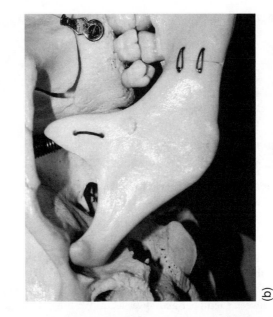

(b)

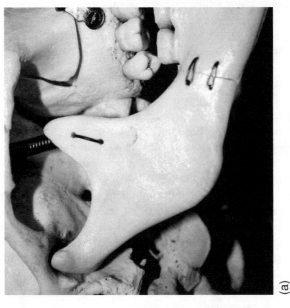

(a)

Figure 14.6   The figure illustrates how, on the left (a), the extruded third upper right molar interferes by preventing the jaw from closing, with the condyle remaining in an optimal position by rotating around the hinge axis without translation. On the right (b), the teeth are in maximal intercuspation and the condyle has been forced into a position anterior to the one on the left.

routine consultations questions about the patient's well-being in areas outside the purview of traditional dentistry. Dentists are not trained to evaluate psychological factors, and asking patients about nail biting has been reported to raise anxiety levels (Wright, Atrash, and Hopkins 1995).

Still, there is general agreement that behavioral and educational modalities are useful and effective in the management of chronic pain conditions (Gramling et al. 1996) and that the management of TMD has benefited from behavioral interventions. As a result, it is reasonable to believe that reducing OPF behaviors may help reduce TMD pain. Kleinrok et al. (1990) hypothesized a relationship between emotional stress and hyperactivity of the masticatory muscles in mandibular parafunctions. Like many other dental therapists, they considered eliminating mandibular parafunctions to be difficult if not impossible. In view of this, they proposed a treatment that substitutes nonharmful motor habits for the parafunctions. They attempted treatment in a group of 222 pupils and obtained good results by arranging adult supervision and cooperation.

Another behavioral treatment modality, habit reversal treatment, has been reported successful in case studies of TMDs, indicating that patient education can sometimes motivate the changes needed in a patient's behavior (Peterson 1993; Sari and Sonmez 2002; Westling 1988; Widmalm, Gunn, and Christiansen 1995).

Conclusions and Summary

Nail biting and other OPFs are common in young children. Consequently, unmanaged parafunctional habits may contribute to the etiology of trauma in the stomatognathic systems of adolescents and adults. (The stomatognathic system refers to all head and neck structures involved in speech, mastication, respiration, and deglutition, including the teeth, temporomandibular joints, and neuromusculature.) Prevention, early detection, and intervention are important clinical activities to diminish the influences of chronic OPFs on the teeth, muscles, and temporomandibular joints. The dentist can assist in detecting OPFs, protecting vulnerable oral and TMJ structures (e.g., with occlusal splints), and making appropriate referrals. Although occlusal splints can protect the oral structures from wear, they have little effect on parafunctional habits. Growing evidence suggests that psychological interventions to address factors contributing to the maintenance of these adverse habits can assist patients in overcoming them. This evidence contradicts the common opinion that longitudinal studies are not warranted because there are no methods to ensure the success of TMD prophylactic procedures and no techniques to guarantee a reduction in parafunctional behaviors. With new studies demonstrating the value of behavioral and educational modalities, new avenues should be pursued, including evaluating young children for parafunctions and intervening to reduce them. The authors believe that such procedures cannot begin too early because chronic habits are difficult to abandon. Unfortunately, many adult patients may have parafunctional habits that are too well established to allow successful treatment.

References

Ash MM Jr. Occlusion, TMDs, and dental education. *Head Face Med* 3:1–4, 2007.

Bayda B, Uslu H, Yavuz I et al. Effect of a chronic nail-biting habit on the oral carriage of Enterobacteriaceae. *Oral Microbiol Immunol* 22:1–4, 2007.

Bohne A, Keuthen N, Wilhelm S. Pathologic hairpulling, skin picking, and nail biting. *Ann Clin Psychiatry* 17:227–232, 2005.

Brehnan K, Boyd RL, Laskin J et al. Direct measurement of loads at the temporomandibular joint in Macaca arctoides. *J Dent Res* 60:1820–1824, 1981.

Castelo PM, Gaviao MB, Pereira LJ et al. Relationship between oral parafunctional/nutritive sucking habits and temporomandibular joint dysfunction in primary dentition. *Int J Pediatr Dent* 15:29–36, 2005.

Dahlström L. Electromyographic studies of craniomandibular disorders: A review of the literature. *J Oral Rehabil* 16:1–20, 1989.

Egermark I, Carlsson GE, Magnusson T. A 20-year longitudinal study of subjective symptoms of temporomandibular disorders from childhood to adulthood. *Acta Odontol Scand* 59:40–48, 2001.

Farsi NM. Symptoms and signs of temporomandibular disorders and oral parafunctions among Saudi children. *J Oral Rehabil* 30:1200–1208, 2003.

Gramling SE, Grayson RL, Sullivan TL et al. Schedule-induced masseter EMG in facial pain subjects vs. no-pain controls. *Physiol Behav* 61:301–309, 1997.

Gramling SE, Neblett J, Grayson R et al. Temporomandibular disorder: Efficacy of an oral habit reversal treatment program. *J Behav Ther Exp Psychiatry* 27:245–255, 1996.

Hylander WL, Bays R. An in vivo strain-gauge analysis of the squamosal-dentary joint reaction force during mastication and incisal biting in *Macaca mulatta* and *Macaca fascicularis*. *Arch Oral Biol* 24:689–697, 1979.

Ito T, Gibbs CH, Marguelles-Bonnet R et al. Loading on the temporomandibular joints with five occlusal conditions. *J Prosthet Dent* 56:478–484, 1986.

Jacobson E. *You Must Relax*, 3rd edition. New York: McGraw Hill, 1948.

Kalamir A, Pollard H, Vitiello AL et al. TMD and the problem of bruxism: A review. *J Bodywork Mov Ther* 11:183–193, 2007.

Kleinrok M, Mielnik-Hus J, Zysko-Wozniak D et al. Investigations on prevalence and treatment of fingernail biting. *Cranio* 8:47–50, 1990.

Macfarlane TV, Blinkhorn AS, Davies RM et al. Association between local mechanical factors and orofacial pain: Survey in the community. *J Dent* 31:535–542, 2003.

Manfredini D, Landi N, Romagnoli M et al. Etiopathogenesis of parafunctional habits of the stomatognathic system. *Minerva Stomatol* 52:339–349, 2003.

Meulen MJ, Lobbezoo F, Aartman IH et al. Self-reported oral parafunctions and pain intensity in temporomandibular disorder patients. *J Orofac Pain* 20:31–35, 2006.

Nilner M. Functional disturbances and diseases in the Stomatognathic system among 7- to 18-year-olds. *Cranio* 3:358–367, 1985.

Odenrick L, Brattström V. The effect of nailbiting on root resorption during orthodontic treatment. *Eur J Orthod* 5:185–188, 1983.

Peterson AL, Dixon DC, Talcott GW et al. Habit reversal treatment of temporomandibular disorders: A pilot investigation. *J Behav Ther Exp Psychiatry* 24:49–55, 1993.

Rugh JD. Association between bruxism and TMD (1991), in *Current Controversies in Temporomandibular Disorders*. Edited by McNeill C. Chicago: Quintessence Books, 1991, pp. 29–31.

Sari S, Sonmez H. Investigation of the relationship between oral parafunctions and temporomandibular joint dysfunction in Turkish children with mixed and permanent dentition. *J Oral Rehabil* 29:108–112, 2002.

Scott, DS, Lundeen TF. Myofascial pain involving the masticatory muscles: An experimental model. *Pain* 8:207–215, 1980.

Ware EM. Tooth loss from fingernail biting. *Tex Dent J* 98:99, 1980.

Westling L. Fingernail biting: A literature review and case reports. *Cranio* 6:182–187, 1988.

Widmalm SE, Gunn SM, Christiansen RL. Oral parafunctions as TMD risk factors in children. *J Craniomandib Pract* 13:242–246, 1995.

Winocur E, Littner D, Adamsusb I et al. Oral habits and their association with signs and symptoms of temporomandibular disorders in adolescents: A gender comparison. *Oral Surg Oral Med Oral Pathol Oral Radiol Endod* 102:482–487, 2006.

Wright V, Atrash B, Hopkins R. Nail biting in rheumatic diseases. *Clin Rheumatol* 14:93–94, 1995.

Section III

Information-Seeking Impulses

15

Problematic Internet Use: Clinical Aspects

Timothy Liu, MD, and Marc N. Potenza, MD, PhD

Over the past decade, the Internet has emerged as a seemingly indispensable part of modern life. The speeding of Internet traffic, the growing varieties of online functions, and the increasing accessibility of wireless connection all enhance Internet use and extend the Internet's worldwide penetration. Despite the initial debate over the validity of diagnosing "Internet addiction" as a distinct disorder, it is clear from clinical experience and the literature that a significant number of individuals experience impairment in multiple realms related to overuse of the Internet. Most research has been done in Asian countries, including South Korea, Taiwan, and China, and problematic Internet use is considered one of the most serious public health issues by the governments of these countries (Block 2008). The phenomenon continues to gain attention from the mental health community in the United States. Recently, the inclusion of problematic Internet use in the forthcoming fifth edition of the *Diagnostic and Statistical Manual of Mental Disorders* (DSM-V) has been proposed (Block 2008; Hollander, Kim, and Zohar 2007).

Among many terms with slightly different connotations, Internet dependency (Scherer 1997), compulsive Internet use (Greenfield 1999), pathological Internet use (Morahan-Martin and Schumacher 2000), and compulsive computer use (Potenza and Hollander 2002) have been used. Internet addiction (Young 1996a) is commonly used for the condition. We have chosen to use "problematic Internet use" in this chapter to remain descriptive and because the term "addiction" is not included in the DSM-IV-TR (text revision) (American Psychiatric Association 2000) and has variable definitions. Moreover, clinicians and researchers reserve the term for excessive patterns of drug use (Potenza 2006). Problematic Internet use can be defined as uncontrolled use of the Internet that (1) leads to significant psychosocial and functional impairments and (2) is not better accounted for by a primary psychiatric disorder such as mania or the physiological effects of a substance.

History of Psychiatric Attention to Problematic Internet Use

Initial interest in human–technology interactions began in the 1930s, when Gordon Allport voiced concerns about the manner in which people used radios (Cantril and Allport 1935). In the 1990s, Griffiths advanced the investigation of and theorizing about technological addictions. He defined them as nonchemical (behavioral) addictions that involve human–machine interaction and distinguished between passive (e.g., watching television) and active (e.g., playing computer games) types (Griffiths 1996). The concept of Internet addiction as a discrete disorder was in part generated by Ivan Goldberg, a New York psychiatrist (Mitchell 2000). In 1995, a year after the introduction of the DSM-IV (American Psychiatric Association 1994), Goldberg combined the criteria for substance use and impulse control disorders and presented them as the criteria for "Internet addiction disorder" on his Web site. His presentation was designed as an exercise to stimulate the mental health profession into critically evaluating the usefulness of creating new disorders (Surratt 1999). However, the

Table 15.1 Young's Internet addiction diagnostic criteria

Five or more of the following:

1. Is preoccupied with the Internet (thinks about previous online activity or anticipates next online session).
2. Needs to use the Internet for increased amounts of time in order to achieve satisfaction.
3. Has made unsuccessful efforts to control, cut back, or stop Internet use.
4. Is restless, moody, depressed, or irritable when attempting to cut down or stop Internet use.
5. Has stayed online longer than originally intended.
6. Has jeopardized or risked the loss of a significant relationship, job, or educational or career opportunity because of the Internet.
7. Has lied to family members, therapists, or others to conceal the extent of involvement with the Internet.
8. Uses the Internet as a way of escaping from problems or of relieving a dysphoric mood (e.g., feelings of helplessness, guilt, anxiety, depression).

Source: Young (1996a).

media subsequently began to publicize the notion of Internet addiction (Warden, Phillips, and Ogloff 2004). Thus, the concept of Internet addiction was socially constructed before substantial scientific or clinical research had been performed.

Academic investigation expanded after the publication of clinical case studies by Young (1996b) and Griffiths (1997). Reported cases had similar constellations of symptoms and included adolescent and middle-aged subjects. Individuals in these reports all spent large amounts of time online and experienced adverse consequences such as marital discord and financial crisis. They reported various mood symptoms such as depression, anxiety, and irritability when access to the Internet was interrupted, consistent with an effect of withdrawal.

A survey of the changing conceptualizations of problematic Internet use highlights the complex and incompletely understood relationships among substance dependence, impulse control disorders, and obsessive-compulsive disorder. Problematic Internet use has been likened to all of these conditions. In the 1990s, Griffiths conceptualized problematic Internet use as a subtype of behavioral addictions, a group of disorders sharing core elements of addictions that include salience, euphoria, tolerance, withdrawal, conflict, and relapse (Griffiths 1997). The first set of diagnostic criteria used by Young (1996b) in a case report of problematic Internet use was also modeled from the DSM-IV (American Psychiatric Association 1994) substance dependence criteria because of presumed similarities between the clinical features of problematic Internet use and substance addiction. Subsequently, problematic Internet use was conceptualized as an impulse control disorder, and the DSM-IV criteria for pathological gambling were adopted to become the suggested Internet addiction diagnostic criteria (Table 15.1) (Young 1996a).

Impulse control disorders such as pathological gambling have been conceptualized not only as behavioral addictions but also as lying within an obsessive-compulsive spectrum (Hollander and Wong 1995). In an analogous fashion, problem Internet use has also been called compulsive-impulsive Internet usage disorder to encompass the impulsive features (arousal) that may initiate the behavior and the compulsive drive that may cause it to persist (Dell'Osso et al. 2006b). Related empirical research is scarce, and only one small-scale study showed that adolescents with problematic Internet use had higher impulsivity than controls on psychometric testing (Cao et al. 2007). Other studies produced mixed results (Lavin et al. 2000; Lin and Tsai 2002; Treuer, Fabian, and Furedi 2001). Finally, a body of research on adolescents' Internet use has posited that the behavior is a coping strategy for responding to adverse family dynamics and interpersonal relationships, social anxieties, and depression (Ha et al. 2007; Liu and Kuo 2007; te Wildt et al. 2007; Yen et al. 2007a).

Table 15.2 Diagnostic criteria for problematic Internet use

A. Maladaptive preoccupation with Internet use, as indicated by at least one of the following.
   1. Preoccupations with use of the Internet that are experienced as irresistible.
   2. Excessive use of the Internet for periods of time longer than planned.
B. The use of the Internet or the preoccupation with its use causes clinically significant distress or impairment in social, occupational, or other important areas of functioning.
C. The excessive Internet use does not occur exclusively during periods of hypomania or mania and is not better accounted for by other Axis I disorders.

Source: Shapira et al. (2003).

Diagnosis

There are no specific formal diagnostic criteria for, nor mention of, problematic Internet use in either the DSM-IV-TR (American Psychiatric Association 2000) or the *International Statistical Classification of Diseases and Related Health Problems,* 10th edition (ICD-10) (World Health Organization 2003). Individuals with problematic Internet use can be given a DSM-IV-TR diagnosis of impulse control disorder not otherwise specified (Code 312.30) (American Psychiatric Association 2000). This category was created for disorders of impulse control that do not meet the criteria for any specific impulse control disorder or for another mental disorder having features involving impulse control described elsewhere in the manual (e.g., substance dependence, a paraphilia) (American Psychiatric Association 2000). The ICD-10 has a very similar diagnosis of habit and impulse disorder, unspecified (Code F63.9) (World Health Organization 2003).

Specific diagnostic criteria are needed for consistent identification of problematic Internet use in clinical settings and to encourage carefully designed investigations. Young (1996b) modeled the first set of proposed diagnostic criteria on the DSM-IV criteria for substance dependence because it was observed that patients had symptoms of Internet use tolerance and withdrawal as well as manifesting profound adverse social consequences (Young 1996b). Subsequently, problematic Internet use was conceptualized as an impulse control disorder without the involvement of an intoxicant, and the DSM-IV criteria for pathological gambling were adopted to become the Young's Internet addiction diagnostic criteria (Table 15.1) (Young 1996a). Three DSM-IV criteria for pathological gambling ("chasing" losses, committing illegal acts to finance gambling, and relying on others for money to relieve a financial situation caused by gambling) were deemed not applicable and were not included. Young's criteria have since become the most widely cited and used criteria in research studies, despite limited empirical support. Some have suggested modifying the criteria by adding a criterion excluding excessive Internet use that can be explained by another Axis I disorder such as mania or hypomania (Table 15.2) (Shapira et al. 2003). Other researchers continue to use DSM-IV-TR substance use disorder criteria to define Internet abuse and Internet dependence (Anderson 2001; Fortson, Scotti, and Chen 2007).

To date, only one study has attempted to develop diagnostic criteria empirically, and this was done by evaluating the diagnostic accuracies of 13 candidate criteria. Diagnostic accuracy of each criterion was measured against the diagnosis made on the basis of a structured psychiatric interview and the subject's Chen Internet Addiction Scale score. However, the sample used was relatively small (fewer than 500 subjects) and was comprised exclusively of Taiwanese adolescents, limiting the applicability of the proposed criteria to the general population (Ko et al. 2005b).

Increasing recognition of the potential harmful effects and public health significance of problematic Internet use has led to the proposal that criteria for problematic Internet use be included in the forthcoming DSM-V (Block 2008). One DSM-V research work group has considered placing this disorder with other compulsive-impulsive disorders in a new category of obsessive-compulsive spectrum disorders (Dell'Osso et al. 2006b). However, because a separate DSM-V research work group focusing on substance use disorders also considered including impulse control disorders such as pathological gambling, the placement of problematic Internet use in the forthcoming DSM, if it is included at all, has not been determined. We anticipate that the debate will continue regarding the validity and usefulness of creating problematic Internet use as a new diagnostic entity (Miller 2007; Mitchell 2000). In addition, societal concerns regarding the medicalization of human behaviors are an important consideration and may influence the next DSM (Conrad 1992). We suggest that formal diagnostic criteria would enhance recognition of and research regarding problematic Internet use. Nonetheless, such criteria will not substitute for a comprehensive evaluation of the patient and the patient's reflection on the Internet's influence on his or her life.

Differential Diagnoses

In some individuals, problematic Internet use is the primary and major problem; in others, it may be accounted for entirely by another disorder (Dell'Osso et al. 2006b). Differentiating problematic Internet use from normal Internet use, excessive Internet use secondary to another Axis I disorder, and other compulsive-impulsive disorders is important.

1. *Normal Internet use.* More than 70% of the U.S. population uses the Internet (Internet World Stats 2008). The Internet is the medium on which computer users spend the most time (32.7 hours/week). This is equivalent to almost half the total time spent each week using all media (70.6 hours) and almost twice as much time as is spent watching television (16.4 hours) (Weide 2007). In that the majority of the population spends considerable time on the Internet, the proportion that experiences problems is small, possibly less than 1% (Aboujaoude et al. 2006). Therefore, the frequency and amount of time spent online may not represent reliable indicators of the effects of Internet use on an individual. Clinicians should carefully evaluate the relationship between the patient's Internet use and emotional distress. Reports by the patient and informants about his or her level of preoccupation, ability to cut down on use, mental state before and after Internet use, and reactions to unavailability of Internet access all represent valuable information.

2. *Other Axis I disorders.* The DSM-IV-TR describes increased participation in goal-directed activities and excessive involvement in pleasurable activities as diagnostic features of manic and hypomanic episodes (American Psychiatric Association 2000). Excessive use of the Internet that occurs exclusively during periods of mania or hypomania thus may be distinct from problematic Internet use that occurs in the absence of these states. Shapira et al. (2003) included an exclusion criterion in their proposed criteria to rule out excessive Internet use that can be fully explained by another Axis I disorder. Other Axis I disorders that have been hypothesized to explain preoccupation with the Internet in some patients include obsessive-compulsive disorder (Yang et al. 2005), attention deficit and hyperactivity disorder (Yoo et al. 2004), dopaminergic medication treatment (Fasano et al. 2006), and Asperger's syndrome. The relationship between problematic Internet use and these conditions is not well understood. Clinically, it is important to investigate the presence of underlying primary diagnoses and avoid reaching premature conclusions about the nature of a patient's Internet use.

3. *Other compulsive-impulsive behaviors.* Theoretically, in some cases the Internet may be merely the mechanism for administering or gaining access to the object of addiction and may be considered the equivalent of an electronic needle (Miller 2007; Shaffer, Hall, and Vander Bilt 2000). In theory, patients who primarily obtain pornographic materials via the Internet and also engage in offline compulsive sexual activities might be best

diagnosed with compulsive-impulsive sexual behaviors, and patients who problemati-
cally gamble both online and offline might be best diagnosed with pathological gambling.
The same applies to compulsive-impulsive patterns of shopping.

However, the Internet confers on these activities specific experiential qualities such as
perceived anonymity, virtual social connectedness, and incessant novelty, making cybersex,
for example, a very different experience from offline sexual encounters (Griffiths 2001).
In some cases, cybersex replaces real-life sexual intimacy (Schneider 2000). Thus, some
have contended that problematic Internet use should be subtyped into Internet gambling,
online gaming, and Internet pornography addiction (Young 2007). Although it is important
to differentiate among the compulsive-impulsive behaviors, understanding the patient's
unique and complex experience with the problematic behavior will provide richer and
more meaningful information for treatment planning. Because prevention and treatment
of specific impulse control disorders have not been systematically examined with respect
to Internet use, additional studies are needed on which to base recommendations in these
areas.

Clinical Picture

A review of a few illustrative case reports reveals the variety of symptoms associated with
problematic Internet use. In an early case report, a middle-aged homemaker who described
herself as initially "computer illiterate" started to participate in Internet-based chat rooms,
and within 3 months she was spending 50–60 hours/week online, sacrificing household
chores, family time, and social activities (Young 1996b). She reported excitement resulting
from online activities and felt a sense of community with other online participants of a
particular chat room. She felt depressed and irritable whenever she was not in front of her
computer. Eventually, her overuse of the Internet led to estrangement from her daughters
and separation from her husband within one year of purchase of her home computer.

A second case report described an 18-year-old man who spent 12–16 hours/day playing
online role-playing games. He neglected school responsibilities, forewent sleep, and stole
money and credit cards from his parents to purchase gaming supplies. After his parents
took away his computer, he became severely depressed, experienced suicidal ideation, and
was psychiatrically hospitalized (Allison et al. 2006). After graduation from high school, he
did not cut down on his online gaming. He reported social anxiety, never dated, and the
friendships that he felt were meaningful were all Internet-based.

The third illustrative case was a 32-year-old male college student with a complex psychiatric history of bipolar disorder, obsessive-compulsive disorder, and paraphilia (Shapira
et al. 2003). He started to use the Internet for playing multiplayer games and subsequently
spent large amounts of time on chat forums, emailing, and Web surfing. He felt a rising
sense of tension before logging on and a relief of this tension when he used the Internet. He
experienced significant academic problems concurrent with his frequent Internet use. His
Internet use did not occur exclusively during any particular mood state.

The fourth case is a 23-year-old medical student who presented with anxiety and problematic Internet use. He, too, had difficulty controlling his use, experienced a rising sense of
tension before logging on, and described tension relief when he used the Internet. Systematic evaluation revealed no family or past psychiatric history and no comorbid psychiatric
diagnoses (Atmaca 2007).

These cases illustrate that problematic Internet use occurs in a wide variety of individuals –
new and savvy users, adolescent and middle-aged individuals, men and women, those with
comorbid psychiatric disorders and those without, those who cannot function or work and
those who appear to have relatively high functioning. Many clinical features are captured
by the proposed diagnostic criteria mentioned – preoccupation; unsuccessful attempts to

cut back use; staying online longer than intended; withdrawal symptoms in the forms of irritation, depression, and restlessness; and severe psychosocial consequences.

A symptom not included in the proposed criteria is a sense of distortion of time when using the Internet. Problematic Internet users have been found in one study to greatly underestimate the time they spend online (Shapira et al. 2003). The potential role of time distortion in the development of problematic Internet use is not well understood.

These case reports suggest that severe psychosocial consequences may result from problematic Internet use, including marital discord, estrangement from family, academic failure, financial problems, and unemployment. Mild to moderate physical ailments have been reported, including dry eyes, blurred vision, sleep deprivation, fatigue, and musculoskeletal discomfort or pain (Chou 2001). A marathon online-gaming session was implicated in the death of a 28-year-old man (BBC News 2005). Possible psychological impairments associated with excessive Internet use include depression (Kraut et al. 1998; Young and Rogers 1998), loneliness, and social isolation (Kraut et al. 1998).

Whether the symptomatology differs between genders is unclear, but males and females may have different motivations for Internet use. Several studies of college students and adolescents suggest that males may be more prone to developing problematic Internet use, possibly because of their greater involvement in certain activities such as online games, cybersex, and gambling (Chou and Hsiao 2000; Johansson and Gotestam 2004; Ko et al. 2005a; Morahan-Martin and Schumacher 2000). With regard to cultural differences, despite the differences in Internet use habits in Asia and the United States (for example, Internet cafes are frequently used in Asia, while in the United States the Internet is mostly accessed from the home and the workplace), case descriptions appear remarkably similar (Block 2008).

Assessment Instruments

Multiple assessment instruments have been developed by researchers from the West and the East. They are derived from different theoretical underpinnings and do not agree on the underlying dimensions that constitute problematic Internet use (Beard 2005). The most widely used instruments are the Diagnostic Questionnaire (DQ) (Young 1996a) and the Internet Addiction Test (IAT) (Table 15.3) (Young 1998). The DQ is basically the question form of Young's Internet addiction diagnostic criteria (see Table 15.1). The IAT has 20 questions and has the advantages of being easy to understand and administer and having high face validity. There is increasing interest in conducting psychometric testing and factor analysis on these and other instruments to establish their validity and reliability for research and clinical purposes.

The psychometric properties of the Internet Addiction Test were investigated in a study in which 86 subjects recruited online took the IAT and answered other questions about Internet use and demographics (Widyanto and McMurran 2004). Factor analysis extracted six factors from the IAT: salience, excessive use, neglect of work, anticipation, lack of control, and neglect of social life. These six factors strongly correlated with each other and showed good to moderate internal consistency. The factor "salience" explained most of the variance and was found the most reliable as indicated by its Cronbach's Alpha (Widyanto and McMurran 2004). The study was small in scale and recruited subjects exclusively via the Internet, which introduced selection bias. Further research is needed to investigate the IAT as a reliable clinical and research tool and to assess whether its sensitivity to clinical changes is adequate for it to be used to follow the longitudinal course of Internet use behaviors.

Caplan (2002) has described the Generalized Problematic Internet Use Scale (GPIUS), which was reliable and valid in a preliminary study. Davis, Flett, and Besser (2002) described the Online Cognition Scale (OCS), a 36-item questionnaire they recommended for clinical assessment and preemployment screening. Other instruments include Brenner's Internet

Table 15.3 Internet addiction test

Answer the following questions on the Likert scale: 1 = Rarely; 2 = Occasionally; 3 = Frequently; 4 = Often; 5 = Always.

1. How often do you find that you stay online longer than you intended?
2. How often do you neglect household chores to spend more time online?
3. How often do you prefer the excitement of the Internet to intimacy with your partner?
4. How often do you form new relationships with fellow online users?
5. How often do others in your life complain to you about the amount of time you spend online?
6. How often do your grades or schoolwork suffer because of the amount of time you spend online?
7. How often do you check your e-mail before something else that you need to do?
8. How often does your job performance or productivity suffer because of the Internet?
9. How often do you become defensive or secretive when anyone asks you what you do online?
10. How often do you block out disturbing thoughts about your life with soothing thoughts of the Internet?
11. How often do you find yourself anticipating when you will go online again?
12. How often do you fear that life without the Internet would be boring, empty, and joyless?
13. How often do you snap, yell, or act annoyed if someone bothers you while you are online?
14. How often do you lose sleep due to late-night log-ins?
15. How often do you feel preoccupied with the Internet when offline, or fantasize about being online?
16. How often do you find yourself saying "just a few more minutes" when online?
17. How often do you try to cut down the amount of time you spend online and fail?
18. How often do you try to hide how long you have been online?
19. How often do you choose to spend more time online over going out with others?
20. How often do you feel depressed, moody, or nervous when you are offline, which goes away once you are back online?

Total scores:
20–49 points: average online user
50–79 points: occasional or frequent problems because of the Internet
80–100 points: Internet use is causing significant problems

Source: Young (1998).

Related Addictive Behavior Inventory (IRABI) (Brenner 1997) and the Pathological Internet Use Scale (PIUS) (Morahan-Martin and Schumacher 2000). Huang et al. (2007) developed and psychometrically tested the Chinese Internet Addiction Inventory in over 1,000 college students in China and showed that it has high internal consistency and acceptable test–retest reliability. These instruments, tested in different samples, have not been widely accepted. Moreover, a general concern exists about the reliability of these self-report measures because they have no built-in "lie" scale (Beard 2005).

As with the evaluation of any psychiatric disorder, standardized diagnostic instruments supplement but cannot replace the clinical interview. Individuals exhibiting problematic Internet use generally present only for comorbid conditions, and few clinicians specifically screen for problematic Internet use. The questions listed in Table 15.4 will assist clinicians in including Internet use history in routine history taking (Beard 2005; Liu and Potenza 2007). The questions are practical and assess in a structured manner the level of use and its effects on the patient's biological, psychological, and social well-being.

Prevalence

The community prevalence of problematic Internet use has not been established, largely because of the lack of standardized diagnostic criteria and large-scale epidemiological studies. To date, only one nationwide epidemiological study of problematic Internet use has been completed in the United States (Aboujaoude et al. 2006). The point prevalence was 0.7% when problematic Internet use was defined as follows. Diagnosis necessitated that respondents report (1) Internet use that interferes with relationships, (2) feeling preoccupied

Table 15.4 Questions selected and edited from sample questions for a screening interview assessing problematic Internet use by Beard

Presenting problem

1. How much time do you spend on the Internet each day? Week? Month?
2. What is the longest amount of time you have spent using the Internet in one sitting?
3. What Internet sites or applications (e.g., chat rooms, email, MUDS) do you use, and what effect do they have on you?
4. What was going on in your life when you began to have difficulties with your Internet use?
5. Do you ever feel preoccupied with the Internet (e.g., think about previous online activity or anticipate next online session)?
6. How did you feel when attempting to cut down or stop your Internet use?
7. Have you ever lied to family members, a therapist, or others to conceal the extent of your involvement with the Internet?

Biological areas

1. How have your health concerns, if any, been impacted by your Internet use?
2. Does your Internet use interfere with your sleep?
3. Does your Internet use interfere with eating regularly?

Psychological areas

1. How do you feel before, after, and while using the Internet?
2. What are your thoughts before, after, and while using the Internet?
3. Have you ever used the Internet to help improve your mood or change your thoughts?
4. Have you ever felt anxious, depressed, or isolated when offline?

Social area

1. How has your Internet use caused problems or concerns with your family?
2. How has your Internet use caused problems or concerns with your significant other?
3. How has your Internet use caused problems or concerns with your social activities and friendships?
4. How has using the Internet interfered with your performance at school or work?
5. Have you ever been in trouble with the authorities because of your Internet use?

Relapse prevention areas

1. Do you believe that you have a problem with your level of Internet use?
2. What seems to trigger your Internet use?
3. What do you see as the benefits and costs of continued Internet use?
4. What plans have you implemented in the past to deal with your level of Internet use?

Sources: Beard (2005); Liu and Potenza (2007).

with Internet use when offline, (3) having tried unsuccessfully either to cut down or quit, and (4) staying online longer than intended (Aboujaoude et al. 2006). Higher percentages of respondents (3.7% to 13.7%) endorsed one or more of these features consistent with problematic Internet use. The survey used a random-digit dial telephone method and interviewed 2,513 adults (≥ 18 years of age) across all states.

No comparable offline prevalence estimate studies in adults have been performed in other countries. Surveys in other countries mainly focused on prevalence estimates in adolescents because this age group is considered at high risk. Large-scale, offline community studies conducted in Finland, Norway, and South Korea reported similar prevalence estimates of problematic Internet use in adolescents of about 2% (Choi 2007; Johansson and Gotestam 2004; Kaltiala-Heino, Lintonen, and Rimpela 2004). Frequencies in psychiatric or primary care clinical settings are not known and represent important research questions.

A review of online versus offline studies (Liu and Potenza 2007) showed that general surveys conducted online reported higher prevalence estimates than those conducted offline, probably a result of the inherent selection bias of online survey methodologies. Moreover, studies of samples of adolescents or college students generally reported higher prevalence estimates than surveys of the general public, suggesting that adolescents and college students may be at higher risk.

Age at Onset

The age of onset of problematic Internet use is not known. It has been reported in children as young as the age of 6 (Choi 2007). Children and adolescents are often considered to have higher risk, and a large proportion of studies have involved youths (Chou 2001; Chou and Hsiao 2000; Fortson, Scotti, and Chen 2007; Ha et al. 2007; Johansson and Gotestam 2004; Kaltiala-Heino, Lintonen, and Rimpela 2004).

Considering the time of onset relative to the time an individual is first exposed to the Internet is also useful. Patients' Internet use often appears to become problematic soon after they first use the Internet, possibly within 6 months to a year, a time when they feel intimidated as well as fascinated by the new technology. This phenomenon has been termed the "newbie" syndrome (Young 1996a). These observations are largely anecdotal, and broader studies are needed to provide empirical support.

Natural History and Course of Illness

Little is known about the course of problematic Internet use because longitudinal studies are largely lacking. One early longitudinal study, designed to investigate whether Internet use was beneficial or harmful psychologically, found that 2 years after the subjects had signed up for the Internet, more frequent use was associated with declines in social activities and communication within the household and increases in depression and loneliness (Kraut et al. 1998). A recent prospective study surveyed 517 young adolescents in Taiwan with the same instruments at baseline and 1 year later to determine how many had problematic Internet use at each time point. The 1-year incidence was 7.5%. About half the subjects identified as having problematic Internet use at baseline did not meet the criteria 1 year later (Ko et al. 2007). These findings suggest that spontaneous recovery is possible or that problematic Internet use is a chronic disorder with spontaneous remissions and recurrences. Longer longitudinal studies are needed to investigate these possibilities.

Effects of Problematic Internet Use on Quality of Life

Data on the effects of problematic Internet use on quality of life are very limited. A case series of 21 subjects with problematic Internet use reported a specific deficit in general mental health, but functioning was otherwise unimpaired (Black, Belsare, and Schlosser 1999). Considering that problematic Internet use could lead to severe psychosocial and functional impairments, it is important to include quality of life measures in future studies.

Biological Data

No biological data regarding problematic Internet use are available. Research modalities such as neuroimaging would be valuable tools in future studies.

Comorbid Conditions

Problematic Internet use has not been included in large-scale psychiatric epidemiological studies such as the National Comorbidity Study (Kessler et al. 2005). A review of case series and studies from other countries and largely involving limited samples such as adolescents revealed that co-occurrence of other psychiatric conditions is the norm rather than the exception (Liu and Potenza 2007). Identified cases often have multiple comorbidities. Common psychiatric comorbidities include mood disorders, other impulsive control disorders, social phobia, substance use disorders, and attention deficit hyperactivity disorder. Comorbid psychotic disorders appear much less common.

1. *Mood disorders.* In case series and surveys, depression has commonly co-occurred with problematic Internet use. In the United States, two case series systematically evaluated about 20 patients face-to-face and found frequent comorbid mood disorders (Black, Belsare, and Schlosser 1999; Shapira et al. 2000). Frequencies of comorbid current major depression were 10% and 24%, respectively, and lifetime frequencies were 15% and 33%, respectively. In the series of Shapira et al. (2000), 70% of subjects had a lifetime diagnosis of bipolar affective disorder I or II. However, all had a current or recent depressive or mixed episode, and none had current or recent mania. These findings suggest a strong association between depressive symptoms and problematic Internet use, consistent with results from community surveys from other countries (Ha et al. 2007; Kim et al. 2006; Yen et al. 2007a). In a Korean series of 12 adolescents with problematic Internet use, major depressive disorder meeting DSM-IV criteria was found in 25% (Ha et al. 2006). Severity of depression may correlate with severity of problematic Internet use (Ha et al. 2007). One longitudinal study suggested that excessive Internet use may lead to depression (Kraut et al. 1998), but Internet use may have also started as a coping strategy for depression and progressed to become problematic in the absence of effective treatment of the depression.

2. *Obsessive-compulsive disorder (OCD) and impulse control disorders* have been hypothesized to lie along the same spectrum (Dell'Osso et al. 2006b). Although an association between OCD and problematic Internet use has been proposed, patient reports suggest that problematic Internet use is probably more closely related to impulse control disorders. Patients often report that their Internet use is more impulsive and ego-syntonic rather than compulsive and ego-dystonic. In the two U.S. case series of problematic Internet use, frequencies of current OCD were 0% and 15% and lifetime OCD frequencies were 10% and 20% (Black, Belsare, and Schlosser 1999; Shapira et al. 2000). The percentages of individuals with any impulse control disorder were considerably higher (38% and 50%) in both series (Black, Belsare, and Schlosser 1999; Shapira et al. 2000). A variety of impulse control disorders were identified in the patients, including intermittent explosive disorder, kleptomania, pathological gambling, pyromania, compulsive buying, compulsive sexual behavior, and compulsive exercising. Surveys among adolescents that showed associations between problematic Internet use and obsessive-compulsive symptoms did not attempt to make a diagnosis of OCD and did not evaluate impulse control disorders (Ha et al. 2007; Yang et al. 2005).

3. *Social phobia.* In the case series of Shapira et al. (2000), concurrent and lifetime social phobia were found in 40% and 45% of subjects, respectively. Social phobia was the most common anxiety disorder in this series. Some have contended that the anonymity of the Internet draws the socially fearful to participate in low-risk social interactions via the Web (Campbell, Cumming, and Hughes 2006). A large-scale epidemiological study in Taiwan found an association between problematic Internet use and social phobia, but social phobia did not predict problematic Internet use in the study's regression model (Yen et al. 2007a). The rate of co-occurring social phobia and problematic Internet use in the general population is not known.

4. *Attention deficit hyperactivity disorder (ADHD).* In a sample of over 500 elementary school students, 22.5% of those identified as problematic Internet users had co-occurring ADHD (Yoo et al. 2004). Those with ADHD and problematic Internet use had significantly higher scores on parental, teacher, and self ratings of ADHD symptoms than those with ADHD alone (Yen et al. 2007a; Yoo et al. 2004). Children with problematic Internet use used

the Internet mainly to play online games. Impaired impulse control may represent a link between ADHD and problematic Internet use.

5. *Substance abuse.* Substance abuse was a common co-occurring condition in both case series discussed (Black, Belsare, and Schlosser 1999; Shapira et al. 2000). Co-occurring estimates of any current substance abuse were 10% and 14%, and lifetime estimates were 38% and 55%. Types and patterns of substance use behaviors should be assessed in future epidemiological studies of problematic Internet use.

Treatments

Given the recent recognition of problematic Internet use as a psychiatric problem, little research has evaluated the safety and efficacy of treatments for the disorder. No double-blind, controlled trials of pharmacotherapies or psychotherapies have been published. However, treatments for problematic Internet use are gradually being developed. Multiple treatment centers and groups have emerged, both online and offline. For example, outpatient treatment services for problematic Internet use are available at the Illinois Institute for Addiction Recovery at Proctor Hospital and McLean Hospital of Harvard Medical School. In some instances, patients have been admitted for inpatient rehabilitation. In China, a halfway house was recently opened for adolescents with problematic Internet use (Watts 2006).

1. *Pharmacotherapy.* Selective serotonin reuptake inhibitors are effective in the treatment of OCD. Studies of the use of SSRIs in impulse control disorders have shown mixed results (Bhatia and Sapra 2004; Gadde et al. 2007; Grant and Potenza 2006; Koran et al. 2007a, 2007b). Problematic Internet use appears to have compulsive and impulsive qualities, and treatment with escitalopram, an SSRI, has been studied recently. An open-label study in 19 subjects showed significant decreases after 10 weeks of escitalopram, 20 mg/day, in weekly hours spent online (from a mean of 36.8 hours to 16.5 hours) and in measures of impulsivity and compulsivity, and improvement in global functioning (Dell'Osso et al. 2006a). After 10 weeks, subjects were blindly randomized to continue treatment with escitalopram or a placebo. After another 9 weeks, therapeutic gains achieved at week 10 were maintained in both treatment groups, and no further gain was shown for either group. The medication was well tolerated. The most frequently reported side effects were drowsiness and nausea, which were modest and self-limited (Dell'Osso et al. 2006a).

   In a case report, an adult patient with an online gaming problem who was also very depressed on presentation responded to escitalopram (Sattar and Ramaswamy 2004). Another case study reported the successful use of an atypical antipsychotic (quetiapine) as augmentation for citalopram in the treatment of a subject who had problematic Internet use (Atmaca 2007). This augmentation strategy has also been used in treating OCD. Further clinical trials are needed to establish the efficacy and effectiveness of medication monotherapy and augmentation strategies.

2. *Psychotherapy.* Among the proposed modalities of therapy, only cognitive-behavioral therapy has been empirically examined, and the outcomes appear favorable. Most patients achieved effective symptom management by the eighth session, and thera-peutic gains were sustained on a 6-month follow-up (Young 2007). Techniques such as keeping a daily Internet log, teaching of time management skills and coping strategies, assertiveness training, and correcting cognitive distortions and rationalizations such as "Just a few more minutes won't hurt" appear helpful (Young 2007). Some clinicians have adopted psychotherapeutic strategies from drug and alcohol treatments. Support groups, although frequently conducted online, often resemble the model of Alcoholics Anonymous. Abstinence recovery models may not be practical because computers have

become a salient part of everyday life. Moderated and controlled use of the Internet may be most appropriate.

3. *Other treatments.* For children and adolescents, family-based interventions such as skills training for parents to improve communication with children and family monitoring of the use of the Internet can be considered (Yen et al. 2007b). Parental and teacher participation in the recognition of and interventions for problematic Internet use is important. Software is available to restrict Internet access and can act as an external control and support when the patient has difficulty controlling his or her use. Online treatment centers such as The Center for Online Addiction (http://www.netaddiction.com) offer E-counseling, self-help books and tapes, and online support groups.

In summary, clinicians should be aware of the clinical features of problematic Internet use and its potential consequences and be equipped to assess Internet use history in the clinical interview. Comprehensive clinical evaluation should reveal the patient's experience with the Internet, its relations to his or her emotional distress and psychiatric symptoms, and the patient's own understanding of the Internet's influences on his or her life. Co-occurring psychiatric disorders should be identified and appropriately treated. Problematic Internet use may respond to serotonin reuptake inhibitors, although larger and longer controlled trials are needed to investigate this possibility. Time management and other life skills may help empower the patient and increase his or her sense of control. In this manner, individuals may be helped to achieve moderated use of the Internet and to benefit from the technology without being consumed by it.

References

Aboujaoude E, Koran LM, Gamel N et al. Potential markers for problematic Internet use: A telephone survey of 2,513 adults. *CNS Spectr* 11:750–755, 2006.

Allison SE, Von Wahlde L, Shockley T et al. The development of the self in the era of the Internet and role-playing fantasy games. *Am J Psychiatry* 163:381–385, 2006.

American Psychiatric Association. *Diagnostic and Statistical Manual of Mental Disorders*, 4th edition. Washington, DC: American Psychiatric Association, 1994.

American Psychiatric Association. *Diagnostic and Statistical Manual of Mental Disorders*, 4th edition, text revision. Washington, DC: American Psychiatric Association, 2000.

Anderson KJ. Internet use among college students: An exploratory study. *J Am Coll Health* 50:21–26, 2001.

Atmaca M. A case of problematic Internet use successfully treated with an SSRI-antipsychotic combination. *Prog Neuropsychopharmacol Biol Psychiatry* 31:961–962, 2007.

BBC News. S Korean Dies after Games Session [BBC News Web site]. August 10, 2005. Available at http://news.bbc.co.uk/2/hi/technology/4137782.stm. Accessed March 21, 2008.

Beard KW. Internet addiction: A review of current assessment techniques and potential assessment questions. *Cyberpsychol Behav* 8:7–14, 2005.

Bhatia MS, Sapra S. Escitalopram in trichotillomania. *Eur Psychiatry* 19:239–240, 2004.

Black DW, Belsare G, Schlosser S. Clinical features, psychiatric comorbidity, and health-related quality of life in persons reporting compulsive computer use behavior. *J Clin Psychiatry* 60:839–844, 1999.

Block JJ. Issues for DSM-V: Internet Addiction. *Am J Psychiatry* 165:306–307, 2008.

Brenner V. Psychology of computer use: XLVII. Parameters of Internet use, abuse and addiction: The first 90 days of the Internet Usage Survey. *Psychol Rep* 80(3 pt 1): 879–882, 1997.

Campbell AJ, Cumming SR, Hughes I. Internet use by the socially fearful: Addiction or therapy? *Cyberpsychol Behav* 9(1): 69–81, 2006.

Cantril H, Allport GW. *The Psychology of Radio*. New York: Harper & Bros., 1935.

Cao F, Su L, Liu T et al. The relationship between impulsivity and Internet addiction in a sample of Chinese adolescents. *Eur Psychiatry* 22:466–471, 2007.

Caplan SE. Problematic Internet use and psychosocial well-being: Development of a theory-based cognitive-behavioral measurement instrument. *Comput Hum Behav* 18:553–575, 2002.

Choi YH. Advancement of IT and seriousness of youth Internet addiction, in *2007 International Symposium on the Counseling and Treatment of Youth Internet Addiction*. Seoul: National Youth Commission, 2007, p. 20.

Chou C. Internet heavy use and addiction among Taiwanese college students: An online interview study. *Cyberpsychol Behav* 4:573–585, 2001.

Chou C, Hsiao MC. Internet addiction, usage, gratification, and pleasure experience: The Taiwan college students' case. *Comput Educ* 35:65–80, 2000.

Conrad P. Medicalization and social control. *Annu Rev Sociol* 18:209–232, 1992.

Davis RA, Flett GL, Besser A. Validation of a new scale for measuring problematic Internet use: Implications for pre-employment screening. *Cyberpsychol Behav* 5:331–345, 2002.

Dell'Osso B, Altamura AC, Allen A et al. Epidemiologic and clinical updates on impulse control disorders: A critical review. *Eur Arch Psychiatry Clin Neurosci* 256(8): 464–475, 2006b.

Dell'Osso B, Altamura AC, Hadley SJ et al. An open-label trial of escitalopram in the treatment of impulsive-compulsive Internet usage disorder. *Eur Neuropsychopharmacol* 16(suppl 1): S82, 2006a.

Fasano A, Elia AE, Soleti F et al. Punding and computer addiction in Parkinson's disease. *Mov Disord* 21:1217–1218, 2006.

Fortson BL, Scotti JR, Chen YC. Internet use, abuse, and dependence among students at a southeastern regional university. *J Am Coll Health* 56:137–144, 2007.

Gadde KM, Wagner HR 2nd, Connor KM et al. Escitalopram treatment of trichotillomania. *Int Clin Psychopharmacol* 22:39–42, 2007.

Grant JE, Potenza MN. Escitalopram treatment of pathological gambling with co-occurring anxiety: An open-label pilot study with double-blind discontinuation. *Int Clin Psychopharmacol* 21:203–209, 2006.

Greenfield DN. Psychological characteristics of compulsive Internet use: A preliminary analysis. *Cyberpsychol Behav* 2:403–412, 1999.

Griffiths M. Gambling on the Internet: A brief note. *J Gambl Stud* 12:471–473, 1996.

Griffiths M. Technological addictions: Looking to the future. Paper presented at the 105th Annual Convention of the American Psychological Association, Chicago, IL, 1997.

Griffiths M. Sex on the Internet: Observations and implications for Internet sex addiction. *J Sex Res* 38:333–342, 2001.

Ha JH, Kim SY, Sujeong CB et al. Depression and Internet addiction in adolescents. *Psychopathology* 40:424–430, 2007.

Ha JH, Yoo HJ, Cho IH et al. Psychiatric comorbidity assessed in Korean children and adolescents who screen positive for Internet addiction. *J Clin Psychiatry* 67(5): 821–826, 2006.

Hollander E, Kim S, Zohar J. OCSDs in the forthcoming DSM-V. *CNS Spectr* 12:320–323, 2007.

Hollander E, Wong CM. Obsessive-compulsive spectrum disorders. *J Clin Psychiatry* 56(suppl 4): 3–6: discussion 53–55, 1995.

Huang Z, Wang M, Qian M et al. Chinese Internet addiction inventory: Developing a measure of problematic Internet use for Chinese college students. *Cyberpsychol Behav* 10:805–811, 2007.

Internet World Stats. Internet usage and population in North America [Internet World Stats Web site], 2008. Available at http://www.internetworldstats.com/stats14.htm#north. Accessed March 29, 2008.

Johansson A, Gotestam KG. Internet addiction: Characteristics of a questionnaire and prevalence in Norwegian youth (12–18 years). *Scand J Psychol* 45(3): 223–229, 2004.

Kaltiala-Heino R, Lintonen T, Rimpela A. Internet addiction? Potentially problematic use of the Internet in a population of 12–18 year-old adolescents. *Addict Res Theory* 12:89–96, 2004.

Kessler RC, Chiu WT, Demler O et al. Prevalence, severity, and comorbidity of 12-month DSM-IV disorders in the National Comorbidity Survey Replication. *Arch Gen Psychiatry* 62:617–627, 2005.

Kim K, Ryu E, Chon M et al. Internet addiction in Korean adolescents and its relation to depression and suicidal ideation: A questionnaire survey. *Int J Nurs Stud* 43:185–192, 2006.

Ko CH, Yen JY, Chen CC et al. Gender differences and related factors affecting online gaming addiction among Taiwanese adolescents. *J Nerv Ment Dis* 193:273–277, 2005a.

Ko CH, Yen JY, Chen CC et al. Proposed diagnostic criteria of Internet addiction for adolescents. *J Nerv Ment Dis* 193:728–733, 2005b.

Ko CH, Yen JY, Cheng-Fang Y et al. Factors predictive for incidence and remission of Internet addiction in young adolescents: A prospective study. *Cyberpsychol Behav* 10:545–551, 2007.

Koran LM, Aboujaoude EN, Gamel N et al. Escitalopram treatment of kleptomania: An open-label trial followed by double-blind discontinuation. *J Clin Psychiatry* 68:422–427, 2007a.

Koran LM, Aboujaoude EN, Solvason B et al. Escitalopram for compulsive buying disorder: A double-blind discontinuation study. *J Clin Psychopharmacol* 27:225–227, 2007b.

Kraut R, Patterson M, Lundmark V et al. Internet paradox: A social technology that reduces social involvement and psychological well-being? *Am Psychol* 53:1017–1031, 1998.

Lavin M, Marvin K, McLarney V et al. Sensation seeking and collegiate vulnerability to Internet dependence. *Cyberpsychol Behav* 2:425–430, 2000.

Lin SSJ, Tsai CC. Sensation seeking and Internet dependence of Taiwanese high school adolescents. *Comput Hum Behav* 18:411–426, 2002.

Liu CY, Kuo FY. A study of Internet addiction through the lens of the interpersonal theory. *Cyberpsychol Behav* 10:799–804, 2007.

Liu T, Potenza MN. Problematic Internet use: Clinical implications. *CNS Spectr* 12:453–466, 2007.

Miller MC. Questions & answers: Is "Internet addiction" a distinct mental disorder? *Harv Ment Health Lett* 24:8, 2007.

Mitchell P. Internet addiction: Genuine diagnosis or not? *Lancet* 355:632, 2000.

Morahan-Martin J, Schumacher P. Incidence and correlates of pathological Internet use among college students. *Comput Hum Behav* 16:13–29, 2000.

Potenza MN. Should addictive disorders include non-substance-related conditions? *Addiction* 101:142–151, 2006.

Potenza MN, Hollander E. Pathological gambling and impulse control disorders, in *Neuropsychopharmacology: The Fifth Generation of Progress*, 5th edition. Edited by Davis KL, Charney D, Coyle J, et al. Baltimore: Lippincott Williams & Wilkins, 2002, pp. 1736–1737.

Sattar P, Ramaswamy S. Internet gaming addiction. *Can J Psychiatry* 49:869–870, 2004.

Scherer K. College life on-line: Healthy and unhealthy Internet use. *Journal of College Student Development* 38:655–665, 1997.

Schneider JP. A qualitative study of cybersex participants: Gender differences, recovery issues, and implications for therapists. *Sex Addict Compulsivity* 7:249–278, 2000.

Shaffer HJ, Hall MN, Vander Bilt J. "Computer addiction": A critical consideration. *Am J Orthopsychiatry* 70:162–168, 2000.

Shapira NA, Goldsmith TD, Keck PE et al. Psychiatric features of individuals with problematic Internet use. *J Affect Disord* 57:267–272, 2000.

Shapira NA, Lessig MC, Goldsmith TD et al. Problematic internet use: Proposed classification and diagnostic criteria. *Depress Anxiety* 17:207–216, 2003.

Surratt CG. *Netaholics? The Creation of a Pathology*. New York: Nova Science Publishers, 1999.

te Wildt BT, Putzig I, Zedler M et al. Internet dependency as a symptom of depressive mood disorders. *Psychiatr Prax* 34(suppl 3): S318–322, 2007.

Treuer T, Fabian Z, Furedi J. Internet addiction associated with features of impulse control disorder: Is it a real psychiatric disorder? *J Affect Disord* 66:283, 2001.

Warden NL, Phillips JG, Ogloff JRP. Internet addiction. *Psychiatry Psychol Law* 11:280–295, 2004.

Watts J. China Opens Internet Addicts' Shelter [*The Guardian* Web site]. August 24, 2006. Available at http://www.guardian.co.uk/technology/2006/aug/24/news.media. Accessed April 30, 2008.

Weide K. **U.**S. Online Consumer Behavior Survey Results 2007, Part I: Wireline Internet Usage. [IDC Web site]. December 2007. Available at http://www.idc.com/getdoc.jsp?containerId=210097. Accessed March 29, 2008.

Widyanto L, McMurran M. The psychometric properties of the Internet addiction test. *Cyberpsychol Behav* 7:443–450, 2004.

World Health Organization. *International Statistical Classification of Diseases and Related Health Problems*, 10th edition. Geneva: World Health Organization, 2003.

Yang CK, Choe BM, Baity M et al. SCL-90-R and 16PF profiles of senior high school students with excessive Internet use. *Can J Psychiatry* 50:407–414, 2005.

Yen JY, Ko CH, Yen CF et al. The comorbid psychiatric symptoms of Internet addiction: Attention deficit and hyperactivity disorder (ADHD), depression, social phobia, and hostility. *J Adolesc Health* 41:93–98, 2007a.

Yen JY, Yen CF, Chen CC et al. Family factors of Internet addiction and substance use experience in Taiwanese adolescents. *Cyberpsychol Behav* 10:323–329, 2007b.

Yoo HJ, Cho SC, Ha MA et al. Attention deficit hyperactivity symptoms and Internet addiction. *Psychiatry Clin Neurosci* 58:487–494, 2004.

Young KS. Internet addiction: The emergence of a new clinical disorder. *Cyberpsychol Behav* 1:237–244, 1996a.

Young KS. Psychology of computer use: XL. Addictive use of the Internet: A case that breaks the stereotype. *Psychol Rep* 79:899–902, 1996b.

Young KS. Internet Addiction Test (IAT) [Center for Internet Addiction Recovery Web site]. 1998. Available at http://www.netaddiction.com/resources/internet_addiction_test.htm. Accessed March 28, 2008.

Young KS. Cognitive behavior therapy with Internet addicts: Treatment outcomes and implications. *Cyberpsychol Behav* 10:671–679, 2007.

Young KS, Rogers RC. The relationship between depression and Internet addiction. *Cyberpsychol Behav* 1:25–28, 1998.

16

Virtual Violence: The Games People Play

Vladan Starcevic MD, PhD, FRANZCP, and
Guy Porter BA, MBBS (Hons)

Video games are played by millions around the world, with the majority of players being children, adolescents, and young adults. Many of these games are violent in nature and content, and some are disturbingly so. There are probably different reasons for playing violent video games. For some people, the gaming activity itself is most appealing, and violence is secondary. For others, playing violent video games may be a socially acceptable outlet for expressing aggressive tendencies. Some players apparently enjoy this activity because of the "buzz" generated by the images and "atmosphere" of danger, akin to the feelings elicited by watching horror films. Regardless of the underlying reason, playing violent video games has caused concern, which has often been exploited by the media. One concern about violent video games has been a highly publicized but difficult to prove link between gaming and subsequent criminal behavior; the other concern pertains to the assumption that violent video games are "addictive."

The focus of this chapter is on the link between playing violent video games and exhibiting aggressive behavior. The research examining this relationship is reviewed and an attempt is made to shed more light on it.

Does Playing Violent Video Games Lead to Violent Behavior?

It is astounding how much controversy has been generated by this question. Perhaps the question has not been posed correctly, in which case an effort to come up with an answer might have been wasted. In many other instances, behaviors are usually not explained on the basis of one personality trait or a previous behavioral pattern. Likewise, it seems too simplistic to blame playing violent video games for episodes of aggressive or criminal behavior. Why then is this link often presumed to exist?

A large part of the reason may lie in the nature of the behavior under consideration. Rare cases of extreme violence, such as school mass shootings, have frequently been blamed on violent video games played by the perpetrators. Society cannot ignore these horrific acts and, in the search for answers, both the public and the media have a tendency to make a link with whatever preceded them. It is a simple exercise in assuming causality: if there seems to be a thematically and temporally "logical" link, as between playing violent video games and subsequently committing a crime, the causal relationship between the two is automatically assumed.

There is nothing unusual about assuming that this causality exists. The media are not expected to espouse scientific principles and do not feel obliged to provide any "hard" evidence of causality. The onus is on social psychology and mental health investigators to scrutinize the link between playing violent video games and subsequent aggression and ascertain whether they are causally related. As a result of research, two basic hypotheses about this relationship have been proposed:

1. Playing violent video games increases the risk of the subsequent aggression. This risk may be particularly heightened in individuals who are already predisposed to aggressive behavior (e.g., through high levels of anger or hostility) and in young children.
2. There is no relationship between playing violent video games and subsequent aggression.

These hypotheses are presented in more detail and examined more closely in the sections that follow. This is followed by a discussion of the possible mechanisms linking exposure to violent video games with aggressive behavior.

Hypothesis 1: Playing Violent Video Games Increases the Risk of Subsequent Aggression

Experimental and correlational studies have reported that playing violent video games is associated with increased levels of physiological arousal, decreased prosocial behaviors, greater hostility, more frequent arguments with teachers and poorer school performance, and more frequent physical fights and aggressive or antisocial behavior (Anderson and Dill 2000; Anderson et al. 2004; Bartholow, Sestir, and Davis 2005; Bushman and Anderson 2002; Gentile et al. 2004; Sheese and Graziano 2005; Silvern and Williamson 1987; Uhlmann and Swanson 2004). In one longitudinal study, exposure to violent video games was related to increased aggressive behavior, but participants were also exposed to other media violence and the effect from violent video game exposure alone could not be ascertained (Slater et al. 2003). Two meta-analyses of experimental and correlational studies concluded that exposure to violent video games was linked to more prominent hostile feelings, hostile attitudes, and aggressive behavior, and to decreased prosocial behavior (Anderson 2004; Anderson and Bushman 2001). The same conclusion was reached in a literature review of the effects of violent video games on children and adolescents (Gentile and Stone 2005).

This research has been criticized on methodological grounds, including arbitrary criteria for dividing games into "violent" and "nonviolent," questionable or inadequate measures of aggressive behavior, failure to control for potentially confounding variables (e.g., genetic predisposition, parenting style, exposure to family violence, socioeconomic status, substance abuse, psychiatric disorders), general lack of follow-up, and retrospective design with inherent recall bias (e.g., Ferguson 2007b; Porter and Starcevic 2007). Also, these studies have merely established an association between playing violent video games and aggression; the finding of an association does not imply a causal relationship.

Despite these criticisms and limitations, the research does suggest that there is a link between playing violent video games and the subsequent aggression. In an attempt to better understand this link, the general aggression model has been put forward (Anderson and Bushman 2001; Anderson and Ford 1986; Bushman and Anderson 2002), and it quickly became the most influential account of how playing violent video games might make aggression more likely. Briefly, this theory postulates that the person's cognition, affect, and arousal determine the relationship between exposure to violent video games and aggression, proposing that "aggressive cognitive scripts" formed as a result of exposure to violent video games cause subsequent aggression. In its original form, the theory suggested a mechanism of passive modeling, so that even persons without a preexisting inclination toward aggression become aggressive simply as a result of repeated exposure to violent video games and media violence in general.

This "blank slate" or "tabula rasa" approach (Pinker 2002) was changed in a modification of the general aggression model, which proposes that anger makes a person more likely to be affected by violent video games in a way that lowers inhibition against aggressive acts and makes aggression more likely (Anderson and Bushman 2002). The combined role of anger and exposure to violent video games was confirmed by a study in which only angry individuals exposed to violent video games behaved aggressively, whereas they were less aggressive when exposed to nonviolent video games (Giumetti and Markey 2007).

However, in another study, children with low trait hostility who played more violent video games were more likely to get into physical fights than children with high trait hostility who played less violent games, suggesting a greater role for playing violent video games than that of trait hostility (Gentile et al. 2004).

The modified general aggression model provides a more plausible explanation of the link between exposure to violent video games and subsequent aggression: instead of a simplistic notion that playing video games inevitably causes aggression, this model takes into account personality characteristics, especially anger and hostility, of persons playing violent video games. These characteristics may make it more likely that playing violent video games *precipitates* aggressive behavior. It would also be important to know to what extent persons with high levels of anger and hostility or antisocial traits are "attracted" to violent video games in the first place (e.g., Funk et al. 2002; Lemmens and Bushman 2006) because in such cases playing violent video games might *facilitate* the expression of anger and hostility and the preexisting propensity toward aggression.

Hypothesis 2: Playing Violent Video Games Is Not Related to Subsequent Aggression

Numerous video games contain some degree of violence, frequently with the player's character as both protagonist and perpetrator of the violence. However, many video gamers state that their participation in violent acts in a virtual environment has no bearing on their behavior in the "real" world and that they are not violent people. This common video gamer assertion is supported by the failure of several studies to show a relationship between playing violent video games and heightened aggression, especially when potential confounders (e.g., presence of "aggressive personality" and exposure to family violence) have been controlled for (Ferguson et al. 2008; Weigman and van Schie 1998; Williams and Skoric 2005). Likewise, several meta-analyses were also unable to confirm a causal link between exposure to violent video games and subsequent aggression (Ferguson 2007a, 2007b; Sherry 2001, 2007).

The findings of these studies have been accounted for by the significant "bias" in research suggesting the causal link between exposure to violent video games and the subsequent aggression (Ferguson 2007a, 2007b). This refers to the various methodological issues already mentioned. In addition, a model of violent behavior – the catalyst model – was proposed to explain the lack of a relationship between exposure to violent video games and the subsequent violent behavior (Ferguson et al. 2008). According to this model, acts of violence occur as a result of an "innate propensity" (e.g., through genetic predisposition or brain injury) in combination with family violence exposure, which then leads to a formation of an "aggressive personality." People with such a personality, usually males, are more likely to exhibit violent behavior at times of stress, which act as "catalysts." Also, these individuals tend to be directed to or choose to be exposed to violent media, including violent video games, which act as "stylistic catalysts." Thus, the model proposes that violent video games do not cause aggression but may determine the form or "style" of aggression. In other words, people with an aggressive personality are more likely to commit acts of violence regardless of whether they are exposed to violent video games, and they may only adopt a pattern or a form of violent behavior based on the violence that they see in video games.

Interestingly, the catalyst model and the modified general aggression model share one important feature, although they use different terminology, emphasize different elements, and appear very different on the surface. Both models suggest that hostility, anger, or aggressive personality traits may make it more likely for individuals, especially children and adolescents, to be attracted to playing violent video games. This gaming activity may then facilitate the expression of anger, hostility, or aggressive personality traits and precipitate aggression, with aggressive behavior possibly being modeled on the violence seen in video games. Indeed, the bidirectional model proposes that while exposure to violent video games may make an individual more aggressive, individuals with higher hostility and anger may preferentially choose to play violent video games (Porter and Starcevic 2007), so that the two processes interact and the direction of causality becomes difficult to determine.

A radically different approach, often espoused by video game developers and pro–video-game lobbyist groups, suggests that, instead of encouraging violence, playing violent video games may actually reduce aggressive behavior by acting as an outlet for "repressed" aggression (e.g., Emes 1997) or by allowing aggressive tendencies to be expressed in a socially acceptable way (e.g., the "catharsis hypothesis"; see Sherry 2007). Although it is difficult to test these propositions, mainly because of the obstacles in measuring the underlying concepts and designing studies adequately, they deserve full attention from investigators. For example, it would be important to ascertain the conditions under which playing violent video games by individuals with similar levels of anger or hostility results in less aggression, as opposed to more aggression. This could provide an answer to an intriguing question of whether playing violent video games might in some cases "protect" players (and others) against acts of violence.

Linking exposure to violent video games with real-world crime is fraught with legal difficulties. Numerous cases filed against video game developers alleging that their games have caused individuals to commit specific crimes have been dismissed on the basis of lack of evidence or other legal technicalities. Furthermore, in the United States, sales of video games (most of which are violent) have increased rapidly since the mid-1990s, while rates of serious violent crime over the same period have declined (U.S. Department of Justice – Office of Justice Programs – Bureau of Justice Statistics). Clearly, many factors other than exposure to violent video games affect the prevalence of crime.

Mechanisms Through Which Playing Violent Video Games Might Facilitate Aggression

When exposure to violent video games in some studies seems to be linked with heightened aggression, the mechanisms through which this happens need to be elucidated. The mechanism that has most commonly been invoked here is a desensitization to violence (e.g., Carnagey, Anderson, and Bushman 2007; Funk 2005), that is, a loss of an aversive response to violent cues.

In an attempt to minimize the conceptual confusion, Carnagey, Anderson, and Bushman (2007) proposed a narrow definition of desensitization to violence as "a reduction in emotion-related physiological reactivity to real violence" (p. 490). The same authors reported that individuals who previously played a violent video game had a lower heart rate and decreased galvanic skin response while watching real violence on a film, thus demonstrating a physiological desensitization to real violence. This finding was interpreted using yet another modification of the general aggression model. In this version of the model, desensitization was described as a physiologically based extinction of fear/anxiety reactions to violence, which is made possible by presenting initially fearful, violence-related stimuli in a positive emotional context (e.g., by making "cartoonish" characters and providing rewards for acting violently in video games). The consequences of such desensitization are decreased perception of injury severity, decreased attention to violent events, decreased sympathy for violence victims, increased belief that violence is normative, and decreased negative attitudes toward violence, which ultimately lead to increased aggression and decreased tendency to intervene to prevent violence or help the victims.

Desensitization to violence and the subsequent aggression may also occur as a result of decreased empathy (e.g., Bartholow, Sestir, and Davis 2005; Funk et al. 2004). While certain video games, such as online multiplayer games, require some degree of collaboration or teamwork, the majority of violent video games place the player in a "kill or be killed situation." In this simplified scenario, the player has to act quickly and has no time or opportunity to empathize with opponents. Repeated exposure to such games may decrease empathy. If the level of empathy was low before exposure to violent video games, playing the games may reinforce a notion that empathizing is unnecessary or even a hindrance for survival. In this way, decreased empathy or a primary deficit in empathy facilitates desensitization to violence among violent video game players.

A high disgust propensity may decrease the likelihood of aggressive behavior involving a body envelope violation (e.g., stabbing) and/or seeing blood, injured tissues, or mutilated body parts. If disgust propensity undergoes habituation and decreases substantially during repeated exposure to violent video games and the person desensitizes to the violence-related disgust content, that may increase an inclination toward violent behavior.

Other aspects of violent video games may also make subsequent aggression more likely, for example, the moral message that violent video games send to young people. In the virtual world of violent video games, the player may kill or injure computer-generated characters or other online gamers without any consequence, including punishment. While many video games provide a story that primes the player to kill, there is very rarely any room for moral consideration of killing, and proceeding to kill invariably benefits the player more than exercising restraint. Indeed, the players are likely to be rewarded for killing by means of points, more powerful weapons, or their own survival. Furthermore, enemies are dehumanized, subtleties do not exist, and reflection on the meaning of the violence is not encouraged. The player is groomed as a "virtual psychopath" with no remorse or compassion when committing acts of extreme violence. A child or an adolescent exposed repeatedly to this kind of virtual world may learn that aggression is necessary, appropriate, desirable, rewarding, effective, and not punishable, and that victims of aggression do not deserve pity, as they are real or potential enemies. This learning interferes with a crucial developmental task of decreasing aggressive potential through incorporation of the societal norms of behavior and cultivation of compassion.

Conclusion

The debate about the relationship between playing violent video games and the subsequent aggression is reminiscent of the controversy about the effects on children of exposure to television and film violence. Numerous studies, including those in which confounding variables were controlled for and children were followed for periods of up to 17 years, have generally supported the notion that watching violence on television and films (exposure to "passive" media violence) is related to the subsequent aggressive and antisocial behavior (e.g., Huesmann et al. 2003; Johnson et al. 2002). If so, there is no reason to expect more benign effects from exposure to much more "active" (or "interactive") media violence, as in violent video games.

Indeed, despite the methodological shortcomings of research and regardless of one's theoretical position, the link between playing violent video games and the subsequent aggression cannot be denied; at the same time, this link should be neither minimized nor exaggerated. While exposure to violent video games is certainly not the only factor determining aggressive behavior, there is evidence to suggest that it can facilitate such behavior and that aggressive behavior can be modeled on the violence seen in video games. In other words, violent video games may *promote* or *condone* violence without necessarily causing it. This causes legitimate concerns about violent video games and raises the question of what should be done.

A hypothetical analogy may be useful here: how would society treat video games that portray child abuse (physical or sexual)? Although exposure to such video games would not necessarily cause one to abuse children, these games would be considered to promote or condone child abuse, perhaps in a way that child pornography does. As a result, such video games would probably be illegal in most countries, as is child pornography. If exposure to most violent video games also promotes or condones aggression without necessarily causing it, why should these video games be legal and held to a different standard? This is a paradox that is ultimately related to societal attitudes and values. Video games that depict particularly extreme forms of violence such as decapitation and dismemberment or feature violence directed against defenseless women are less socially acceptable and are frequently banned or censored in some countries. However, many modern Western societies consider "ordinary" aggressive behavior to be to some extent socially acceptable and tolerate it, while (at least publicly) showing zero tolerance for aggressive behavior toward children. As a reflection of these societal norms, in the realm of video games, killing an adult might seem more acceptable than hitting a child. This double standard sends conflicting and confusing messages about the type and amount of aggression that is or that could be tolerated by the society.

The prevention of aggression is a very broad enterprise that involves various initiatives targeting numerous factors that make this behavior more likely. Tighter regulation and control of the commercially produced and distributed violent video games might be only one such initiative. Its chief goal is to ensure that extremely violent games cannot be made legally available to those most vulnerable; that is, to children and adolescents under a certain age. Although such legal regulation is already in place in many countries, it may need to be reviewed and new policies may need to be introduced to enforce it. These changes, along with campaigns to educate parents and caregivers about the potentially detrimental effects of violent video games, might help efforts to decrease the promotion of violence in video games. Parental involvement is particularly important to ensure that children and adolescents with high levels of anger and hostility, conduct disorder, or antisocial behavior have restricted or no access to violent video games and other violent media.

While episodes of aggression seen in the context of clinical psychiatric practice are typically related to a range of etiologies, including substance intoxication, psychosis, personality disorders, and situational crises, mental health professionals should routinely inquire about exposure to violent media when assessing younger individuals with aggressive behavior. Finally, there is a need for better longitudinal studies to definitively establish the nature of the link between exposure to video game violence and subsequent aggressive behavior and/or crime.

References

Anderson CA. An update on the effects of playing violent video games. *J Adolesc* 27:113–122, 2004.

Anderson CA, Bushman BJ. Effects of violent video games on aggressive behavior, aggressive cognition, aggressive affect, physiological arousal, and prosocial behavior: A meta-analytic review of the scientific literature. *Psychol Sci* 12:353–359, 2001.

Anderson CA, Bushman BJ. Human aggression. *Annu Rev Psychol* 53:27–51, 2002.

Anderson CA, Carnagey NL, Flanagan M et al. Violent video games: Specific effects of violent content on aggressive thoughts and behavior. *Adv Exp Soc Psychol* 36:199–249, 2004.

Anderson CA, Dill KE. Video games and aggressive thoughts, feelings, and behavior in the laboratory and in life. *J Pers Soc Psychol* 78:772–790, 2000.

Anderson CA, Ford CM. Affect of the game player: Short-term effects of highly and mildly aggressive video games. *Pers Soc Psychol Bull* 12:390–402, 1986.

Bartholow BD, Sestir MA, Davis EB. Correlates and consequences of exposure to video game violence: Hostile personality, empathy, and aggressive behavior. *Pers Soc Psychol Bull* 31:1573–1586, 2005.

Bushman BJ, Anderson CA. Violent video games and hostile expectations: A test of the General Aggression Model. *Pers Soc Psychol Bull* 28:1679–1686, 2002.

Carnagey NL, Anderson CA, Bushman BJ. The effect of video game violence on physiological desensitization to real-life violence. *J Exp Soc Psychol* 43:489–496, 2007.

Emes CE. Is Mr. Pac Man eating our children? A review of the effect of video games on children. *Can J Psychiatry* 42:409–414, 1997.

Ferguson CJ. Evidence for publication bias in video game violence effects literature: A meta-analytic review. *Aggress Violent Behav* 12:470–482, 2007a.

Ferguson CJ. The good, the bad and the ugly: A meta-analytic review of positive and negative effects of violent video games. *Psychiatr Q* 78:309–316, 2007b.

Ferguson CJ, Rueda SM, Cruz AM et al. Violent video games and aggression: Causal relationship or byproduct of family violence and intrinsic family motivation? *Crimin Justice Behav* 35:311–332, 2008.

Funk JB. Children's exposure to violent video games and desensitization to violence. *Child Adolesc Psychiatr Clin N Am* 14:387–404, 2005.

Funk JB, Baldacci HB, Pasold T et al. Violence exposure in real life, video games, television, movies, and the Internet: Is there desensitization? *J Adolesc* 27:23–39, 2004.

Funk JB, Hagan J, Schimming J et al. Aggression and psychopathology in adolescents with a preference for violent electronic games. *Aggress Behav* 28:134–144, 2002.

Gentile DA, Lynch PJ, Linder JR et al. The effects of violent video game habits on adolescent hostility, aggressive behaviors, and school performance. *J Adolesc* 27:5–22, 2004.

Gentile DA, Stone W. Violent video game effects on children and adolescents: A review of the literature. *Minerva Pediatr* 57:337–358, 2005.

Giumetti GW, Markey PM. Violent video games and anger as predictors of aggression. *J Res Pers* 41:1234–1243, 2007.

Huesmann LR, Moise-Titus J, Podolski CL et al. Longitudinal relations between children's exposure to TV violence and their aggressive and violent behavior in young adulthood: 1977–1992. *Dev Psychol* 39:201–221, 2003.

Johnson JG, Cohen P, Smailes EM et al. Television viewing and aggressive behavior during adolescence and adulthood. *Science* 295:2468–2471, 2002.

Lemmens JS, Bushman BJ. The appeal of violent video games to lower educated aggressive adolescent boys from two countries. *Cyberpsychol Behav* 9:638–641, 2006.

Pinker S. *The Blank Slate: The Modern Denial of Human Nature.* New York: Penguin, 2002.

Porter G, Starcevic V. Are violent video games harmful? *Australas Psychiatry* 15:422–426, 2007.

Sheese BE, Graziano WG. Deciding to defect: The effects of video-game violence on cooperative behavior. *Psychol Sci* 16:354–357, 2005.

Sherry J. The effects of violent video games on aggression: A meta-analysis. *Hum Commun Res* 27:409–431, 2001.

Sherry J. Violent video games and aggression: Why can't we find links? in *Mass Media Effects Research: Advances Through Meta-analysis*. Edited by Preiss R, Gayle B, Burrell N, Allen M, Bryant J. Mahwah, NJ: Erlbaum, 2007, pp. 231–248.

Silvern SB, Williamson PA. The effects of video game play on young children's aggression, fantasy and prosocial behavior. *J Appl Dev Psychol* 8:453–462, 1987.

Slater MD, Henry KL, Swaim R et al. Violent media content and aggression in adolescents: A downward-spiral model. *Commun Res* 30:713–736, 2003.

Uhlmann E, Swanson J. Exposure to violent video games increases automatic aggressiveness. *J Adolesc* 27:41–52, 2004.

U.S. Department of Justice – Office of Justice Programs – Bureau of Justice Statistics. Key Crime & Justice Facts at a Glance – Serious violent crime levels declined since 1993. Available at http://www.ojp.usdoj.gov/bjs/glance.htm. Accessed June 15, 2009.

Weigman O, van Schie E. Video game playing and its relations with aggressive and prosocial behaviour. *Br J Soc Psychol* 37:367–378, 1998.

Williams D, Skoric M. Internet fantasy violence: A test of aggression in an online game. *Commun Monogr* 72:217–233, 2005.

17

Counseling in Cyberspace: Your E-Therapist Is on Call

John H. Greist, MD

When the ingenious Sumerian who invented writing first carved those cuneiform symbols in stone along the Tigris River some 6000 years ago, a skeptic standing nearby predicted with concerned countenance that people would soon stop talking to each other.

Warner Slack (2000)

Slack, who conducted the first patient–computer interview in 1965 (Slack et al. 1966), wrote with gentle irony about continued resistance to the intrusion of computer interviews into privileged clinician–patient communications. Having ventured into the sacrosanct domain of psychotherapy (Slack and Slack 1972), he reaped a whirlwind of criticism from psychotherapists. Whence this reaction, echoing the more dramatic and enduring reactions to Copernicus, Darwin, and Freud? Computer–patient interactions were yet another wound to mankind's ego. At a most heretical level, how dare one further diminish man's resemblance to God's image. How dare indeed! Humanitarian and scientific forces are answering that challenge.

What Computer-Based Therapy Is Available for Impulse Control Disorders?

The short answer is, "precious little." In their comprehensive 2007 review, "*Hands-On Help*," Isaac Marks and his colleagues found 97 computer therapy systems (Marks, Cavanagh, and Gega 2007) targeting disorders ranging from generalized anxiety disorder, panic disorder, and OCD to depression, substance abuse, and schizophrenia. Many programs had been studied in randomized controlled trials (RCTs), and some were in clinical use. No program addressed an impulse control disorder such as pathological gambling, kleptomania, trichotillomania, or pyromania.

Some computer programs to treat impulse control disorders are commercially available, however. Stoppicking.com and Stoppulling.com offer interactive help for skin picking and trichotillomania via the Web for "a dollar a day." Employing principles of habit reversal, neither appears to have been subjected to an RCT, and both remain confined to the never-never land of testimonial belief. A recent open-label evaluation of Stoppulling.com reports encouragingly:

Preliminary data from 265 users of the program during the first year of public availability suggested significant improvement in symptoms, with some evidence that duration of program use accounted for reductions in symptom severity. Response rates were comparable to long-term follow-up after more intense cognitive behavioral treatment. Stoppulling.com may provide a potentially useful self-help alternative or adjunctive strategy for repetitive hair pulling. (Mouton-Odum et al. 2006)

Stoppulling.com has been accessed by individuals in 40 countries, demonstrating the great potential reach of Web-based programs (Mouton-Odum, personal communication, 2008).

Web technology permits self-help versions of therapies to travel where no therapists are available.

Stoppingovershopping.com offers a Web-based treatment program for compulsive buying. The program includes a cognitive-behavior therapy (CBT) workbook, CD, reminder card, shopping diary, and instructions for how to apply these elements of the program. Three 1-hour telephone consultations are available as part of the program. Though the program is not completely standardized, it does illustrate use of the Web to deliver structured, evaluatable CBT. As with Stoppicking.com and Stoppulling.com, the program has not been subjected to scientific evaluation.

Because clinician-administered CBT for impulse control disorders has been demonstrated effective in RCTs, development of computer-assisted therapy programs is appropriate. But determining how well these programs work and in what models they are most effective will require additional RCTs. The considerable prevalence of impulse control disorders and the paucity of proven treatments make these disorders attractive opportunities for entrepreneurs. Still, many early computer-delivered treatment programs even when proven efficacious, have languished in the "valley of death" between creation and commercial viability.

Why Develop Computer-Based Psychotherapies for Impulse Control Disorders?

First, To Increase the Availability of Treatment

The problems in advancing the care of sufferers with impulse control disorders are the same as those for all medical disorders: frequent unavailability of any care; limited accessibility to care; poor standardization; cost; and prominently, a large gap between what is known and what is practiced. Historically, changes in medical practice occur slowly, even glacially, despite evidence of their benefit. Max Planck's maxim holds true for medicine as well as for other science-based professions: "A new scientific truth does not triumph by convincing its opponents and making them see the light, but rather because its opponents eventually die and a new generation grows up that is familiar with it." It is not surprising that psychotherapists, purveying the most interpersonal of treatments, might resist the implementation of therapies such as CBT that emphasize the preeminence of the patient as therapist, thereby relegating psychotherapists to the roles of educator, coach, and motivator.

We can first try to make high-quality CBT for impulse control disorders widely available by trying to train more CBT therapists, a worthwhile goal because skilled human therapists will always be needed. But this approach will continue to bump against the quality and quantity limits of human therapists. Second, self-help books written by some of these skilled therapists will help additional patients and additional therapists, who will refine their techniques after reading these patient guides.

However, transformative technologies offer the most hope for making CBT widely available. We have moved from land-line telephones to cell phones, from faxing to emailing and text messaging, and with miniaturized cameras, to sending individual video and audio information. All forms of communication are rapidly becoming available via small hand-held devices. To predict the future of technologies is hazardous, as shown by the following 1876 view from Western Union: "The telephone has too many shortcomings to be seriously considered as a means of communication." Nonetheless, computer-administered CBT can be provided via these new media. The World Wide Web is more accessible than ever. And the telephone, used as a computer terminal in interactive voice response (IVR) applications, can overcome the functional illiteracy of the more than 20% of the U.S. population who have difficulty reading but understand what they hear and can respond by speaking answers or pressing telephone number keys.

As described throughout this volume, cognitive-behavior therapy (CBT) is an effective treatment for many impulse control disorders. And as with OCD, where few receive CBT, few patients with impulse control disorders receive this form of treatment. Even for OCD, which is more commonly treated than most if not all impulse control disorders, the considerable attractions of CBT have proven insufficient – two NIMH-sponsored OCD treatment studies indicated that CBT has short-term efficacy twice that of FDA-approved serotonin reuptake inhibitor (SRI) medications for adults and children (Foa et al. 2005; POTS 2004), and another demonstrated long-lasting benefit (Marks 1997) compared with the frequent early relapse that follows SRI discontinuation (Pato et al. 1988).

Computer-administered self-help programs for impulse control disorders can easily be widely distributed. Unlike clinicians, they can be available 24/7, at times patients find convenient but therapists prefer not to be working. In the BT STEPS OCD program administered by telephone using IVR, 61% of calls occurred between 5 PM and 9 AM or on weekends, outside usual office hours; in COPE^{TM}, a companion depression program, 68% of contacts occurred in the same time span (Osgood-Hynes, Greist, and Marks 1998). Patients appreciate not having to commute to therapists' offices. They also appreciate the privacy of computer therapy as well as the greater comfort in disclosing sensitive subject matter to a nonhuman interviewer while recognizing its relevance for their care.

Second, To Overcome the Variable Quality of Clinician-Delivered Psychotherapy

For any form of therapist-delivered psychotherapy, the actual treatment is quite variable. As therapists move along in their careers, they innovate and improvise in attempts to improve results for their patients. This extensive and inevitable series of studies with an n of 1 yields idiosyncratic psychotherapeutics, sometimes better and sometimes worse than the mean, but inescapably variable. Fundamental tenets of science (accurate measurement, reliability, replication) are easily breached in clinical practice. Partly because even manualized therapies are at best variably applied (and because some psychotherapy is truly psychobabble), payment, even for CBT with proven efficacy, has been difficult to obtain. This lack of insurance coverage extracts a high social cost. But, reproducibly delivering effective psychotherapy is most challenging. Even idealistic internists were (McDonald 1976) and remain (Dexter et al. 2001, 2004) unable to implement proven medical practice algorithms such as influenza immunization without computer reminders, leading McDonald to his classic article's subtitle, "The Nonperfectability of Man."

Computer therapy programs can deliver reproducible treatments. The programs can be "trained" by recognized experts, who specify precisely what the program will do not only generally but across a host of situations and nuances, modeling the computer's responses on the responses of an expert therapist. Program branching is contingent on present and previous patient responses as well as changes in severity scores, passage of time, and other variables specified by the program's authors. Once programmed, computer therapy is standardized, including the built-in, tailored personalization.

Third, To Facilitate the Evaluation of Therapy Effectiveness

Programs can assess patient status with inherently blinded measures as well as via assessments possible only in this medium, such as Memory Enhanced Retrospective Evaluation of Treatment (MERET^{TM}), where the patient's voice, vernacular, and affects are recorded at baseline to anchor a later retrospective evaluation of change (Mundt et al. 2007). Programs document every interaction and the path of interactions. Data are ready for analyses at any time.

Fourth, To Improve Outcome

Paced by the patient, though with encouragement from the program, computer therapies can employ several communications media that increase treatment-effect size (Gould and Clum 1993). Electronic data capture makes ordinary and alarm reports to clinicians routine (Nierenberg et al. 2004).

Computer-administered therapies, like all therapies, are most beneficial when integrated into a stepped care treatment program. In stepped care, self-help that is not occurring (poor adherence is a major limiting factor with all treatments) or is occurring without expected benefits can be rapidly augmented by coaching to encourage program use to troubleshoot problems with CBT techniques. A single clinician can supervise computer-assisted self-help therapy for many patients, intervening directly with the few adherent patients who fail to improve by means of computer-assisted and clinician-monitored CBT alone.

Of course, no therapy works for everyone, and computer therapies are no exception. In the COPE depression program (Osgood-Hynes, Greist, and Marks 1998), 80% of those who, after sampling the program, thought it was "very logical" had a 50% or greater reduction in 17-item Hamilton Depression Scale scores, compared with 40% of those who rated COPE as "moderately logical" and none who rated COPE as "OK, not that logical (or) not at all logical."

Fifth, To Reduce the Cost of Psychotherapy

Costs for program development while substantial, are miniscule compared with those for medications, and once the program is developed, delivery costs are modest. Costs are also small compared with training clinicians, who then practice with variable abilities, algorithms, affects, and dialogues. Ongoing program evaluation in RCTs is facilitated by structured module creation and dismantling studies. When program improvements are made, updates are universally available, in striking contrast to the difficulty of delivering effective continuing education to clinicians.

Obstacles to Computer-Administered Self-Help Treatment

The situation with regard to CBT for OCD, for which the evidence base is large, provides some perspective. In more than three decades, little progress has been made in training therapists to provide CBT for OCD. The failure of clinicians to adopt proven new treatments is difficult to understand except as a part of humankind's difficulty in embracing new beliefs and paradigms. Many therapists practice what they were preached, more or less, for the rest of their careers. Beyond inertia, many therapists and their teachers are uncomfortable with the prospect of making anxious patients more anxious and uncomfortable in the short term with exposure and ritual prevention (ERP), the essential components of this form of CBT, even when the prospect of long-term gains is high. They forget that surgeons cut into patients, causing short-term injury and postoperative pain in order to excise or correct an underlying pathology. Also, remuneration for CBT may not be as great as for other psychotherapies because the CBT recommended by experts is time limited. Patients either benefit and move on to infrequent relapse prevention monitoring or ineffective therapy is discontinued after a few sessions. Habituation occurs in the patient – not in a psychotherapy dyad – and in order to benefit, the patient must carry out ERP homework sessions. Cognitive-behavior therapy is a true self-help therapy guided by the clinician.

The state of affairs in OCD led to development of BT STEPS™, a nine-step computer-administered, self-help, IVR CBT program. Its authors concluded wryly that it was easier to train a computer than therapists.

In an RCT for OCD (Greist et al. 2002), unaided use of BT STEPS was compared with 12 hours of CBT provided by well-trained CBT therapists at eight sites that were independent of the BT STEPS authors. Both treatments were compared with relaxation as a control treatment. In intent-to-treat analyses, clinician-treated patients reduced their Yale-Brown Obsessive-Compulsive Scale (Y-BOCS) scores more (mean $= 8.0$ points) than did BT STEPS patients (mean $= 5.6$ points), and both treatments were more effective than relaxation (mean $= 1.7$ points). For 63% of BT STEPS patients and 92% of therapist-treated patients who completed at least one ERP session, Y-BOCS scores decreased similarly in the

BT STEPS and the clinician-treated groups (a mean of 7.8 and 8.1 points, respectively). Both groups were more improved than the relaxation condition patients (with a 1.8 point mean decrease), of whom 78% had been compliant. Importantly, the intent-to-treat analysis showed that time spent obsessing and ritualizing decreased a mean of 3 hours 24 minutes *daily* for both BT STEPS and clinician-treated patients compared with a mean of 36 minutes for the relaxation controls.

Payment for development, evaluation, and implementation is another obstacle to developing computer-based self-help therapies. Excellent clinicians who might prepare programs are appropriately daunted by the time and monetary costs involved, as well as by the anticipated difficulties of mastering computer technologies and commercialization. Technology obstacles have largely disappeared, however, with the advent of excellent Web and interview-authoring languages or outsourcing to those facile in their use. Grants can pay for development and evaluation, but rarely for implementation. Developers and researchers are seldom effective at business development. Proven programs with grant-supported development and high projected commercial value have failed to reach the marketplace. For example, the RCT of the IVR BT STEPS program for OCD was completed in 1997, but the program languished until 2008, when it emerged as Web-based CT STEPS™, provided by Jazz Pharmaceuticals in conjunction with their launch of extended-release fluvoxamine (Luvox CR) for OCD. Nevertheless, the commoditization of interview-authoring languages permits face-valid therapy programs to be developed at comparatively low cost and launched on the strength of testimonials rather than RCTs. The FDA does not regulate psychotherapy.

Insurers have been reluctant to embrace computer-based therapies, stating that they will not pay for nonhuman therapy even when human therapy is rationed and often less effective. Many patients are reluctant to pay for psychotherapy, expecting it to be provided at no cost as part of their health care plan.

What Qualities Are Needed in Computer Therapies?

It is early in the course of the design, development, study, and dissemination of computer therapies. Early innovation invites and encourages variety. As one wit put it, the best way to learn is to make mistakes as fast as you can. Remembering Thomas Carlyle's dictum that our duty is "not to see what lies dimly at a distance but to do what lies clearly at hand," available technologies offer opportunities that were impossible a few years ago. Assuming a psychotherapy is of proven efficacy – and a few do pass scientific scrutiny – its presumed essential elements need to be specified in detail so that they can be communicated clearly to the patient and built into computer programs. At bottom, all psychotherapies are self-help therapies, depending on the acceptance of agreed principles and their application by the patient in his or her life.

Elements of effective human therapy that seem worthy of emulation in computer-assisted therapy include clarity, interactivity, flexibility, empathy, brevity, assessment and monitoring, and reinforcement of attempts at and accomplishment of therapeutic change. The extent to which the medium is the message remains uncertain. Many people prefer text, but while text is faster than voice, some cannot read; others prefer voice and the affect it conveys; at times, a picture may be worth many words. These communication opportunities are merging rapidly in hand-held devices, whose computing power doubles, according to Moore's law, about every 18 months, while their cost is halved. The check preventing the misapplication of this marvelous technology in psychotherapy will be the scientific method applied in RCTs. Large population studies with dismantling designs promise that the psychotherapy researcher's dream may be realized in our lifetime. Effective psychotherapies, tailored to the individual patient's needs and communication styles, will be widely available and easily evaluated.

Dr. Greist shares intellectual property rights in BT STEPS™, CT STEPS™, and COPE™ systems described in this chapter as well as other treatment programs that are not.

References

Dexter PR, Perkins SM, Maharry KS et al. Inpatient computer-based standing orders vs physician reminders to increase influenza and pneumococcal vaccination rates: A randomized trial. *JAMA* 292:2366–2371, 2004.

Dexter PR, Perkins S, Overhage JM et al. A computerized reminder system to increase the use of preventive care for hospitalized patients. *N Engl J Med* 345:965–970, 2001.

Foa EB, Liebowitz MR, Kozak MJ et al. Randomized, placebo-controlled trial of exposure and ritual prevention, clomipramine, and their combination in the treatment of obsessive-compulsive disorder. *Am J Psychiatry* 162:151–161, 2005.

Gould RA, Clum GA. A meta-analysis of self-help treatment approaches. *Clin Psychol Rev* 13:169–186, 1993.

Greist JH, Marks IM, Baer L et al. Behavior therapy for obsessive-compulsive disorder guided by a computer or by a clinician compared with relaxation as a control. *J Clin Psychiatry* 63:138–145, 2002.

Marks IM. Behaviour therapy for obsessive-compulsive disorder: A decade of progress. *Can J Psychiatry* 42:1021–1027, 1997.

Marks IM, Cavanagh K, Gega L. *Hands-On Help: Computer-Aided Psychotherapy*. Maudsley Monographs no. 49. New York: Psychology Press, 2007.

McDonald CJ. Protocol-based computer reminders, the quality of care and the non-perfectability of man. *N Engl J Med* 295:1351–1355, 1976.

Mouton-Odum S, Keuthen NJ, Wagener PD et al. Stoppulling.com: An interactive, self-help program for trichotillomania. *Cognit Behav Pract* 13:215–226, 2006.

Mundt JC, DeBrota DJ, Greist JH et al. Anchoring perceptions of clinical change on accurate recollection of the past: Memory enhanced retrospective evaluation of treatment (MERET®). *Psychiatry* 4:39–45, 2007.

Nierenberg AA, Trivedi MH, Ritz L et al. Suicide risk management for the sequenced treatment alternatives to relieve depression study: Applied NIMH guidelines. *J Psychiatr Res* 38:583–589, 2004.

Osgood-Hynes DJ, Greist JH, Marks IM. Self-administered psychotherapy for depression using a telephone-accessed computer system plus booklets: An open U.S.-U.K. study. *J Clin Psychiatry* 59:358–365, 1998.

Pato MT, Zohar-Kadouch R, Zohar J et al. Return of symptoms after discontinuation of clomipramine in patients with obsessive-compulsive disorder. *Am J Psychiatry* 145:1521–1525, 1988.

Pediatric OCD Treatment Study (POTS) Team. Cognitive-behavior therapy, sertraline, and their combination for children and adolescents with obsessive-compulsive disorder: The Pediatric OCD Treatment Study (POTS) randomized controlled trial. *JAMA* 292:1969–1976, 2004.

Slack WV. Patient–computer dialogue: A review, in *Yearbook of Medical Informatics 2000: Patient-Centered Systems*. Edited by van Bemmel J, Mccray A. Stuttgart: Schattinauer, 2000, pp. 71–78.

Slack WV, Hicks GP, Reed CE et al. A computer-based medical-history system. *N Engl J Med* 274:194–198, 1966.

Slack WV, Slack CW. Patient–computer dialogue. *N Engl J Med* 286:1304–1309, 1972.

Sexual and Aggressive Impulses

18

Hypersexuality: Clinical Aspects

Peer Briken, MD, Andreas Hill, MD, and Wolfgang Berner, MD

History of Psychiatric Attention to the Disorder

This chapter focuses on nondeviant sexual behaviors in men and women that escalate into serious consequences for the individual or others. Following Kafka (2000), we will call them "paraphilia-related disorders" (PRDs). However, models of sexual normality are constructed within a cultural discourse that changes over time (Klein 2002; Sigusch 1998). Sigusch (1998), for example, opines that during the period of "sexual revolution" (i.e., the 1960s), sex was mystified in a positive sense, as ecstasy and transgression, but has now taken on a negative aura characterized by abuse, violence, and lethal infection. Because expressions of sexuality are at special risk of being normalized, stigmatized, or medicalized, a clinically useful model has to consider the cultural, phenomenological, and political contexts alongside clinical aspects (Klein 2002).

Historically, the terminology and definitions regarding excessive sexual behavior have varied widely. Early references to such conditions can be found in the work of Hippocrates, Erasistratus, Plutarch, and Galen, each using different terms. For example, the expression "erotomania," also called de Clérambault's syndrome, after the French psychiatrist Gaëtan Gatian de Clérambault (1872–1934), has been used in different ways. Berrios and Kennedy (2002) describe four convergences in the history of erotomania. According to the first, erotomania was seen from classical times to the early eighteenth century as a general disease caused by unrequited love. According to the second convergence, which remained in use up to the nineteenth century, erotomania was a disease of excessive physical love (nymphomania). The third (twentieth-century) convergence focused on the view that erotomania is a form of mental disorder. The fourth and current definition sees erotomania as the delusional belief of being loved by someone else. So, under the current definition, erotomania would be part of a differential diagnosis but would not describe what we now understand as a PRD (see later).

In German-speaking countries, the terminology for a kind of addiction to sexual impulses has a long tradition that follows Richard von Krafft-Ebing's (1903) description of "hyperaesthesia sexualis," which shows similarities to morphinism and alcoholism. Giese (1962), a prominent German sex researcher, used an analogy to addictions for his diagnostic guidelines for sexual perversions (both for deviant forms such as sexual sadism and nondeviant sexual expressions such as Don Juanism). The guidelines he used included a decline to pure sensuality; an increase in frequency accompanied by a decrease in satisfaction; increasing promiscuity and anonymity of contacts; the elaboration of fantasy, practice, and refinement; a self-description of feeling compulsively addicted; and periodic restlessness. This definition was found to be useful not only clinically but also for decisions about criminal responsibility, and it is still integrated into the German penal code.

In the international literature, Carnes' description (1983, 1991) of "out-of-control" sexual behavior as an "addiction" was followed by an ongoing and controversial debate (Briken et al. 2007). Quadland (1985) characterized this behavior as "sexual compulsivity," whereas Barth and Kinder (1987) suggested the term "sexual impulsivity" and proposed to reserve the term "addiction" only for substance-related disorders. Schwartz (1992), noting the high rates of sexual victimization during childhood in persons who later show sexual addictive symptoms, regarded these symptoms as an aspect of posttraumatic stress disorder. According to Coleman, Raymond, and McBean (2003), "sexual compulsivity" may represent a variant of obsessive-compulsive disorder. Levine and Troiden (1988) criticized the whole concept of sexual addiction as being a stigmatizing myth.

Diagnosis

As we have already described, problematic forms of excessive sexual behavior have in recent years been given several terms, including compulsive sexual behavior, hypersexuality, excessive sexual drive, paraphilia-related disorder, nonparaphilic sexual addiction, sexual impulsivity, and impulsive-compulsive sexual behavior (Coleman, Raymond, and McBean 2003; Mick and Hollander 2006). The *Diagnostic and Statistical Manual of Mental Disorders*, 3rd edition (DSM-III-R) (American Psychiatric Association 1987), included the term "sexual addiction" under the category of "psychosexual disorders not otherwise specified," but this was dropped in the fourth edition (DSM-IV) (American Psychiatric Association 1994) and was not integrated into its later text revision (DSM-IV-TR) (American Psychiatric Association 2001). Currently, a PRD can be classified as an "impulse control disorder, not otherwise specified" or as a "sexual disorder, not otherwise specified."

In the tenth revision of the *International Classification of Diseases* (ICD-10; World Health Organization 1992), "excessive sexual drive" (Code F52.8) is part of the sexual dysfunction section. However, diagnostic criteria for this disorder are not specified. To our knowledge, investigations of cross-cultural aspects or comparisons of ICD-10 (World Health Organization 1992) and DSM-IV-TR (American Psychiatric Association 2000) concepts of PRDs have not been carried out.

Problematic forms of excessive sexual behavior may be classified in the upcoming DSM-V in a new category of disorders named behavioral and substance addictions (Mick and Hollander 2006). This tentative category may include several impulse control disorders (pathological gambling, pyromania, and kleptomania), as well as others currently included in the category of impulse control disorders not otherwise specified (Internet addiction and compulsive buying).

Goodman (1998) proposed a set of diagnostic criteria for addictive disorders that could be applied to either behavior disorders or substance abuse. Under his definition of addiction, any behavior used to produce gratification and to escape internal discomfort can become compulsive and constitute an addictive disorder. In his opinion, two key features distinguish sexual addiction from other patterns of sexual behavior: (a) the individual is not able to control the sexual behavior, and (b) the sexual behavior has significant harmful consequences but continues despite these outcomes. The addictive process is thus characterized by three major components: (a) aberrant functioning of the motivational reward system, (b) impairment of the self-regulation system, and (c) a tendency to use sexually related, external actions to cope with the effects of impaired self-regulation. Although this theory is supported by empirical data, it does not confirm the labeling of the behavior as an addiction. John Bancroft and his colleagues (Bancroft et al. 2003; Bancroft and Vukadinovic 2004) have found that the relationship between negative mood states and sexuality can be paradoxical – increased sexual desire and behavior may occur during negative mood states such as depression in some individuals (more often in men than in women and more often in those with relatively low levels of sexual inhibition and high levels of arousability). However, in view of the limited and variable data concerning etiology and treatment approaches, this group prefers to use the term "out of control sexual behavior."

Kafka et al. (Kafka 2000; Kafka and Hennen 1999, 2002) described the concept of PRDs, which they defined as "sexually arousing fantasies, urges or activities that are culturally sanctioned aspects of normative sexual arousal and activity but which increase in frequency or intensity (for more than six months duration) so as to preclude or significantly interfere with the capacity for reciprocal affectionate activity" (Kafka and Hennen 1999). In contrast to paraphilias, a group of sexual conditions characterized by deviant sexual arousal, PRDs were defined as disinhibited or excessive expressions of normal (i.e., nondeviant) adult heterosexual or homosexual object choice. According to Kafka and Hennen (1999, 2002), PRDs can occur as distinct disorders or as comorbid with paraphilias. The advantage of this concept seems to be that it uses a descriptive term without characterizing the putative underlying mechanisms (such as impulsivity, compulsivity, or addiction). Another strength may be that individuals with paraphilias and those with PRDs share many clinical characteristics (Kafka 2000). On the other hand, patients without paraphilic symptoms may feel stigmatized by the use of "paraphilia" as part of the term PRD. We have found Kafka's concept useful for research as well as for clinical purposes. However, we (Briken et al. 2007) recommend a more dynamic and course-related distinction between paraphilic and nonparaphilic forms of problematic excessive sexual behavior.

Differential Diagnosis
Paraphilias and Paraphilia-Related Disorders

Nonparaphilic problematic forms of excessive sexual behavior can occur in the context of other psychiatric disorders, most commonly in individuals with paraphilias. We proposed an algorithm (Briken, Hill, and Berner 2005; Briken et al. 2007) to distinguish comorbid nonparaphilic disorders from paraphilias. Diagnosis starts with the criterion of a recurrent failure to control sexually arousing fantasies, sexual urges, or behaviors over a period of at least 6 months. These sexual fantasies, urges, or behaviors cause clinically significant distress or impairment in social, occupational, or other areas of functioning. The disturbance is not better accounted for by another mental disorder (e.g., a manic episode) and is not caused by a general medical condition. The main distinction between the two types is that the paraphilic type involves unconventional sexual behaviors and the nonparaphilic type involves conventional, or at least nondeviant, ones. Within each type, several subtypes exist. Like Kafka and Hennen (1999, 2002), we use the term PRDs for the nonparaphilic type. Comorbidity between the paraphilic and the nonparaphilic types should only be diagnosed if nonparaphilic symptoms occur independently from paraphilic ones and are not a sign of a progressive course of a paraphilia. Many researchers and clinicians agree that symptomatology in paraphilias can worsen over time (Briken, Hill, and Berner 2005; Giese 1962; Goodman 1998). For example, if a paraphilic behavior is accompanied by an increase in masturbation frequency with paraphilic fantasies or behaviors and a decrease in satisfaction, excessive masturbation should not be diagnosed as a distinct disorder but viewed as a symptom of progression.

Other Disorders

Sexual obsessive thoughts are common in obsessive-compulsive disorder (OCD). However, the content of these thoughts consists most often of acting on violent sexual impulses or of fears of being a pervert or a homosexual that are not accompanied by sexual arousal and do not lead to sexual activities. Sexual impulsivity and increased libido or sexual drive are sometimes a symptom of manic or hypomanic episodes in bipolar disorder or an accompanying symptom of schizophrenia. If restricted to symptomatic phases of these disorders, these symptoms should not be diagnosed as a comorbid disorder. Delusional disorder (erotomania) can also lead to sexual impulsivity and stalking behavior and can be accompanied by a comorbid paraphilia or nonparaphilic PRD (Briken et al. 2005b).

Table 18.1 Differential diagnosis for paraphilia-related disorders (PRDs)

Differential diagnosis for PRDs
DSM-IV Axis I Psychiatric Disorders
Paraphilias
Bipolar affective disorder (type I or II)
Posttraumatic stress disorder
Adjustment disorder
Delusional disorder (erotomania)
Obsessive-compulsive disorder
Organic pathology
Brain lesions
Seizure disorder
Degenerative neurological disorders (e.g., Alzheimer's
    disease, Huntington's chorea, Parkinson's disease)

Although sexual impulsivity can be a symptom of borderline personality disorder (BPD), empirical evidence of an association between PRD and BPD is unclear. Lloyd et al. (2007), studying 85 patients with "compulsive sexual behavior," found only one who met full criteria for BPD, although many showed impulsivity, affective instability, and feelings of emptiness. In other therapeutic or forensic psychiatric contexts, however, this association may be stronger (Briken et al. 2006, 2007). For differentiating sexual impulsivity in BPD from PRD, the time criterion (symptoms for at least 6 months) seems to be the most useful distinction.

Symptoms of uncontrolled sexual behavior can also occur in the context of neuropsychiatric disorders (most commonly in frontal and temporolimbic brain lesions, as in multiple sclerosis, Wilson's disease, and Huntington's chorea). Altered sexual behavior is also common after L-dopa therapy in patients with Parkinson's disease (Briken et al. 2005a; Stein et al. 2000). When this behavior is caused by a medical condition, it should not be diagnosed as a PRD. Table 18.1 summarizes the differential diagnosis for PRDs.

Clinical Picture

Although the terminology used for expressions of sexual impulsivity varies considerably, the described symptoms, behaviors, or conditions are very similar and consistent (Briken, Hill, and Berner 2005, 2008; Coleman, Raymond, and McBean 2003; Kafka 2000). There is no specific category for these disorders in the DSM-IV-TR, and these symptoms and behaviors are not described. Table 18.2 gives an overview of these conditions adapted from Kafka (2000).

It seems important to recognize that there is a wide range of normal sexual expression (Coleman, Raymond, and McBean 2003) and no clear dichotomy between healthy and nonhealthy expressions of sexual behavior. For all these symptoms, and especially for forms of promiscuity and desire incompatibility, normative ideas can lead to confusion between (a) variants of behavior, (b) problematic behavior, and (c) pathologic behavior. Thus, looking at the behavior patterns alone without reflecting on underlying motivational contexts, negative consequences, and the course over time seems insufficient. Many of the observed motivational, emotional, behavioral, and relationship patterns are probably maintained through positive and negative reinforcement cycles that make clearly distinguishing causes, correlates, and consequences difficult.

Paraphilia-related disorders are often accompanied by loneliness and emotional distance from others (Briken et al. 2006; Hill, Briken, and Berner 2007). However, loss of friendships and family relationships may also result from the problematic sexual behavior. Partners of individuals with PRD may develop depressive, psychosomatic, or sexual symptoms as a

Table 18.2 Symptoms of paraphilia-related disorders (PRDs)

Symptom, Behavior, Condition	Objective for Sexual Arousal
Compulsive masturbation	Masturbation is the primary sexual activity even during a stable intimate relationship, most commonly at least once per day
Protracted promiscuity	Frequent one-night stands, use of prostitutes, brief sex affairs
Pornography, telephone sex, cybersex dependence	Persistent, repetitive, time-consuming patterns of use of pornographic material, telephone sex, and sexual chat rooms, with different levels of sexual arousal
Severe sexual desire incompatibility	Excessive sexual desire in one partner produces sexual demands on the other partner (who does not suffer from hypoactive sexual desire)
Other	Excessive prostitution, sexual harassment, and time-consuming and ego-dystonic sexual fantasizing

consequence of the individual's PRD. Financial problems may arise directly from the costs for the behavior (e.g., going to prostitutes or using telephone sex) or indirectly via decreased productivity or loss of employment (e.g., as a consequence of using the Internet for the sexual behavior at work and being fired). In a subgroup of individuals with PRDs, sexual behavior may result in a higher risk of sexually transmitted diseases (HIV/AIDS, herpes, syphilis, gonorrhea), genital injury, or the use of sexual enhancement drugs (e.g., "poppers" such as amylnitride or PDE-5 inhibitors such as sildenafil) (Coleman, Raymond, and McBean 2003).

Comorbid paraphilic behaviors (but also the PRDs) can be accompanied by illegal activities such as the use of child or animal pornography or sexual violence or offenses. Loss of professional status, financial problems, and even incarceration may result (Briken et al. 2006; Hill, Briken, and Berner 2007). Although PRDs may worsen the quality of life of individuals and their relatives, studies systematically focusing on this subject remain to be done.

The development of the World Wide Web has increased the availability of pornography and facilitated communication with people who have peculiar sexual interests. The possibility of reaching sexual gratification by a mouse click from home has reduced the social barriers against the use of pornography, especially in men, and has increased the proportion of people feeling a strong demand for regular consumption in an addictive manner (Hill, Briken, and Berner 2007). Specialized clinical departments report a steady increase in men seeking treatment because they feel addicted to such forms of consumption (Hill, Briken, and Berner 2007). A similar increase in prevalence is true for telephone sex, peep shows, and different forms of prostitution (Briken, Hill, and Berner 2005), which are legally and easily available in some countries and forbidden in others. Whether social regulations influence only the relation between open forms of consumption and secret forms or are able to suppress the PRD behavior as a whole is unknown. It seems reasonable to believe that the relationship may be similar to that observed in the realms of alcoholism and gambling, where strong regulations of available possibilities for consumption may reduce related activities for the greater part of the population but may motivate a small proportion to pursue dangerous and criminal activities.

Assessment Instruments

Several authors have formulated screening questions or questionnaires (Coleman, Raymond, and McBean 2003; Kafka 2000). The questions of Coleman, Raymond, and McBean (2003) (Table 18.3) seem particularly useful and clinically relevant. However, a

Table 18.3 Screening questions for paraphilia-related disorders (PRDs)

Do you, or others who know you, find that you are overtly preoccupied or obsessed with sexual activity?

Do you find yourself compelled to engage in sexual activity in response to stress, anxiety, or depression?

Have serious problems developed as a result of your sexual behavior (e.g., loss of a job or relationship, sexually transmitted infections, injuries or illnesses, or sexual offenses)?

Do you feel guilty and shameful about some of your sexual behaviors?

Do you fantasize or engage in any unusual or what some would consider "deviant" sexual behavior?

Do you find yourself constantly searching or "scanning" the environment for a potential sexual partner?

Do you ever find yourself sexually obsessed with someone who is not interested in you or does not even know you?

Do you think your pattern of masturbation is excessive, driven, or dangerous?

Do you find yourself compulsively searching for erotica for sexual stimulation?

Do you find yourself spending excessive amounts of time on the Internet engaging in various sexual pursuits?

Have you had numerous love relationships that are short-lived, intense, and unfulfilling?

Do you feel a constant need for sex or expressions of love in your sexual relationship?

Source: Coleman, Raymond, and McBean (2003).

positive response to these screening questions does not justify diagnosing a patient with a PRD. It can only suggest the need for a more detailed evaluation.

Tests

The Multiphasic Sex Inventory (MSI; Nichols and Molinder 1984) is a 300-item, true–false, self-report questionnaire consisting of statements about sexual activities, problems, and experiences. It is primarily intended to be used in assessing sexual offenders to develop treatment plans and to assess progress during treatment. The MSI has 20 scales, which include a variety of measures for sexual deviance and also a sexual obsession subscale. Test–retest reliability studies have shown the MSI to be stable over time. This instrument seems useful, especially in the context of evaluating paraphilic symptoms and sexual offenses.

Carnes (1991) developed a Sexual Addiction Screening Test as a self-assessment tool. This scale consists of 25 questions, with 13 or more positive responses indicating the presence of sexual addiction. The scale exhibited good reliability in an initial developmental study.

Kalichman et al. (1994) developed a scale by adapting items from a self-help guide for persons with "sexual addictions" for predicting sexually risky behaviors, in particular behaviors that put individuals at risk for HIV infection. This Sexual Compulsivity Scale (SCS) correlates with rates of unprotected sex and numbers of sexual partners.

The Compulsive Sexual Behavior Inventory (Coleman et al. 2001) contains three factors: control, abuse, and violence. Lower scores indicate higher levels of compulsive sexual behavior. A recent study (Miner et al. 2007) revealed validity for a two-structure model (control and violence).

Other than these questionnaires, no instrument or clinical interview has been developed to allow a reliable diagnosis of PRDs.

Prevalence

No systematic epidemiological or cross-cultural studies of this condition have been performed. This clearly has to do with the controversy about the disorders, the lack of officially accepted diagnostic criteria, and the lack of a validated diagnostic instrument. However, it has been estimated that 5% to 6% of the general population may be affected (Carnes 1991). This figure seems an overestimate because no studies have been undertaken. Small studies suggest that PRDs are more common in men than women (3–5:1 ratio) (Kafka 2000), but they may be affected by ascertainment bias. We observed a similar gender ratio in a German clinical outpatient sample (Briken et al. 2007). Langström and Hanson (2006) studied 2,450 men and women aged 18–60 years from a 1996 Swedish national survey of sexuality and health to identify correlates of "hypersexuality" (not hypersexual disorder in a clinical sense) in a representative, non-clinical population. First, indicators for "hypersexual" behavior were identified (e.g., rates of masturbation and pornography use). In the second step, the population was classified into three groups (low, moderate, or high) according to their hypersexual sexual behavior. The cutoff for the "high group" was set at three or more indicators for hypersexuality to identify as closely as possible the 90th percentile separately for each gender (12% of the men and 7% of the women). For both women and men, high rates of impersonal sex were related to separation from parents during childhood, relationship instability, sexually transmitted disease, tobacco smoking, substance abuse, dissatisfaction with life in general, and paraphilic sexual interests. The authors concluded that elevated rates of impersonal sex are associated with a range of negative health indicators in the general population. Although this study cannot clarify the causality of the observed correlations and should not be misinterpreted as a study of sexual disorders in the general population, it supports the importance of social (e.g., relationship aspects) and psychological factors in considering the observed behavior patterns.

Age at Onset

Remarkable or inappropriate sexual behavior in children and adolescents sometimes leads to child and adolescent psychiatric evaluations and treatment. Important diagnoses to rule out, especially in children, include neurological diseases such as Klüver Bucy syndrome. Excessive or impulsive sexual behavior may also be a reaction to difficult developmental factors, such as a self-soothing response to a nonsexual discomfort or an overstimulating environment (El-Gabalawi and Johnson 2007). Sometimes attention deficit hyperactivity disorder (ADHD) or mania in children and adolescents can be associated with problematic sexual behavior patterns.

The typical patient presenting with a PRD is in the mid-twenties to thirties, more often male, whose sexual behavior (increasingly related to Internet pornography consumption) has led to relationship, workplace, or financial problems. In the case of women, some seek help because they experience a "binge-starve" quality to their sexual behavior comparable to eating disorders. In one study (Briken et al. 2007), women were more likely to suffer from problems associated with promiscuity than men and less likely to experience compulsive masturbation or pornography dependence.

Another typical group of patients are self-identified "sex addicts," many of whom have serious problems in their personal relationships, with feelings of shame and guilt related to their sexual behavior. Some of these individuals fulfill the criteria for a PRD. Others do not suffer from any sexual or psychiatric disorder, but their moral ideas lead them to misinterpret and stigmatize their sexual behavior as pathological. Many of these individuals do not need PRD-specific psychotherapeutic treatment but rather informative and destigmatizing counseling.

Disinhibition caused by neurodegenerative diseases, including Alzheimer's disease, can lead to unusual, excessive sexual behavior in the elderly that can endanger their social status and respect. In this circumstance, a PRD should not be diagnosed.

Natural History and Course of Illness

The natural short-term and long-term courses of PRDs have not been studied. In clinical reports, many authors describe early imprinting sexual experiences, such as traumas, extreme oversexualization or sexual scruples in relationships to caregivers, and overstimulation by primary caregivers. The psychoanalytical theory that "perverse" expressions of sexual behavior in adults represent a "reversal of a defeat in childhood" (Stoller 1975) has been offered as one explanation for why sex becomes the "drug of choice" (Schneider and Irons 2001) as a coping strategy. Alternatively, Carnes (1991) describes the development of an addictive cycle that consists of preoccupation, ritualization, and sexual acting out followed by despair, shame, and guilt, which in turn are alleviated by renewed sexual preoccupation. Over time, the symptomatology may show progression.

Because age is one of the main variables affecting sexual drive, and because there is a decline in sexual desire and activity in middle-aged and elderly individuals compared with adolescents or young adults (Levine 2003), problematic sexual behavior expressions may lose some of their intensity (in the sense of biological drive) during the life span. Goodman (1998, p. 241) states that "while sexual addiction tends to be a chronic, lifelong disorder, the frequency of addictive sexual behavior typically peaks between the ages of 20 and 30, and then gradually declines." However, understanding PRDs as a form of coping with personal distress (anxiety, depression) (Bancroft and Vukadinovic 2004; Briken, Hill, and Berner 2008) makes it plausible that, even with decreased biological drive, the individual's behavioral coping patterns do not change automatically if motives, wishes, and psychological coping mechanisms have not changed.

Biological Data
Sexual Drive

Androgens (testosterone and dihydrotestosterone) play an important role in the hormonal regulation of male and female sexuality. In men, sexual activity may increase testosterone levels (Jannini et al. 1999). No studies have evaluated testosterone levels in individuals with PRDs. However, results from studies in sexual offenders and men with paraphilias do not support a hypothesis of relatively high testosterone levels associated with paraphilic behavior (Briken, Hill, and Berner 2003). Despite this, testosterone levels may be associated with aggression, violent behavior, or dominance. On the other hand, a normal testosterone level seems to be a necessary precondition for normal sexual drive or libido (Meston and Fröhlich 2000). Assuming that men with PRDs do not have an abnormal increased sexual drive but instead are using sexuality to cope with negative mood states, pharmacological agents that suppress testosterone production or action should be considered only in extreme cases (e.g., risk of harm to others) where suppressing the general sexual drive seems necessary.

Vulnerability of the Motivation–Reward System

It has been hypothesized that sexual fantasies and behaviors in men with PRDs are more strongly (positively or negatively) reinforced by the associated activation of the reward system. Blum et al. (2000) postulate dysfunctional brain reward cascades (caused by certain genetic variants) associated with hypodopaminergic traits. In such cases, the brain would require relatively high dopamine levels to allow the afflicted person to feel good. This may increase the risk for multiple addictive, impulsive, and compulsive behavioral propensities in areas such as drug use and sexual patterns. According to Berridge and Robinson's (2003) model, manipulation of the mesolimbic dopamine system may change the intensity of an individual's wanting of drugs. While "wanting" means the expectation of pleasure, the term "liking" describes the experience of pleasure, possibly mediated by endogenic opioids. However, many other neurotransmitters and neuropeptides may influence an aberrant reward system (for a review, see Goodman 2008). An opioid hypothesis, however, could support a rationale for using medications that influence the reward system (e.g., naltrexone).

Impaired Affect Regulation

Impaired affect regulation (Bancroft and Vukadinovic 2004; Briken, Hill, and Berner 2008; Goodman 1998, 2008) in individuals with PRDs could explain the relatively high prevalence of comorbid affective and anxiety disorders and the emotional instability that the individual may attempt to cope with by means of sexual behavior. Preexisting vulnerabilities or (traumatic) stress-induced dysregulations of the hypothalamic-pituitary-adrenal (HPA) system, as well as alterations in the norepinephrine and serotonin systems, may increase the risk for anxiety and affective disorders in these individuals. This hypothesis supports the use of mood stabilizing, anxiolytic, and antidepressant medications as therapies.

Impaired Behavior Inhibition, Impulsivity

Serotonin has been recognized as the main neurotransmitter associated with impulsivity in the sense of impaired inhibition of behavior (Briken and Kafka 2007). Despite evidence that supports the hypothesis of impaired behavioral inhibition in individuals with PRDs, no dysfunction of serotonin metabolism or receptors has been established. Data regarding pedophilic patients (Maes et al. 2001), and more indirectly from the suggested efficacy of selective serotonin reuptake inhibitors (SSRIs) (Briken and Kafka 2007; Hill et al. 2003), support this theory. Serotonin also inhibits sexual arousal and reduces orgasmic and ejaculatory capacity (Meston and Fröhlich 2000). However, the effects of serotonin vary for different serotonin receptors; for example, activation of 5-HT1A receptors accelerates ejaculation and activation of 5-HT2C receptors inhibits ejaculation (Waldinger 2008). Interestingly, the 5-HT2C receptor is the only receptor inhibiting many addiction-related behaviors (Goodman 2008).

Comorbid Conditions

The estimated prevalence and range of comorbid conditions varies widely because different concepts, definitions, instruments, behavior patterns, and study populations have been investigated. It appears that the more severe the symptoms and consequences of the PRD (especially their negative influence on relationships), the higher the psychiatric comorbidity.

Most studies have found high present as well as lifetime rates of other psychiatric disorders of up to 40% for anxiety disorders (especially social phobia), 70% for mood disorders (especially dysthymic disorder) and 30%–50% for substance abuse disorders (especially alcohol abuse) (Briken et al. 2007; Coleman, Raymond, and McBean 2003; Kafka and Hennen 2002). Men may also present with comorbid sexual dysfunctions (Briken et al. 2007). In an anonymous survey of 75 persons suffering from sexual addiction problems (Schneider and Schneider 1990), 39% reported substance abuse problems, 32% had an eating disorder, 13% characterized themselves as compulsive spenders, and 5% as compulsive gamblers. In addition, attention deficit hyperactivity disorder (ADHD) can be a comorbid condition in up to 18% of patients with PRDs (Kafka and Hennen 2002). Individuals with PRDs may also present with physical health problems, such as sexually transmitted diseases or abuse of sexual performance enhancers (e.g., "poppers") (Briken et al. 2008; Coleman, Raymond, and McBean 2003).

Treatments

Most experts agree that multimodal approaches, including various modalities (individual, group, family, and couples therapy; medication; self-help groups) and theoretical backgrounds (psychodynamic, cognitive behavioral, systemic) are most helpful (Briken, Hill, and Berner 2005; Briken et al. 2008; Delmonico, Griffin, and Carnes 2002; Kafka 2000). However, it is difficult to obtain empirical outcome data for such multimodal and individualized treatment approaches. Almost no short-term outcome data on therapeutic strategies for the treatment of PRDs fulfill higher criteria of evidence-based medicine (e.g., randomized controlled studies). Data on the long-term outcome are completely absent.

Treatment goals and the development of a treatment plan for PRDs vary with the predominating symptomatology, comorbidity, and the underlying hypothesis regarding the cause of the disorder. Most experts propose stage models with first-, second-, and third-order goals for the treatment (e.g., Briken, Hill, and Berner 2005; Delmonico, Griffin, and Carnes 2002; Goodman 1998; Kafka 2000).

First-Order Treatments

The first step in treatment includes a thorough diagnostic process and an evaluation of the sexual history. Exploring the patient's sexuality requires experience and empathy to avoid an atmosphere of shame. Issues that should be addressed in addition to the assessment of symptoms are:

> Sexual education
> First sexual experiences (e.g., playing doctor)
> Role of sexuality and intimacy in the family (shame, oversexualization, sexuality of parents)
> Physical development (e.g., puberty, menarche, urogenital surgery due to any medical condition, self-injurious behavior concerning the genitals)
> Development of sex role and identity
> Sexual fantasies (e.g., paraphilic interests)
> Beginning, frequency, and practices of masturbation; fantasies associated with masturbation
> Sexual contacts and relationships
> Sexual dysfunctions (these are very common in relationships in patients with PRDs)
> Pornography use (frequency, content)
> Use of the Internet for sexual purposes
> Prostitution (frequency, special interests, financial problems)
> Use of sexual enhancement drugs or other psychotropic substance use during sexual activities
> High-risk sexual behaviors, sexually transmitted diseases
> Traumatic sexual experiences
> Previous treatment experiences

In addition to obtaining formal diagnoses using DSM-IV-TR or ICD-10 criteria, this process should lead to an estimation of the relative importance of sexual interests and performance for the individual (general sexual drive and libido) across the life span (including in less problematic times) and of the former and present ability to control sexual urges and behaviors. The evaluation should also address whether positive (e.g., stimulation against boredom) or negative reinforcement (coping with anxiety or depression) strategies support the sexual behavior or whether the sexual behavior is even a form of pre- or parasuicidality (Goodman 1998; Hand 2004). A biaxial classification and monitoring of the symptomatology on two motivational continua of of (a) pleasure-seeking and (b) painful-affect-relieving behavior allows a distinction between more compulsive (motivated more by negative reinforcement) or impulsive (motivated more by positive reinforcement) forms (Goodman 1998).

The evaluation should also lead to a hypothesis about the psychic structure, the integration of sexuality into the personality, and the attachment style and capacity to build (not only sexual but also intimate) relationships. Evaluation should specifically address the centrality of splitting processes in self and object representations, evidence of dissociation, denial, affect isolation, and externalization of conflicts.

Goodman (1998, p. 158) suggests that the process in PRDs can be "understood as compulsive dependence on external action as a means of regulating one's internal (or subjective) states, one's feelings and sense of self." By using defense mechanisms such as splitting, denial, and affect isolation, the individual believes that he or she can control the behavior. Perhaps some individuals with a history of traumatizing experiences involving loss of situational control regain power with their sexual fantasies and behavior until this defense mechanism loses its ego-stabilizing function. Dissociative tendencies may be relevant by disrupting one's ability to focus on time (e.g., spent online) or on downstream consequences of behavior (Bancroft and Vukadinovic 2004). To assess these psychodynamic aspects, diagnostic instruments such as operationalized psychodynamic diagnostic systems (Cierpka et al. 2007) may be useful.

Many patients are ambivalent and need information and motivational help. Taking a history with a special focus on the sexual behavior and its negative and positive consequences is helpful. Doing this helps the clinician formulate treatment goals together with the patient and to inform the patient about the therapeutic options and strategies. Treatment goals in this first order should be realistic and short-term. The most problematic issues, like suicidality or harm to others, should be addressed first. Reducing access to the "drug of choice" is extremely helpful if possible, especially for those patients who use the Internet for their behavior. The Internet has been called a "triple-A engine" (Cooper 2002; Hill, Briken, and Berner 2007) because of its accessibility, affordability, and anonymity. Sex on the Internet (e.g., pornography, sex-focused chat rooms) is a very strong reinforcement trigger. Self-limiting time, changing to a provider that prefilters the content, installing screening software, and moving the computer to a location where others can see it may be concrete and helpful first steps (Delmonico, Griffin, and Carnes 2002).

Outpatient treatment for patients with PRDs is generally preferable (Goodman 1998) because it facilitates confrontation with the patient's real-life impulses and encourages reintegration into reality. However, indications for a hospitalization or admission to a specialized treatment facility may arise. These include (Goodman 1998):

Significant medical difficulty
Risk of harm to self or others
Inability to provide self-care
Unavailability of a living arrangement in which improvement can occur
Need to interrupt a cycle of behavior when outpatient treatment has been unsuccessful

It is also generally agreed that, no matter what the primary impulse control disorder or behavioral addiction is, a substance use disorder, if present, should be treated first (Schneider and Irons 2001).

Goodman (1998), during stage I, suggests using motivational and support techniques, as well as affect-regulating medications (SSRIs). Because of the limited data on positive effects and because of significant side effects, we believe that antiandrogens (cyproterone acetate, medroxyprogesterone acetate, GnRH agonists) should be restricted to dangerous cases in severe paraphilias (pedophilia or sexual sadism) or used as a transient option in patients with severe PRDs where suicidality or harm to others is related to a high sexual drive and an inability to control sexual fantasies or behaviors (Briken, Hill, and Berner 2003; Briken and Kafka 2007). There are no systematic outcome data regarding the use of antiandrogens in PRDs.

The effectiveness of SSRIs in depression, anxiety, and OCD has been demonstrated in many controlled, double-blind clinical studies. Since the early 1990s, SSRIs have also been used in the treatment of paraphilias and PRDs. Case histories have been followed by retrospective and prospective clinical studies (Briken et al. 2007; Hill et al. 2003). Recently, the first controlled study in 28 gay and bisexual men with a symptomatology similar to PRD revealed some positive results. Citalopram given at 20–60 mg/day led to a significant decrease in sexual drive, frequency of masturbation, and pornography use (Wainberg et al. 2006).

Possible mechanisms of action of SSRIs are (a) general inhibition of sexual activity; (b) reduction of impulsiveness; (c) relief of underlying depressive symptoms or anxiety disorders; and (d) an indirect reduction of testosterone serum levels (Hill et al. 2003). Thus, it seems reasonable to prescribe SSRIs, particularly in patients with underlying negative reinforcement strategies (escape from negative affects) and impaired behavior inhibition (impulsivity). Different SSRIs have been used (fluoxetine, fluvoxamine, paroxetine, sertraline, citalopram), as well as the primarily serotonergic tricyclic antidepressant clomipramine. No differences in treatment outcome have been found. Symptom improvement is generally seen after 2–4 weeks (maximum after 2 to 3 months). The SSRI doses are the same as those for depressive disorders; in some patients, however, increasing the doses to those used in OCD is necessary. If delayed ejaculation leads to increased use of sexual fantasies to reach orgasm, the dosage should be individually titrated; smaller doses are often sufficient to reduce symptoms. The side effects of SSRIs are the same as for other indications.

Studies on treating PRDs with anticonvulsants and atypical antipsychotics are lacking. Such medications could ameliorate sexual impulsive behaviors that are associated specifically with bipolar spectrum disorders, however (Briken and Kafka 2007).

Combining psychostimulants with SSRIs to treat both ADHD and sexual impulsivity has been reported (Kafka and Hennen 2000). However, the diagnosis of comorbid ADHD must first be firmly established because psychostimulants could increase sexual symptoms in individuals with a PRD without comorbid ADHD.

Finally, case reports and case series report the use of naltrexone (150–200 mg) for compulsive sexual behavior (for an overview, see Briken and Kafka 2007). The hypothesized mechanisms of action are an endogenous opiate receptor blockade, a subsequent accumulation of endogenous opioids, or the inhibition of dopamine release in the nucleus accumbens. These hypothesized mechanisms suggest that naltrexone may benefit patients in whom positive reinforcement strategies seem to be relevant (Hand 2004) or patients with a PRD and comorbid substance use disorder. Studies that investigate these issues are clearly needed.

Second-Order Treatments

Stage II treatment (stabilization of behavior and affect) uses relapse prevention techniques to distinguish between forms of sexual behavior that are high-risk and low-risk and to help the patient refrain from engaging in high-risk forms. Typical situational factors (e.g., the abuse of alcohol or conflicts with a partner), concomitant affect states (e.g., anxiety, depression, rage), cognitions, and consequential (sexual) behaviors should be monitored regularly. Keeping a daily diary concerning these factors may facilitate this. A diary helps identify early warning signs (Goodman 1998) and helps the patient avoid them. The development of alternative coping strategies or skills appears to be more successful than focusing on enhancement of control. Dialectical behavioral therapy (DBT) skills training (Linehan et al. 2006), stress and anger management, social competence training, and relaxation techniques can be helpful. Lapses and relapses should be discussed as soon as possible, reframed as a part of the disorder (if they do not include risk of self-harm or harm to others), and used to improve coping and relapse prevention strategies. Patients should develop ideas about which healthy rather than problematical form of sexuality they want in their lives. General lifestyle changes (e.g., balance between work and recreation) should be considered.

Relapse prevention may be conducted most effectively in a group setting. This resource is efficient and offers opportunities to establish meaningful relationships and to learn from identification and confrontation with others suffering from similar problems. Also, shame and guilt may be treated better in groups, where others can provide support.

Second-order treatment should also further address the psychological and pharmacological treatments of comorbid disorders discussed earlier.

Third-Order Treatments

During Stage III treatment, the therapeutic focus shifts from working on the behavioral level to the underlying or accompanying affects. Frequently, these often-painful affects seem to be isolated from behavior. Triggering situations should be identified, and affects and concomitant cognitions should be clarified. Another focus is on integration of sexuality and personality pathology. Therapy should enhance the capacity to build meaningful sexual as well as intimate interpersonal relationships (Goodman 1998). A transference-focused psychotherapy (TFP) approach that works mainly with current relationships (the relationship with the therapist or important emotional relationships outside therapy) may be useful. The most important issues to address here are again the analysis of splitting (e.g., a perception of others as all good or all bad) and denial. The precondition is a safe therapeutic relationship that allows the patient to explore these issues. Developmental aspects such as family dysfunctions and traumatic experiences or neglect may be addressed at this point. Sometimes, involving family members or couples therapy is useful, too. Couples therapy focusing on sexual problems using a sensate focus technique – such as Masters and Johnson's therapy or modified versions such as the Hamburg model of couples therapy for sexual dysfunction (Hauch 2006) – can help reestablish satisfactory sexual contact in emotionally meaningful relationships and to avoid more anonymous and promiscuous sexual behaviors.

If the PRD arose in a patient with a comorbid personality disorder such as borderline personality disorder (BPD) or narcissistic or antisocial personality disorder, programs for the treatment of these disorders should be applied. For borderline personality disorder, this may be DBT (Linehan et al. 2006) or TFP according to Kernberg (Clarkin et al. 2007; Critchfield, Levy, and Clarkin 2007). In cases of antisocial personality disorder, special facilities with experience in less compliant patients may be necessary. For narcissistic personality disorder, group and individual psychotherapy can be offered in cognitive behavioral as well as psychodynamically oriented forms. No clear empirical data show clear advantages for these different options.

The general indications for medication in treatment of personality disorders should be applicable. Some symptoms seem more medication-responsive in borderline personality disorder: affective symptoms appear to respond best; impulsivity second best; and aggressive behavior, dependency, and emotional emptiness least (Oldham 2001).

A special challenge for treatment are those PRDs that are comorbid with paraphilias. Literature on the treatment of sexual offenders very clearly shows that preoccupation with sexual themes (and PRD may represent such a preoccupation) is much more difficult to treat by means of sexual offender treatment programs normally used inside and outside prison to reduce the probability of relapses (Hanson, Morton-Bourgon, and Harris 2003).

The 12-steps program of Alcoholics Anonymous has been adapted in programs for sexual addiction (Sex Addicts Anonymous, SAA; Sex and Love Addicts Anonymous, SLAA; Sexaholics Anonymous, SA; etc.), as have programs modeled after Al-Anon (the mutual-help program for families and friends of alcoholics). Most of these self-help groups offer platforms on the Internet where concerned persons receive information material and can complete screening questionnaires. Self-help groups offer a support network, a free membership, and a framework for help for addictive problems (Goodman 1998). Not all patients will benefit from such groups, however. Patients posing a possible risk of harm to others, for instance, would be problematic for these groups. In addition, these patients may not benefit. Furthermore, large differences between the groups may exist depending on the particular members. Finally, some patients cannot accept the spiritual approach that many self-help groups follow. However, the system of self-help groups is important, and therapists should have the knowledge to advise their patients about this opportunity and about how to evaluate the safety and suitability of a particular group.

References

American Psychiatric Association. *Diagnostic and Statistical Manual of Mental Disorders*, 3rd edition. Washington, DC: American Psychiatric Association, 1987.

American Psychiatric Association. *Diagnostic and Statistical Manual of Mental Disorders*, 4th edition. Washington, DC: American Psychiatric Association, 1994.

American Psychiatric Association. *Diagnostic and Statistical Manual of Mental Disorders*, 4th edition, text revision. Washington, DC: American Psychiatric Association, 2001.

Bancroft J, Janssen E, Strong D et al. The relation between mood and sexuality in heterosexual men. *Arch Sex Behav* 32:217–230, 2003.

Bancroft J, Vukadinovic Z. Sexual addiction, sexual compulsivity, sexual impulsivity, or what? Toward a theoretical model. *J Sex Res* 41:225–234, 2004.

Barth RJ, Kinder BN. The mislabeling of sexual impulsivity. *J Sex Marital Ther* 13:15–23, 1987.

Berridge KC, Robinson TE. Parsing reward. *Trends Neurosci* 29:507–513, 2003.

Berrios GE, Kennedy N. Erotomania: A conceptual history. *Hist Psychiatry* 13:381–400, 2002.

Blum K, Braverman ER, Holder JM et al. Reward deficiency syndrome: A biogenetic model for the diagnosis and treatment of impulsive, addictive, and compulsive behaviours. *J Psychoactive Drugs* 32(suppl i–iv): 1–112, 2000.

Briken P, Habermann N, Berner W et al. The influence of brain abnormalities on psychosocial development, criminal history and paraphilias in sexual murderers. *J Forensic Sci* 50:1204–1208, 2005a.

Briken P, Habermann N, Berner W et al. Diagnosis and treatment of sexual addiction: A survey among German sex therapists. *Sex Addict Compulsivity* 14:131–143, 2007.

Briken P, Habermann N, Kafka MP et al. The paraphilia-related disorders: An investigation of the relevance of the concept in sexual murderers. *J Forensic Sci* 51:683–688, 2006.

Briken P, Hill A, Berner W. Pharmacotherapy of paraphilias with long-acting agonists of luteinizing hormone-releasing hormone: A systematic review. *J Clin Psychiatry* 64:890–897, 2003.

Briken P, Hill A, Berner W. Sexuelle Sucht: Diagnostik, Ätiologie, Behandlung. *Z Sexualforsch* 18:185–197, 2005.

Briken P, Hill A, Berner W. Kann Sex süchtig machen? [Can sex become addictive?] *MMW Fortschr Med* 150:32–34, 2008.

Briken P, Hill A, Nika E et al. Obszöne Telefonanrufe – Beziehungen zu Paraphilien, Paraphilie verwandten Störungen und "Stalking." [Obscene telephone calls – relation to paraphilias, paraphilia related disorders and stalking.] *Psychiatr Prax* 32:304–307, 2005b.

Briken P, Kafka MP. Pharmacological treatments for paraphilic patients and sexual offenders. *Curr Opin Psychiatry* 20:609–613, 2007.

Carnes PJ. *Out of the Shadows: Understanding Sexual Addiction.* Minneapolis, MN: CompCare Publications, 1983.

Carnes PJ. *Don't Call It Love: Recovery from Sexual Addiction.* New York: Bantam Books, 1991.

Cierpka M, Grande T, Rudolf G et al. The operationalized psychodynamic diagnostics system: Clinical relevance, reliability and validity. *Psychopathology* 40:209–220, 2007.

Clarkin JF, Levy KN, Lenzenweger MF et al. Evaluating three treatments for borderline personality disorder: A multiwave study. *Am J Psychiatry* 164:922–928, 2007.

Coleman E, Miner M, Ohlerking F et al. Compulsive sexual behavior inventory: A preliminary study of reliability and validity. *J Sex Marital Ther* 27:325–332, 2001.

Coleman E, Raymond N, McBean A. Assessment and treatment of compulsive sexual behaviour. *Minn Med* 86:42–47, 2003.

Cooper A. *Sex and the Internet.* New York: Brunner-Routledge, 2002.

Critchfield KL, Levy KN, Clarkin JF. The Personality Disorders Institute / Borderline Personality Disorder Research Foundation randomized control trial for borderline personality disorder: Reliability of Axis I and II diagnoses. *Psychiatr Q* 78:15–24, 2007.

Delmonico DL, Griffin E, Carnes PJ. Treating online compulsive sexual behavior: When cybersex is the drug of choice, in *Sex and the Internet.* Edited by Cooper A. New York: Brunner-Routledge, 2002, pp. 147–167.

El-Gabalawi F, Johnson RA. Hypersexuality in inpatient children and adolescents: Recognition, differential diagnosis, and evaluation. *CNS Spectr* 12:821–827, 2007.

Giese H. *Psychopathologie der Sexualität.* Stuttgart: Enke, 1962.

Goodman A. *Sexual Addiction: An Integrated Approach.* Madison, CT: International Universities Press, 1998.

Goodman A. Neurobiology of addiction: An integrative review. *Biochem Pharmacol* 75:266–322, 2008.

Hand I. Negative und positive Verstärkung bei pathologischem Glücksspielen: Ihre mögliche Bedeutung für die Theorie und Therapie von Zwangsspektrumsstörungen. [Negative and positive reinforcement in pathological gambling: Their potential impact on theory and therapy of obsessive-compulsive spectrum disorders.] *Verhaltenstherapie* 14:133–144, 2004.

Hanson RK, Morton-Bourgon K, Harris AJR. Sexual offender recidivism risk: What we know, and what we need to know. *Ann NY Acad Sci* 989:151–166, 2003.

Hauch M. *Paartherapie bei sexuellen Störungen.* Stuttgart: Thieme, 2006.

Hill A, Briken P, Berner W. [Pornography and sexual abuse in the Internet.] *Bundesgesundheitsblatt Gesundheitsforschung Gesundheitsschutz* 50:90–102, 2007.

Hill A, Briken P, Kraus C et al. Differential pharmacological treatment of paraphilias and sex offenders. *Int J Offender Ther Comp Criminol* 47:407–421, 2003.

Jannini EA, Screponi E, Carosa E et al. Lack of sexual activity from erectile dysfunction is associated with a reversible reduction in serum testosterone. *Int J Androl* 22:385–392, 1999.

Kafka MP. The paraphilia-related disorders, in *Principles and Practice of Sex Therapy.* Edited by Leiblum SR, Rosen RC. New York: The Guilford Press, 2000.

Kafka MP, Hennen, J. The paraphilia-related disorders: An empirical investigation of nonparaphilic hypersexuality disorders in outpatient males. *J Sex Marital Ther* 25:305–319, 1999.

Kafka MP, Hennen J. Psychostimulant augmentation during treatment with selective serotonin reuptake inhibitors in men with paraphilias and paraphilia-related disorders: A case series. *J Clin Psychiatry* 61:664–670, 2000.

Kafka MP, Hennen J. A DSM-IV Axis I comorbidity study of males ($n = 120$) with paraphilias and paraphilia-related disorders. *Sex Abuse* 14:349–366, 2002.

Kalichman SC, Johnson JR, Adair V et al. Sexual sensation seeking: Scale development and predicting AIDS-risk behavior among homosexually active men. *J Pers Assess* 62:385–397, 1994.

Klein M. Sexual addiction: A dangerous clinical concept. 2002. Available at http://www.ejhs.org/volume5/SexAddiction.htm.

Krafft-Ebing R. *Psychopathia sexualis.* Stuttgart: Enke, 1903.

Långström N, Hanson RK. High rates of sexual behavior in the general population: Correlates and predictors. *Arch Sex Behav* 35:37–52, 2006.

Levine MP, Troiden RR. The myth of sexual compulsivity. *J Sex Res* 25:347–363, 1988.

Levine SB. The nature of sexual desire: A clinician's perspective. *Arch Sex Behav* 32:279–285, 2003.

Linehan MM, Comtois KA, Murray AM et al. Two years randomized controlled trial and follow-up of dialectical behavior therapy vs. therapy by experts for suicidal behaviors and borderline personality disorder. *Arch Gen Psychiatry* 63:757–766, 2006.

Lloyd M, Raymond N, Miner M et al. Borderline personality traits in individuals with compulsive sexual behavior. *Sex Addict Compulsivity* 14:187–206, 2007.

Maes M, van West D, De Vos N, Westenberg H et al. Lower baseline plasma cortisol and prolactin together with increased body temperature and higher mCPP-induced cortisol responses in men with pedophilia. *Neuropsychopharmacology* 24:37–46, 2001.

Meston CM, Frohlich PF.The neurobiology of sexual function. *Arch Gen Psychiatry* 57:1012–1030, 2000.

Mick TM, Hollander E. Impulsive-compulsive sexual behavior. *CNS Spectr* 11:944–955, 2006.

Miner MH, Coleman E, Center BA et al. The compulsive sexual behavior inventory: Psychometric properties. *Arch Sex Behav* 36:579–587, 2007.

Nichols HR, Molinder I. *Manual for the Multiphasic Sex Inventory.* Tacoma, WA: Crime and Victim Psychology Specialists, 1984.

Oldham JM. Integrated treatment planning for borderline personality disorders, in *Integrated Treatment of Psychiatric Disorders.* Edited by Kay J. Washington, DC: American Psychiatric Publishing, 2001, pp. 51–77.

Quadland MC. Compulsive sexual behavior: Definition of a problem and approach to treatment. *J Sex Marital Ther* 11:121–132, 1985.

Schneider JP, Irons RR. Assessment and treatment of addictive sexual disorders: Relevance for chemical dependency relapse. *Substance Use Misuse* 36:1795–1820, 2001.

Schneider JP, Schneider BH. Marital satisfaction during recovery from self-identified sexual addiction among bisexual men and their wives. *J Sex Marital Ther* 16:230–250, 1990.

Schwartz MF. Sexual compulsivity as post-traumatic stress disorder: Treatment perspectives. *Psychiatr Ann* 22:333–338, 1992.

Sigusch V. The neosexual revolution. *Arch Sex Behav* 27:331–359, 1998.

Stein DJ, Hugo F, Oosthuizen P et al. Neuropsychiatry of hypersexuality. *CNS Spectr* 5:36–46, 2000.

Stoller RJ. *Perversion: The Erotic Form of Hatred.* New York: Pantheon, 1975.

Wainberg ML, Muench F, Morgenstern J et al. A double-blind study of citalopram versus placebo in the treatment of compulsive sexual behaviors in gay and bisexual men. *J Clin Psychiatry* 67:1968–1973, 2006.

Waldinger MD. Premature ejaculation: Different pathophysiologies and etiologies determine its treatment. *J Sex Marital Ther* 34:1–13, 2008.

World Health Organization. Tenth revision of the *International Classification of Diseases*, Chapter V (F): Mental and behavioural disorders. Diagnostic criteria for research. Geneva: World Health Organization, 1992.

19

The Sex Industry: Public Vice, Hidden Victims

William M. Spice, MRCP

Introduction

Commercial sex work encompasses a highly heterogeneous range of activities. It may act as the sole source of income for an individual or be used to augment earnings derived from other activities. Equally diverse is the range of individuals who engage in sex work, whether female, male, or transgendered. Although this chapter focuses on the health costs to female sex workers, many of the same principles also apply to those who are male or transgendered.

The basic transaction that underlies all sex work is the exchange of sexual services for economic compensation, usually in the form of money or drugs. Historically, such exchanges have been taken to involve direct physical contact between the worker and the client. However, in recent years, communications technology has allowed other "noncontact" forms of sex work, for example telephone sex lines and Internet webcams to proliferate. The Internet has also been the vehicle for a massive expansion in pornography in which, again, both sex workers and customers are anonymous and topographically remote (Ward and Aral 2006). The worker and the client come into closer proximity in striptease and lap-dancing venues, but direct contact remains minimal, ensuring little if any risk of physical harm (Harcourt and Donovan 2005). While women in these occupations are undoubtedly at risk of exploitation and coercion, exploring these aspects is beyond the scope of this chapter. Here we will deal with the factors that are most important in determining the level of risk that accrues from direct physical contact between the sex worker and the client.

Sex workers are some of the most marginalized and stigmatized members of society and suffer from a correspondingly high level of morbidity and mortality compared with other groups. Risks to the health and well-being of sex workers fall into four interrelated categories: physical violence, the sequelae of injected drug use, acquisition of blood-borne viruses and other sexually transmitted diseases, and injury to mental health. The physical, social, and economic setting in which sex work takes place defines the extent to which these risks come into play and hence the overall jeopardy suffered by the individual.

Violence

Violence or the threat of violence, whether sexual, physical, or verbal, is an almost universal experience for sex workers. Because of the illegal nature of sex work in the majority of settings, workers are less likely to report assaults, and clients may feel that sex workers are "fair game" (Barnard 1993). In a questionnaire survey of 115 outdoor and 125 indoor workers in three British cities (Leeds, Glasgow, and Edinburgh), Church et al. (2001) found that only one-third of sex workers had ever reported an assault to the police. Sex workers are at risk of violence not only from clients but also from pimps, vigilantes, nonpaying partners, and, in some countries, the police themselves (Alexander 1998; El Bassel et al. 2001).

In a study of 475 sex workers in five countries (South Africa, Thailand, Turkey, the United States, and Zambia), Farley et al. (1998) found that between 50% and 78% had been raped during their time as sex workers. Ward, Day, and Weber (1999) reported a mortality rate of 5.93 per 1,000 person years in a prospective study of London sex workers (12 times the expected rate for women of a similar age), half of which was due to murder. Potterat et al. (2004) studied mortality in a cohort of Colorado sex workers between 1967 and 1999 and calculated a crude mortality rate for death by homicide of 229 per 100,000, many times the rate for women in the general population. Male taxicab drivers in comparison had a murder rate of 29 per 100,000. The extreme dangers of street sex work were brought into sharp focus by the murder of five women by a serial killer in Ipswich, United Kingdom, in 2006 (Ipswich Murder Probe Amnesty Call, http://news.bbc.co.uk, December 11, 2006). The following subsections discuss the factors associated with increased risk of violence.

Physical Setting

Venues for sex work range from outdoor settings such as the street and truck stops to massage parlors, brothels, private apartments, and hotels. It is generally accepted that outdoor workers are at higher risk of violence, particularly when working alone. In a study by Church et al. (2001), 50% of street workers had experienced violence over the previous 6 months, compared with 26% of those working from premises. Outdoor sex work was associated with a risk several times as great as indoor work in most categories examined. Assaults ranged from kicking, punching, and slapping to rape, strangulation, and stabbing. A higher incidence of violence in street as opposed to indoor sex work was also reported in studies by Farley et al. (1998), Pyett and Warr (1997), and Sanders (2004). A study of flat-working women in London conducted by Whittaker and Hart (1996) highlighted the advantages of having a maid who helps to vet clients, look after money, and call for assistance if needed.

Criminalization and the Law

Street sex work is criminalized in almost every part of the world. The added pressures placed on workers to avoid detection can increase the risk of violence. For example, the likelihood of arrest may lead workers to operate in less visible or familiar settings (Alexander 1998). The worker's ability to negotiate a transaction and to size up potentially dangerous clients may be compromised by the need to get into the client's car as quickly as possible (Alexander 1998; Barnard 1993). Making up for income lost as a result of detention or fines may increase the pressure to agree to unprotected sex for more money or to take on "dodgy" clients who might otherwise have been declined.

In contrast, the law affords sex workers a degree of protection if they operate in a regulated setting. For example, legalized brothels in Victoria, Australia, and Nevada in the United States provide a more secure, managed environment and the possibility of legal redress in the event of assault (Brents and Hausbeck 2005; Pyett and Warr 1997). Drawbacks of legalized brothels have been cited, however, in terms of loss of the worker's freedom to refuse clients or to leave the premises when they choose (Farley et al. 1998).

Drug Use

The use of cocaine, crack cocaine, and heroin is both common among street sex workers and integrally linked to an increased risk of violence from commercial clients and pimps (Kurtz et al. 2004; Pyett and Warr 1997). The study of New York street workers by El-Bassel et al. (1997) showed that the use of injected heroin predicted violence with an odds ratio of 9.81, which was more statistically significant than other factors, including homelessness and visiting crack houses. Surratt et al. (2004) reported similar findings in a study of street-based sex workers in Miami. Use of crack or heroin while working was strongly predictive of violence, along with other indicators, including financial hardship and having sex in the client's car. Pyett and Warr (1997) attributed the greater risk of violence among sex workers who use drugs to their reduced capacity to recognize and manage potentially dangerous situations. Other authors have suggested that the known effects of crack cocaine in increasing verbal aggression may precipitate violent responses from the client or the pimp, in addition to the irritability associated with coming down from a "high" (Sterk and Elifson 1990). Furthermore, clients may be more inclined to abuse sex workers who are known to be using drugs as a result of the additional stigma attached to the habit or seeing them as "soft targets" (El-Bassel et al. 2001).

Sexually Transmitted Disease

The historical portrayal of commercial sex workers as reservoirs of infection, particularly HIV, is well documented (Cameron 1998; D'Costa et al. 1985; McCarthy, Khalid, and El Tigani 1995; Padian 1988; Rosenberg and Weiner 1988). This assumption has been challenged by a number of studies showing that rates of sexually transmitted infections (STI) are low in many sex worker groups and that these low rates are strongly linked to the use of condoms. Furthermore, as the rate of female-to-male transmission of HIV is approximately one-half the rate from male to female, it could be argued that sex workers are at higher risk than their clients.

Ward et al. (1993) reported an HIV prevalence of 0.9% among 228 London sex workers recruited between 1989 and 1991 who reported condoms being used for 98% of all commercial transactions. The incidence of other acute sexually transmitted infections including gonorrhea, chlamydia, trichomonas, and primary genital herpes was strongly associated with nonpaying partners, for whom condom use was only 12%. In the 1999 study by Ward, Day, and Weber, 320 sex workers recruited between 1985 and 1991 were followed for a total of 675 person years up to 1994. Baseline prevalence rates were 1.3% for HIV, 2.3% for syphilis, 3.0% for gonorrhea, and 8.2% for chlamydia. Condom use with paying clients increased significantly over the study period. Viral infections were associated with injecting drugs and bacterial infections with noncommercial partners.

These results were reinforced by a comparison of STI rates in London sex workers studied over the periods 1985–1992 and 1996–2002 (Ward et al. 2004). A significant decline from 80% to 32% occurred in those reporting any previous STI, and the proportion of participants with a current STI fell from 25% to 8%. This was against the background of a rising incidence in the general population and was again attributed largely to increased condom use with commercial clients. For comparison, a study of 783 sex workers (female, male, and transgendered) in San Francisco (Cohan et al. 2006) yielded rates of 1.8% for syphilis, 12.4% for gonorrhea, and 6.8% for chlamydia.

The most important factors affecting the risk of STI are considered in the following subsections.

Use of Condoms

Condoms remain the most effective measure for preventing sexually transmitted infections. In the context of sex work, the likelihood of effective condom use is critical in determining the burden of morbidity from infections acquired by this route. The highest rates of condom use are found in controlled environments such as massage parlors and brothels. A prospective study of 41 state-registered sex workers in three licensed Nevada brothels found that condoms had been used for vaginal intercourse in 100% of the 353 transactions analyzed (Albert et al. 1995). There were no cases of condoms breaking, and reports of slippage were infrequent, suggesting that sex workers are able to maintain a high level of protection in situations where condom use is the norm.

Pyett, Haste, and Snow (1996) also reported little occupation-related risk in a survey of sex workers in the legalized brothels of Victoria, Australia. The main risk factors were related to having unprotected sex with noncommercial partners and injected drug use (IDU). A further study of 388 Melbourne brothel workers undertaken by Lee et al. in 2005 showed a low incidence of STI, with 0.61 cases of chlamydia per 100 person months. Adherence to the use of condoms with paying clients was 100%. Again, the main risk was unprotected sex with noncommercial clients: those who reported no intimate partners for the previous 3 months had an incidence of 0.15 per 100 person months, whereas the incidence among those with one or more intimate partners was 0.87.

In settings where sex work is unregulated, such as the street, condom use may be patchy and inconsistent for several reasons. First, workers who are suffering economic hardship or supporting expensive drug habits may have a low threshold for agreeing to unprotected sex for more money (Alexander 1998; Baker, Case, and Policiccio 2003; Barnard 1993; Jeal and Salisbury 2004). Secondly, women operating on their own may have unprotected sex forced on them, amounting to rape (Barnard 1993; El-Bassel et al. 2001; Sanders 2004). Thirdly, police in some countries regard possession of condoms as evidence of sex work and pursue a policy of confiscation (Alexander 1998).

Drug Use

Injected drug use (IDU) is the second most common route of HIV infection after sexual transmission, and consequently sex workers who share injection equipment are at heightened risk. This was evident in a study of incarcerated sex workers in Connecticut. Those who had practiced IDU were found to have an HIV rate of 28%, compared with 8% in those who had not (Blakenship et al. 1996). Among street sex workers in Ho Chi Minh City in Vietnam, IDU carried an odds ratio of 66 for HIV acquisition in a univariate analysis (Tuan et al. 2004). The epidemic of HIV infection in Russia since 1995 has accompanied a similar rise in injected drug use, with rates of infection among sex workers in different cities ranging from 15% to 65% (Lowndes, Alary, and Platt 2003). Seroprevalence for HIV type 1 in a group of 71 female sex workers operating in a range of indoor and outdoor settings in southern Catalonia, Spain, was 11.3%, most of which could be accounted for by IDU (Casabona et al. 1990). Similarly, the prevalence of HIV among 6,400 injected drug users in 16 U.S. municipalities was 12.7% (Kral et al. 1998).

Injected drug use and HIV are not so strongly linked in situations where needle and syringe exchange facilities are available. A study of 206 street sex workers in Glasgow (McKeganey et al. 1992) revealed that 147 (71%) were injecting drugs, a considerably higher proportion than reported elsewhere in the United Kingdom. Of the 115 workers tested for HIV, however, only 4 (3.5%) were positive (2.5% overall). Condom use was reported to be universal. The relatively low HIV seroprevalence in this group was attributed to the availability of clean injection equipment and condoms from a drop-in clinic operating within the red light area.

Hepatitis B and C are two other blood-borne viruses, often resulting in chronic infection, that may be transmitted either sexually or through IDU-related activities (although sexual transmission of hepatitis C appears largely confined to HIV-positive men who have sex with men). A study of 586 IDU female street sex workers in Miami found infection rates of 53.4% and 29.7% for hepatitis B and C, respectively, compared with 22.4% for HIV (Inciardi, Surratt, and Kurtz 2006).

Narcotics

Drug use is extremely widespread among sex workers, particularly in the street context, with the prevalence in New York estimated at over 80% (Plant 1990). Drugs used by sex workers include marijuana, alcohol, cocaine, crack cocaine, heroin, and speed (amphetamines). Some of the most serious health consequences relate to drugs, such as cocaine and heroin, that can be injected. These include skin infections at injection sites, thrombosis, pulmonary embolism, mycotic aneurysm, infective endocarditis, and death through overdose or the presence of contaminating substances. Crack smoking causes a wide range of cardiovascular, neurological, and pulmonary complications, including myocardial dysrhythmias, endocarditis, hypertension, stroke, cerebral hemorrhage, pneumonia, interstitial pneu-monitis, pulmonary edema, hemorrhage, and infarction. Crack smoking also results in skin trauma around the mouth and lips due to the heat generated by the crack pipe. Wallace et al. (1992, 1997) postulated that unprotected oral sex in the presence of perioral trauma is an important route of HIV transmission. They found a significant association between crack smoking and HIV in a study of sex workers in Manhattan.

There is an important distinction between those who do not start using drugs until after starting sex work and those whose primary reason for entering sex work is to support their habit. The first group, sometimes known as "before crack" workers, are regarded as having a more professional approach to sex work, including rigorous adherence to the use of condoms. In contrast, the second group, known as "after crack" workers, are held to be more likely to agree to lower prices for their services, practice unsafe sex for more money, and accept crack as direct payment (Alexander 1998). The exchange of sex for crack is well recognized in U.S. cities, and such women, known as "strawberries," are likely to be homeless and to live in poverty (Elwood et al. 1997). In a study of the relationship between drug use and commercial sex in Houston, Texas, Baseman, Ross, and Williams (1999) found that any lifetime use of drugs was strongly predictive of selling sex, with an odds ratio of 15.45. Current use of crack cocaine had an odds ratio of 6.24, compared with 2.11 for heroin and 1.82 for cocaine.

Mental Health

There are two main issues concerning commercial sex work and mental health. The first is the extent to which psychological problems originate from experiences that precede an individual's entry into sex work as opposed to being a consequence of it. The second is whether adverse experiences such as physical and sexual assault are the main cause of psychological trauma or whether it is the inherent transformation of the worker into a commodity, a sexual object, that causes emotional distress, regardless of the specific context.

A high proportion of sex workers have a history of childhood sexual abuse, which itself is likely to be causal in determining entry into sex work (Bagley and Young 1987; Farley and Barkan 1998; Simons and Whitbeck 1991). It follows that continuing exposure to physical and sexual assaults as a sex worker must add to the preexisting burden of psychological trauma. Furthermore, as a result of prior conditioning, an individual with a history of sexual abuse is likely to have a lower barrier for avoiding or resisting assault and is unlikely to have coping strategies to minimize further injury to mental and physical health. Vanwesenbeeck et al. (1995) found that condom use and risk taking by sex workers in Holland were related to the severity of childhood and adult adverse experiences.

A study of Puerto Rican sex workers found that 70% had high levels of depressive symptoms and exhibited correspondingly greater risk behaviors in terms of condom use and injected drugs (Alegria et al. 1994). Significantly higher symptom rates were observed among street workers (87%) compared with brothel workers (45%), suggesting that the physical context of sex work strongly influences outcomes. In contrast, the study by Farley et al. (1998) on posttraumatic stress disorder (PTSD) among sex workers from five countries reported no difference in levels of PTSD between brothel and street workers, even though those on the street had experienced significantly higher levels of physical violence. This was interpreted to mean that "*psychological trauma is intrinsic to the act of prostitution.*" However, it is known that sex workers do not necessarily confine themselves to one particular type of sex work over the course of their working lives, and therefore the lack of information on these workers' past histories may have confounded this finding.

The question of whether sex work per se is independently associated with mental disorder was tackled by El Bassel et al. (1997) in a study of street workers in Harlem, New York. These investigators matched 176 sex workers with 130 women who were not but whose life experiences were comparable in terms of poverty and other traumatic events. Psychological distress scores based on the Brief Symptom Inventory were significantly higher among sex workers, although the study failed to settle the issue of the extent to which the observed distress was a consequence or precursor of entry into sex work.

Sanders (2004), in interviews with women working mainly in indoor settings, found that emotional and psychological distress related primarily to feelings of depersonalization and loss of self-esteem as well as to the fear of discovery by family and intimate partners. The workers identified the practical and emotional difficulties encountered in keeping their working and private lives separate as a greater threat to their well-being than either violence or infection.

There seems little doubt that sex trading as an occupation has a propensity to cause psychological distress, although common sense also suggests that the context in terms of the physical setting, levels of violence, drug dependence, coercion from pimps, and pressure from police must have a major impact on the extent to which this occurs. Individuals' life experiences prior to entering sex work also undoubtedly affect the levels of distress found in various studies. What is needed to resolve these questions is a study of sex workers whose lives are unencumbered by traumatic past experiences and whose working conditions are free from the negative influences described in this chapter. However, given the extent to which these factors appear to be inextricably woven into the fabric of sex work, the prospects of finding such a sample are remote.

Conclusion

Sex work is a dangerous business. The constant threat of violence, the consequences of sexually transmitted disease, and the cumulative damage to mental health are all compounded by the effects of heroin, crack cocaine, and other drugs. This chapter has sought to demonstrate the interrelatedness of these factors in the lives of female sex workers and the ways in which their impact is modified by the physical setting, the level of control and autonomy workers have over their conditions of work, and the degree to which they are victimized by the authorities.

References

Albert A, Warner D, Hatcher R et al. Condom use among female commercial sex workers in Nevada's legal brothels. *Am J Public Health* 85:1514–1520, 1995.

Alegria M, Vera M, Freeman D et al. HIV infection, risk behaviours and depressive symptoms among Puerto Rican sex workers. *Am J Public Health* 84:2000–2002, 1994.

Alexander P. Sex work and health: A question of safety in the workplace. *J Am Med Womens Assoc* 53:77–82, 1998.

Bagley C, Young L. Juvenile prostitution and child sex abuse: A controlled study. *Can J Commun Ment Health* 6:5–26, 1987.

Baker L, Case P, Policiccio D. General health problems of inner-city sex workers: A pilot study. *J Med Libr Assoc* 91:67–71, 2003.

Barnard M. Violence and vulnerability: Conditions of work for streetworking prostitutes. *Sociol Health Illn* 15:683–705, 1993.

Baseman J, Ross M, Williams M. Sale of sex for drugs and drugs for sex: An economic context of sexual risk behavior for STDs. *Sex Transm Dis* 26:444–449, 1999.

Blankenship K, Thompson A, Khoshnood K et al. Commercial sex work and risk for HIV infection among incarcerated women, in *International Conference on AIDS*, July 7–12, 1996 (abstract no. Tu.C.2654), vol. 11, p. 377.

Brents B, Hausbeck K. Violence and legalised brothel prostitution in Nevada. *J Interpers Violence* 20:270–295, 2005.

Cameron D. Can we reduce HIV transmission by providing healthcare and HIV therapy to commercial sex workers? *J Int Assoc Physicians AIDS Care* 4:24–26, 1998.

Casabona J, Sanchez E, Salinas R et al. Seroprevalence and risk factors for HIV transmission among female prostitutes. *Eur J Epidemiol* 6:248–252, 1990.

Church S, Henderson M, Barnard M et al. Violence by clients towards female prostitutes in different work settings: Questionnaire survey. *BMJ* 322:524–525, 2001.

Cohan D, Lutnick A, Davidson P et al. Sex worker health: San Francisco style. *Sex Transm Infect* 82:418–422, 2006.

D'Costa L, Plummer F, Bowmer I et al. Prostitutes are a major source of sexually transmitted diseases in Nairobi, Kenya. *Sex Transm Dis* 12:64–69, 1985.

El-Bassel N, Schilling R, Irwin K et al. Sex trading and psychological distress among women recruited from the streets of Harlem. *Am J Public Health* 87:66–70, 1997.

El-Bassel N, Witte S, Wada T et al. Correlates of partner violence among female street-based sex workers: Substance abuse, history of childhood abuse, and HIV risks. *AIDS Patient Care Sex Transm Dis* 15:41–51, 2001.

Elwood W, Williams M, Bell D et al. Powerlessness and HIV prevention among people who trade sex for drugs ('strawberries'). *AIDS Care* 9:273–284, 1997.

Farley M, Baral I, Kiremire M et al. Prostitution in five countries: Violence and post-traumatic stress disorder. *Fem Psychol* 8:405–426, 1998.

Farley M, Barkan H. Prostitution, violence and post-traumatic stress disorder. *Womens' Health* 27:37–48, 1998.

Harcourt C, Donovan B. The many faces of sex work. *Sex Transm Infect* 81:201–206, 2005.

Inciardi J, Surratt H, Kurtz S. HIV, HBV and HCV infections among drug-involved, inner-city street sex workers in Miami, Florida. *AIDS Behav* 10:139–147, 2006.

Jeal N, Salisbury C. A health needs assessment of street-based prostitutes: Cross-sectional survey. *J Public Health* 26:147–151, 2004.

Kral A, Blumenthal R, Booth R et al. HIV seroprevalence among street-recruited injection drug and crack cocaine users in 16 US municipalities. *Am J Public Health* 88:108–113, 1998.

Kurtz S, Surratt H, Inciardi J et al. Sex work and date violence. *Violence Against Women* 10:357–385, 2004.

Lee D, Binger A, Hocking J et al. The incidence of sexually transmitted infections among frequently screened sex workers in a decriminalised and regulated system in Melbourne. *Sex Transm Infect* 81:434–436, 2005.

Lowndes C, Alary M, Platt L. Injection drug use, commercial sex work and the HIV/STI epidemic in the Russian Federation. *Sex Transm Dis* 30:46–48, 2003.

McCarthy M, Khalid I, El Tigani A. HIV-1 infection in Juba, southern Sudan. *J Med Virol* 46:18–20, 1995.

McKeganey N, Barnard M, Leyland A et al. Female streetworking prostitution and HIV infection in Glasgow. *BMJ* 305:801–804, 1992.

Padian N. Prostitute women and AIDS: Epidemiology. *AIDS* 2:413–419, 1988.

Plant M. *AIDS, Drugs and Prostitution*. London: Tavistock/Routledge, 1990.

Potterat J, Brewer D, Muth S et al. Mortality in a long-term open cohort of prostitute women. *Am J Epidemiol* 159:778–785, 2004.

Pyett P, Haste B, Snow J. Who works in the sex industry? A profile of female prostitutes in Victoria. *Aust NZ J Public Health* 20:431–433, 1996.

Pyett P, Warr D. Vulnerability on the streets: Female sex workers and HIV risk. *AIDS Care* 9:539–547, 1997.

Rosenberg M, Weiner J. Prostitutes and AIDS: A health department priority? *Am J Public Health* 78:418–423, 1988.

Sanders T. A continuum of risk? The management of health, physical and emotional risks by female sex workers. *Sociol Health Illn* 26:557–574, 2004.

Simons R, Whitbeck L. Sexual abuse as a precursor to prostitution and victimisation among adolescent and adult homeless women. *J Fam Issues* 12:361–379, 1991.

Sterk C, Elifson K. Drug-related violence and street prostitution, in *Drugs and Violence: Causes, Correlates and Consequences*. Edited by de la Rosa M, Lambert E, Gropper B. NIDA Research Monograph no. 103. Rockville, MD: NIDA, 1990, pp. 208–222.

Surratt H, Inciardi J, Kurtz S et al. Sex work and drug use in a subculture of violence. *Crime Delinq* 50:43–59, 2004.

Tuan N, Hien N, Chi P et al. Intravenous drug use among street-based sex workers: A high-risk behaviour for HIV transmission. *Sex Transm Dis* 31:15–19, 2004.

Vanwesenbeeck I, deGraaf R, van Zessen G et al. Professional HIV risk taking, levels of victimisation and well-being in female prostitutes in the Netherlands. *Arch Sex Behav* 24:503–515, 1995.

Wallace J, Porter J, Weiner A et al. Oral sex, crack smoking and HIV infection among female sex workers who do not inject drugs. *Am J Public Health* 87:470, 1997.

Wallace J, Weiner A, Steinberg A et al. Fellatio is a significant risk behavior for acquiring AIDS among New York City streetwalking prostitutes, in *Abstracts of the VIIIth International Conference on AIDS*, vol. 2, 1992, p. C277.

Ward H, Aral S. Globalisation, the sex industry and health. *Sex Transm Infect* 82:345–347, 2006.

Ward H, Day S, Green A et al. Declining prevalence of STI in the London sex industry, 1985 to 2002. *Sex Transm Infect* 80:374–376, 2004.

Ward H, Day S, Mezzone J et al. Prostitution and risk of HIV: Female prostitutes in London. *BMJ* 307:356–358, 1993.

Ward H, Day S, Weber J. Risky business: Health and safety in the sex industry over a 9 year period. *Sex Transm Infect* 75:340–343, 1999.

Whittaker D, Hart G. Managing risks: The social organisation of indoor sex work. *Sociol Health Illn* 18:399–414, 1996.

20

Intermittent Explosive Disorder: Clinical Aspects

Emil F. Coccaro, MD, and Michael S. McCloskey, PhD

History of Psychiatric Attention to Intermittent Explosive Disorder

Intermittent explosive disorder (IED) is a psychiatric diagnosis applied to individuals who repeatedly engage in acts of impulsive aggression. The diagnosis of IED has been a part of the *Diagnostic and Statistical Manual of Mental Disorders* (DSM) only since the introduction of the third edition (DSM-III) in 1980. However, the construct of a "disorder of impulsive aggression" has been a part of the DSM since its inception in 1956.

In the first edition (DSM-I), this construct was referred to as "passive-aggressive personality (aggressive type)" and was characterized as "persistent reaction to frustration with irritability, temper tantrums and destructive behavior." This construct evolved into "explosive personality" in the second edition (DSM-II). Patients with "explosive personality" were characterized as being "aggressive individuals" who display "intermittently violent behavior" and are "generally excitable, aggressive, and over-responsive to environmental pressures" with "gross outbursts of rage or of verbal or physical aggressiveness different from their usual behavior." In DSM-III, "explosive personality" was codified and operationalized as "IED" for the first time and assigned clinical disorder status under Axis I.

The diagnostic criteria, however, were not well operationalized (e.g., Criterion A "assaultive" and "destructive" acts had no specific guidelines regarding which behaviors would satisfy the criteria for severity, frequency, or time frame) and were otherwise problematic. Subjects who were generally aggressive or impulsive in between the ill-defined aggressive episodes were excluded from receiving the diagnosis (Criterion C). Because individuals with recurrent, problematic, impulsive aggression are also generally impulsive and aggressive between more severe outbursts, this exclusion ruled out the vast majority (i.e., about 80%) of individuals who now would be diagnosed with IED (Felthous et al. 1991).

Current IED Criteria Sets

With the introduction of the fourth edition (DSM-IV), the earlier exclusionary "C" criteria that excluded individuals with chronic aggression problems (effectively excluding most subjects now considered IED) was removed. This had the net effect of allowing for more empirical work to take place. The DSM-IV still lacked objective criteria for the intensity, frequency, and nature of aggressive acts to meet criteria for IED (see Table 20.1).

The World Health Organization's (WHO) diagnostic manual, the *International Classification of Mental and Behavioral Disorders* (ICD-10) (World Health Organization 1992), has no IED diagnosis. The closest approximation to IED in the ICD-10 is the diagnosis of "other habit and impulse disorders," which is broadly defined as persistently maladaptive behavior in which there is a "failure to resist impulses to carry out the behavior." In addition, the

Table 20.1 DSM-IV criteria for intermittent explosive disorder

A. Several discrete episodes of failure to resist aggressive impulses that result in serious assaultive acts or destruction of property.
B. The degree of aggressiveness expressed during the episodes is grossly out of proportion to any precipitating psychosocial stressors.
C. The aggressive episodes are not better accounted for by another mental disorder (e.g., antisocial personality disorder, borderline personality disorder, a psychotic disorder, a manic episode, conduct disorder, or attention deficit hyperactivity disorder) and are not a result of the direct physiological effects of a substance (e.g., a drug of abuse, a medication) or a general medical condition (e.g., head trauma, dementia of the Alzheimer's type).

behavior must involve "a prodromal period of tension with a feeling of release at the time of the act" that is not secondary to another psychiatric condition (World Health Organization 1992).

Noting the limitations of the DSM-IV (and ICD-10) criteria for IED, Coccaro and colleagues developed an alternative criteria set that integrated their research findings with the DSM conceptualizations of IED (Coccaro 2003; Coccaro et al. 1998). These "integrated research" criteria for IED (IED-IR), differed from DSM-IV IED criteria on four key points.

First, the IED-IR criteria clearly operationalized the severity and frequency of aggressive behavior required for the diagnosis. Using the IED-IR criteria, individuals could be diagnosed by the presence of frequent low-intensity aggression (e.g., arguments occurring on average twice weekly) and/or of less frequent but higher-intensity aggressive behavior (e.g., physical assault or destruction of property three times in a year). The inclusion of verbal aggression within the IED-IR construct reflected data showing both that frequent verbal aggression occurred in over 85% of subjects with physical aggression and that subjects with frequent verbal aggression in the absence of more severe assaultive acts show the same core deficits and impairment as assaultive subjects (Coccaro 2003; Coccaro et al. 1998; McCloskey et al. 2008a). Furthermore, both groups manifest similar serotonergic deficits and an antiaggressive response to serotonin reuptake inhibitors (Coccaro and Kavoussi 1997; Salzman et al. 1995).

Second, the IED-IR criteria explicitly required the aggressive behavior to be impulsive in nature. This decision was also informed by research showing that psychosocial (Dodge, Pettit, and Bates 1994), biological (Linnoila et al. 1983; Virkkunen et al. 1994) and treatment response data (Barratt et al. 1997; Sheard et al. 1976) differentiated between "impulsive" and "premeditated" aggression.

Third, the IED-IR criteria explicitly required the presence of subjective distress (i.e., in the individual) and/or social or occupational dysfunction in order to clearly link distress/dysfunction to aggressive behavior.

Fourth, the IED-IR criteria allowed subjects with borderline and/or antisocial personality disorder (BPD/AsPD) to receive a comorbid IED diagnosis (i.e., if they otherwise meet the IED-IR criteria). This decision stemmed from the finding that IED subjects with and without BPD/AsPD are similarly aggressive, and both IED groups are much more aggressive, than non-IED subjects with BPD/AsPD. In other words, high levels of aggression were always associated with the presence of IED but not necessarily the presence of BPD/AsPD (see the subsection on "Comorbidity"). These research criteria for IED (Table 20.2) have been used in studies of IED in several sites in the United States (Frankle 2005; Goveas, Csernansky, and Coccaro 2004; Hollander et al. 2003; New et al. 2002, 2004; Siever et al. 1999). Moreover, some suggested changes have been adopted in the text revision edition of the DSM-IV.

Table 20.2 Research criteria for IED: IED-IR

A. Recurrent incidents of aggression manifest as either:
A1. Verbal or physical aggression toward other people, animals, or property occurring twice weekly on average for 1 month
Or
A2. Three episodes involving physical assault against other people or destruction of property over a 1-year period.
B. The degree of aggressiveness expressed is grossly out of proportion to the provocation or any precipitating psychosocial stressors.
C. The aggressive behavior is generally not premeditated (i.e., it is impulsive) *and* is not committed in order to achieve some tangible objective (e.g., money, power, intimidation, etc.).
D. The aggressive behavior causes either marked distress in the individual or impairment in occupational or interpersonal functioning.
E. The aggressive behavior is not better accounted for by another mental disorder (e.g., major depressive/manic/psychotic disorder; ADHD); general medical condition (e.g., head trauma, Alzheimer's disease); or the direct physiological effects of a substance.

Differential Diagnosis

The cardinal symptom of IED is repeated acts of impulsive (affective) aggression that are not better accounted for by another psychiatric disorder, medical condition, or substance. This is true of both DSM and integrated research criteria sets. However, many psychiatric disorders (e.g., mood disorders, personality disorders) and some substances (e.g., alcohol) are both associated with increased aggression and comorbid with IED, making differential diagnosis difficult. In many of these situations, a determination of whether IED is present can be made by assessing the temporal relationship between the disorder, the substance use, and the aggressive behavior.

Bipolar disorder, and to a lesser extent unipolar depression, have been linked to increased agitation and aggressive behavior in some individuals (Fava and Rosenbaum 1999; Swann 1999), but for these individuals the pathological aggressiveness is limited to the manic and/or depressive episodes. For individuals with IED, even if a mood disorder exists, heightened levels of aggressive behavior persist during otherwise euthymic periods.

Similarly, alcohol and other substance use disorders facilitate aggression (Wells, Graham, and West 2000). If individuals abusing these substances display aggressive behavior that would otherwise meet criteria for IED but that only occurs during periods of acute intoxication and/or withdrawal, then they would not receive an IED diagnosis. However, if the individual also engaged in sufficient aggressive behavior when not intoxicated or going through withdrawal, then IED would be diagnosed.

For chronic disorders, differential diagnosis is considerably more difficult. Individuals with IED are more likely to have experienced past traumatic events. They also tend to be hypervigilant and perseverate on perceived injustices; however, they do not share the reexperiencing of symptoms (i.e., flashbacks, highly distressing intrusive thoughts) that occur with posttraumatic stress disorder (PTSD). If a person appears to meet criteria for both PTSD and IED, the clinician should assess whether the level of aggression met IED criteria prior to the trauma. The onset of IED is typically in early adolescence. If the trauma occurred later than adolescence and the aggressive behavior began around the time of other PTSD symptoms, then an additional diagnosis of IED would not be warranted.

DSM-IV criteria for antisocial (AsPD) and borderline (BPD) personality disorders include anger and aggression (though these are not required symptoms as they are for IED). Because the symptoms of AsPD, BPD, and IED all develop in adolescence, determining whether the aggressive behavior in AsPD or BPD is associated with the personality disorder or IED is difficult. Unlike IED patients, some individuals with AsPD primarily engage

Table 20.3 LHA aggression scores (mean ± SD): Relevance to IED not BPD/AsPD

Subjects' Sample Site	Controls		Non-IED Subject		IED
	Healthy Controls	Personality Dx *without* IED	BPD/AsPD *without* IED	IED *without* BPD/AsPD	IED *with* BPD/AsPD
Philadelphia ($n = 437$)	4.9 ± 4.2^a	7.9 ± 5.2^b	10.2 ± 4.9^b	16.4 ± 5.6^c	18.9 ± 5.0^c
Chicago ($n = 352$)	5.3 ± 3.8^a	11.5 ± 5.9^b	10.3 ± 5.2^b	17.7 ± 4.4^c	19.5 ± 3.8^c

$a = p < .05$ from all groups.
$b = p < .05$ from HC & IED subjects.
$c = p < .05$ from HC & non-IED subjects.
BPD/AsPD = borderline personality disorder and/or antisocial personality disorder.
LHA = Lifetime history of aggression.
IED = Intermittent explosive disorder.

in aggression that is motivated by tangible rewards other than revenge (e.g., mugging a person to steal their money). For these individuals, a second diagnosis of IED would not be warranted.

However, for the majority of AsPD and BPD patients, the aggressive behavior is predominately in response to angry feelings. How to diagnose these individuals is a point of variance between the DSM-IV and Research IED criteria sets. While proponents of both IED criteria sets posit that aggressive behavior should "count" toward the diagnosis of AsPD and/or BPD, the DSM-IV criteria allow for an IED diagnosis *only* if the aggressive behavior is not better explained by AsPD and/or BPD. The text of DSM-IV does not explain how to make this determination. However, data suggest that individuals with AsPD and/or BPD who do not otherwise meet criteria for IED are not more aggressive than other patients with non-AsPD/BPD personality disorders (see Table 20.3). Accordingly, the mere presence of AsPD/BPD does not explain the presence of aggressiveness in the individual, and therefore IED should be diagnosed in AsPD/BPD individuals when the criteria for IED are met. This is why the IED-IR criteria allow IED to be comorbid with AsPD and/or BPD.

Clinical Picture and Course of Illness

Prevalence

Since its initial inclusion in the DSM, IED has been described as "rare" (American Psychiatric Association 1994). However, this designation was based on very limited empirical research. Two recently published epidemiological studies found that approximately 4%–6% of individuals met lifetime criteria for IED, depending on the criteria set used (Coccaro et al. 2004; Kessler et al. 2006). One-month and 1-year point prevalences of IED in these studies were reported as 2.0% (Coccaro et al. 2004) and 2.7% (Kessler et al. 2006), respectively. If so, 16.2 million Americans will have IED during their lifetimes and as many as 10.5 million in any year and 6 million in any month. Prevalence was not associated with race in these studies. This result is consistent with a separate epidemiological survey of 2,554 Latinos that found a lifetime IED prevalence of 5.8% (Ortega, Canino, and Alegria 2008). Furthermore, a study of 4,725 respondents in the Ukraine found comparable rates of lifetime IED (4.2%), suggesting that a lifetime prevalence of IED of 4%–6% is not limited to American samples (Bromet et al. 2005).

Symptom Presentation

Aggressive outbursts in IED have a rapid onset (McElroy et al. 1998), often without a recognizable prodromal period (Felthous et al. 1991; Mattes 1990). Episodes are short-lived – less than 30 minutes (McElroy et al. 1998) – and involve verbal assault, destructive and nondestructive property assault, or physical assault (Mattes 1990; McElroy et al. 1998). Aggressive outbursts most commonly occur in response to a minor provocation by a close intimate or associate (Felthous et al. 1991; McElroy et al. 1998), and IED subjects may have less severe episodes of verbal and nondestructive property assault in between more severe episodes (Coccaro 2003; McElroy et al. 1998). Episodes are associated with substantial distress, impairment in social functioning, occupational difficulty, and legal or financial problems (Mattes 1990; McElroy et al. 1998).

In a recent community sample study of more than 9,200 individuals, subjects meeting current IED criteria (defined as three high-severity episodes in the current year) had engaged in direct interpersonal aggression (67.8%), threatened interpersonal aggression (20.9%), and aggression against objects (11.4%). These subjects reported engaging in 27.8 (SD = 4.1) high-severity aggressive acts during their worst year, with two to three lifetime aggressive outbursts requiring medical attention. The mean dollar value of property damage due to lifetime IED aggressive outbursts was $1,603 (SD = $135) (Kessler et al. 2006).

Quality of Life

High levels of hostility and aggression negatively impact quality of life across several dimensions, including interpersonal relationships (Laurent, Kim, and Capaldi 2007; Lawrence and Bradbury 2007), sleep quality (Ireland and Culpin 2006), job satisfaction (Judge, Scott, and Ilies 2006), and health (Miller et al. 1995; Vahtera et al. 1997). Similarly, the limited data suggest that individuals with IED have more health problems (McCloskey et al., submitted), are more impaired in terms of overall functioning, and are less happy than healthy volunteers or psychiatric controls (McCloskey et al. 2006, 2008). Notably, their quality of life improves after successful treatment (McCloskey et al. 2008b). There is a dearth of data on the impact of IED on the quality of life of family members. However, numerous studies have linked witnessing and experiencing aggression in childhood with adverse adult consequences, including intergenerational transmission of aggression (Conger et al. 2003).

Age of Onset, Gender, and SES

Intermittent explosive disorder begins as early as childhood and peaks in mid-adolescence, with a mean age of onset in three separate studies ranging from 13.5 to 18.3 years (Coccaro et al. 2004; Coccaro, Posternak, and Zimmerman 2005; Kessler et al. 2006). In one study, the age of onset occurred at a significantly earlier time in males (Coccaro, Posternak, and Zimmerman 2005). The average duration of symptomatic IED ranges from 12 years to an adult's complete lifetime (Coccaro et al. 2004; Kessler et al. 2006; McElroy et al.1998). Although IED is common in males (Coccaro et al. 1998; Mattes 1990; McElroy et al. 1998), recent data suggest that IED occurs equally among men and women (Coccaro et al. 2004; Coccaro, Posternak, and Zimmerman 2005; Kessler et al. 2005, 2006). In a large epidemiological survey, sociodemographic variables (e.g., sex, age, race, education, marital status, occupational status, family income) did not differ across IED statuses (Kessler et al. 2006).

Comorbidity

Available data suggest that IED is a chronic disorder whose onset *precedes* other comorbid Axis I disorders (Coccaro, Posternak, and Zimmerman 2005; Kessler et al. 2006). If so, it is unlikely that IED evolves into another disorder. It is more likely that IED promotes the development of other disorders by leading to divorce, financial difficulties, and stressful life experiences that promote their onset later in adulthood (Kessler et al. 2006). In clinical samples, IED is highly comorbid with a variety of Axis I disorders, such as mood disorders, anxiety disorders, and alcohol and other substance use disorders (Coccaro, Posternak, and Zimmerman 2005). In community samples, however, the odds ratios for a relationship between current IED and such disorders were significant ($p < .05$) only for generalized anxiety disorder (OR = 2.1; 95% CI: 1.3–3.2), alcohol abuse (OR = 2.6; 95% CI: 1.7–4.2), and any substance use disorder (OR = 2.4; 95% CI: 1.5–3.8). Again, the vast majority of subjects reported that IED began at an earlier age than these comorbid conditions (Coccaro, Posternak, and Zimmerman 2005; Kessler et al. 2006).

For Axis II disorders, only subjects with borderline (BPD) and antisocial (AsPD) personality disorders are more highly represented among IED subjects compared with non-IED ones (Coccaro et al. 1998). This comorbidity is not due to individuals with BPD and/or AsPD in general having high levels of aggression and therefore IED. Data (Table 20.3) indicate that aggression levels among BPD/AsPD subjects *with and without* IED are the same and that levels of aggression in non-IED subjects are significantly less than those in IED subjects regardless of the presence or absence of BPD/AsPD. Accordingly, the key difference between IED subjects *with and without* BPD/AsPD is level of aggression, not the presence or absence of BPD and/or AsPD. In addition, while 40%–50% of IED subjects in these two samples had BPD/AsPD, only about 25% of BPD/AsPD individuals in the community meet criteria for IED (Coccaro et al. 2004).

Familial Correlates

A family history study comparing first-degree relatives of 30 IED and 20 control probands found significantly elevated morbid risk for IED in the IED relatives compared with the control relatives (0.26 vs. 0.08, $p < .01$) (Coccaro 2003). Elevation in the morbid risk for IED was not caused by the presence or absence of comorbid conditions among the IED probands (e.g., history of suicide attempts, major depression, alcoholism, drug use disorder) nor by increases in morbid risk of other non-IED disorders in the relatives (e.g., major depression, alcoholism, drug use disorders, anxiety disorder, or any other disorder). Accordingly, familial aggregation of IED is not the result of an epiphenomenon of the liability of either the proband or the relative to having non-IED comorbid conditions and suggests a clear familial "signal." This finding supports research showing that socially aberrant aggressive behavior reflects a substantial degree of genetic influence (Bergeman and Seroczynski 1998).

Biology

Laboratory studies clearly show a biobehavioral relationship between aggression and selected brain chemicals (e.g., serotonin) (Coccaro and Siever 2002), but studies in IED have been conducted only over the past few years. Published data suggest that IED subjects have altered serotonin function compared with non-IED subjects or healthy controls (Goveas, Csernansky, and Coccaro 2004; New et al. 2002, 2004). Reports of other studies supporting the IED–serotonin link are in preparation by the author (EFC). They demonstrate a reduction in prolactin responses to d-fenfluramine challenge and a difference in platelet 5-HT transporter numbers (measured via H^3-paroxetine binding) in IED subjects compared with non-IED subjects or healthy controls. These findings are supported by imaging studies. Two fluorodeoxyglucose (FDG) PET studies found low FDG utilization after d,l-fenfluramine challenge in frontal cortex areas (Siever et al. 1999) and low FDG utilization after m-CPP challenge in the anterior cingulate in IED subjects compared with healthy controls (New et al. 2002). A third, ligand binding study of the 5-HT transporter also reports reduced 5-HT transporter availability in the anterior cingulate in IED subjects versus controls (Frankle 2005). Finally, an fMRI study (Coccaro et al. 2007) demonstrated increased activation of the amygdala and reduced activation of the orbital medial prefrontal cortex, when viewing angry faces in IED subjects compared with healthy controls. This reduced prefrontal activation may be dependent on the level of emotional information processing (McCloskey et al., submitted).

Assessment of IED

There are no well-validated measures of IED. However, two measures have been developed by the authors: a brief questionnaire that could be used as a screening measure and a semistructured interview to more thoroughly diagnose the disorder.

The Intermittent Explosive Disorder Module (IED-M) is a 20–30 minute structured diagnostic interview developed to obtain systematic information sufficient to make research diagnoses of current and lifetime IED by both DSM-IV and integrated research criteria. The IED-M obtains quantitative information about lifetime and current frequencies of verbal aggression, aggression against property, and physical aggression. Contextual descriptive information about the three most serious episodes of each type of aggression during the 1-year period in which it occurred most frequently (e.g., "what was the provocation?" and "what were the consequences of this outburst?") provide information about the proportionality of the aggressive response. Additional phenomenological information about aggressive acts is also obtained, including but not limited to age of onset and offset of each type of aggression, the effects of the aggressive behaviors on relationships with family and friends, subjective level of distress, emotions and physical symptoms prior to and after an outburst, and frequency of substance use during aggressive outbursts. Preliminary psychometric data suggest that the IED has strong interrater reliability ($k = .83$) when used as part of a full diagnostic battery that includes structured clinical interviews for other Axis I and Axis II disorders. Construct validity for the measure comes from research showing that individuals identified as having IED using the IED-M were more aggressive than psychiatric controls on a behavioral aggression measure (McCloskey et al. 2006).

The Intermittent Explosive Disorder Diagnostic Questionnaire (IED-DQ) is a brief, seven-item, self-report measure of IED according to DSM-IV criteria and research criteria for IED. The IED-DQ contains items that assess aggression frequency, severity, resulting distress from aggressive behavior and exclusionary mental health or medical conditions. Results from our developmental studies using the IED-DQ indicate good psychometric properties (test–retest reliability, construct validity, strong concordance – kappa ~ 0.80), with the best estimated diagnoses of IED established via a clinical interview such as the IED-M. Sensitivity and specificity for the IED-DQ versus the IED-M were 0.86 and 0.91, respectively, for the DSM-IV IED and were 0.85 and 0.95 for the IED by research criteria (McCloskey et al., submitted).

Treatment of IED

Psychopharmacologic Treatment
Impulsive Aggression

Several psychopharmacologic agents appear to have effects on aggression. Classes of agents shown to have "antiaggressive" effects in double-blind, placebo-controlled trials involving individuals with "primary" aggression (i.e., not secondary to psychosis, severe mood disorder, or organic brain syndromes) include mood stabilizers such as lithium (Donovan et al. 2000; Sheard et al. 1976), 5-HT uptake inhibitors such as fluoxetine (Coccaro and Kavoussi 1997; Fava et al. 1993; Salzman et al. 1995), and anticonvulsants such as diphenhydantoin at 300 mg/day or carbamazepine (Barratt et al. 1997; Gardner and Cowdry 1986). While beta-blockers such as propanolol or nadolol (Ratey et al. 1992; Yudofsky, Silver, and Schneider 1987) have also been shown to reduce aggression, these agents have been tested exclusively in patient populations with "secondary" aggression (e.g., mental retardation, organic brain syndromes, etc.). Classes of agents that may have "proaggressive" effects include tricylic antidepressants such as amitriptyline (Soloff et al. 1986), benzodiazepines (Gardner and Cowdry 1985), and stimulant and hallucinatory drugs of abuse such as amphetamines, cocaine, and phencyclidine (Volavka and Citrome 1998). Emerging evidence of differential psychopharmacology is of critical importance, and double-blind, placebo-controlled clinical trials suggest that antiaggressive efficacy is specific to *impulsive* rather than nonimpulsive aggression (Barratt et al. 1997; Sheard et al. 1976).

Intermittent Explosive Disorder

Completed analysis of a double-blind, placebo-controlled trial of fluoxetine on impulsive aggressive behavior in 100 subjects with IED (by research criteria) demonstrates clear antiaggressive efficacy for fluoxetine versus a placebo (Coccaro et al. 2009). This study notes reduction in overt aggressive behavior as reported by subjects, subjective or objective anger or aggression, and a response rate of 70% (CGI scores of "much improved" or "very much improved"). Notably, fluoxetine was not associated with any increase in aggression compared with a placebo. In contrast, compared with fluoxetine, the placebo was associated with a greater frequency of increased aggression, and increased magnitude of aggression, after randomization. While the trial results are positive, only 29% of IED subjects displayed no aggression at the end of the trial, indicating that while fluoxetine can reduce impulsive aggressive behavior, remission of IED symptoms may take more than the drug itself. A placebo-controlled study involving divalproex, titrated to a plasma level of 80–120 mg/day, reported a favorable effect on overt aggression, but only in IED subjects with comorbid Cluster B personality disorder (Hollander et al. 2003).

Psychotherapy
Anger Dyscontrol

Despite the prevalence and burden of IED, no published randomized clinical trials (RCTs) have examined the efficacy of psychosocial treatments for this disorder. The efficacy of psychosocial interventions for the related construct of anger dyscontrol is well documented. Five meta-analytic reviews of anger treatments (Beck and Fernandez 1998; Bowman-Edmondson and Cohen-Conger 1996; Del Vecchio and O'Leary 2004; DiGuiseppe and Tafrate 2003; Tafrate 1995) support the conclusion that cognitive-behavioral therapies (e.g., relaxation training, self-inoculation training, cognitive restructuring, and multicomponent treatments) evidence a moderate to large effect for anger and aggression at the end of treatment, with similar effects at follow-up.

Overall, treatment efficacy was not dependent on the specific cognitive-behavioral intervention used, though multicomponent treatments containing both cognitive and behavioral components were most often employed. Furthermore, one review (Del Vecchio and O'Leary 2004) suggested that multicomponent treatments may be most effective for aggressive behavior. The generalizability of this research to IED is limited in that the anger-treatment literature often fails to discriminate between anger problems with and without pathological aggression. Highly aggressive individuals may be more resistant to treatment.

A meta-analysis of treatment for interpersonal (domestic) violence found that psychosocial interventions had only "small" effects on reducing aggression (Babcock, Green, and Robie 2004). However, the generalizability of this finding is also limited because only a small portion of individuals with IED have a history of domestic violence. One study that compared IED and non-IED aggressive drivers, who received a brief (four 90-minute sessions) cognitive-behavioral program, found that CBT was more effective than self-monitoring overall, but IED subjects tended not to respond as well to treatment. This led the authors to suggest that IED individuals may benefit from longer, more intensive therapy (Galovski and Blanchard 2002).

Intermittent Explosive Disorder

The authors recently completed an IED psychotherapy outcome study ($n = 45$) comparing the efficacy of a 12-week multicomponent CBT intervention presented in either group or individual format to a wait-list control group. The treatment was modeled after the Cognitive Restructuring, Relaxation and Coping Skills Training (CRCST) treatment developed to treat anger (Deffenbacher and Mckay 2000) but was modified to serve as a more appropriate treatment for aggressive individuals (e.g., extend treatment from 8 to 12 sessions, include a time-out technique, and increase emphasis on aggression and relapse prevention). Aggression, anger, and associated symptoms were assessed at baseline, midtreatment, posttreatment, and 3-month follow-up. Both group and individual CRCST reduced aggression, anger, hostile thinking, and depressive symptoms, while improving anger control relative to wait-list participants. Posttreatment effect sizes were large and were maintained at 3-month follow-up, providing initial support for the efficacy of CBT in the treatment of IED (McCloskey et al. 2008b).

Other Issues Regarding Treatment of IED

No studies have examined the optimal length of treatment for IED. Our experience is that impulsive aggression is a trait that can be suppressed, but not eliminated, by medication. We have found that within about one month of discontinuing fluoxetine, patients with impulsive aggressive behavior experience a return of impulsive aggressive behavior to pretreatment levels. The one study that examined the effect of lithium on impulsive aggression in prison inmates found that impulsive aggressive behavior returned to pretreatment levels within 1 month of a switch to a placebo (Sheard et al. 1976). This is in contrast to our findings regarding the effects of CRCST, which continue at least 3 months after active treatment has ended (McCloskey et al., in press). This is probably because the treatment elements (relaxation training, cognitive restructuring, and coping skills training) have been incorporated into the individual's life and are still active. In contrast, once medication leaves the body, its effects on behavior end.

In addition, no published studies have investigated the effect of combining modalities of treatment. Examining our own data with fluoxetine and CRCST in IED subjects, we are struck by the observation that both modalities yield a similar magnitude of improvement in outcome measures (e.g., ~ 30% remission and ~ 15% partial remission from IED). Because these two modalities work through different mechanisms, we hypothesize that together they would be more effective than either is alone. Our clinical experience is consistent with this idea, but these data are anecdotal. Whether medication or CRCST should be first-line probably depends on the patient because some prefer medication (some individuals perceive this as easier) whereas others prefer psychotherapeutic treatment (some individuals wish to avoid medications). Severity of aggression also affects the choice of modality, and combining medication and CRCST could be a first-line treatment in cases of severe aggressive behavior.

Helpful resources for victims of intimate partner violence can be found in Chapter 22 of this volume.

References

American Psychiatric Association. *Diagnostic and Statistical Manual of Mental Disorders*, 4th edition. Washington, DC: American Psychiatric Association, 1994.

Babcock JC, Green CE, Robie C. Does batterers' treatment work? A meta-analytic review of domestic violence treatment. *Clin Psychol Rev* 23:1023–1053, 2004.

Barratt ES, Stanford MS, Felthous AR et al. The effects of phenytoin on impulsive and premeditated aggression: A controlled study. *J Clin Psychopharmacol* 17:341–349, 1997.

Beck R, Fernandez E. Cognitive-behavioral therapy in the treatment of anger. *Cognit Ther Res* 22:62–75, 1998.

Bergeman C, Seroczynski A. Genetic and environmental influences on aggression and impulsivity, in *Neurobiology and Clinical Views on Aggression and Impulsivity*. Edited by Maes M, Coccaro E. London: Wiley, 1998, pp. 63–80.

Bowman-Edmondson C, Cohen-Conger J. A review of treatment efficacy for individuals with anger problems: Conceptual, assessment and methodological issues. *Clin Psychol Rev* 16:251–275, 1996.

Bromet EJ, Gluzman SF, Paniotto VI et al. Epidemiology of psychiatric and alcohol disorders in Ukraine: Findings from the Ukraine World Mental Health survey. *Soc Psychiatry Psychiatr Epidemiol* 40:681–690, 2005.

Coccaro E, Siever L. Pathophysiology and treatment of aggression, in *Neurosychopharmacology: The Fifth Generation of Progress*. Edited by Davis KL, Charney D, Coyle JT et al. Nashville, TN: American College of Neuropsychopharmacology, 2002, pp. 1709–1723.

Coccaro EF. *Intermittent Explosive Disorder*. New York: Marcel Dekker, 2003.

Coccaro EF, Kavoussi RJ. Fluoxetine and impulsive aggressive behavior in personality-disordered subjects. *Arch Gen Psychiatry* 54:1081–1088, 1997.

Coccaro EF, Kavoussi RJ, Berman ME et al. Intermittent explosive disorder-revised: Development, reliability, and validity of research criteria. *Compr Psychiatry* 39:368–376, 1998.

Coccaro EF, Lee R, Kavoussi RJ. A double-blind, placebo-controlled, trial of fluoxetine in impulsive aggressive patients with Intermittent Explosive Disorder. *J Clin Psychiatry* 70:653–662, 2009.

Coccaro EF, McCloskey MS, Fitzgerald DA et al. Amygdala and orbitofrontal reactivity to social threat in individuals with impulsive aggression. *Biol Psychiatry* 62:168–178, 2007.

Coccaro EF, Posternak MA, Zimmerman M. Prevalence and features of intermittent explosive disorder in a clinical setting. *J Clin Psychiatry* 66:1221–1227, 2005.

Coccaro EF, Schmidt CA, Samuels JF et al. Lifetime and 1-month prevalence rates of intermittent explosive disorder in a community sample. *J Clin Psychiatry* 65:820–824, 2004.

Conger RD, Neppl T, Kim K et al. Angry and aggressive behavior across three generations: A prospective, longitudinal study of parents and children. *J Abnorm Child Psychol* 31:143–160, 2003.

Deffenbacher JL, Mckay M. *Overcoming Situational and General Anger*. Oakland, CA: New Harbinger Publications, 2000.

Del Vecchio T, O'Leary KD. Effectiveness of anger treatments for specific anger problems: A meta-analytic review. *Clin Psychol Rev* 24:15–34, 2004.

DiGuiseppe R, Tafrate RC. Anger treatment for adults: A meta-analytic review. *Clin Psychol: Sci Pract* 10:70–84, 2003.

Dodge KA, Pettit GS, Bates JE. Socialization mediators of the relation between socioeconomic status and child conduct problems. *Child Dev* 65(2 spec no): 649–665, 1994.

Donovan SJ, Stewart JW, Nunes EV et al. Divalproex treatment for youth with explosive temper and mood lability: A double-blind, placebo-controlled crossover design. *Am J Psychiatry* 157:818–820, 2000.

Fava M, Rosenbaum JF. Anger attacks in patients with depression. *J Clin Psychiatry* 60 (suppl 15): 21–24, 1999.

Fava M, Rosenbaum JF, Pava JA et al. Anger attacks in unipolar depression, Part 1: Clinical correlates and response to fluoxetine treatment. *Am J Psychiatry* 150:1158–1163, 1993.

Felthous AR, Bryant SG, Wingerter CB et al. The diagnosis of intermittent explosive disorder in violent men. *Bull Am Acad Psychiatry Law* 19:71–79, 1991.

Frankle WG, Lombardo I, New AS et al. Brain serotonin transporter distribution in subjects with impulsive aggressivity: A positron emission study with [11C]McN 5652. *Am J Psychiatry* 162:915–923, 2005.

Galovski T, Blanchard EB. The effectiveness of a brief psychological intervention on court-referred and self-referred aggressive drivers. *Behav Res Ther* 40:1385–1402, 2002.

Gardner DL, Cowdry RW. Alprazolam-induced dyscontrol in borderline personality disorder. *Am J Psychiatry* 142:98–100, 1985.

Gardner DL, Cowdry RW. Positive effects of carbamazepine on behavioral dyscontrol in borderline personality disorder. *Am J Psychiatry* 143:519–522, 1986.

Goveas JS, Csernansky JG, Coccaro EF. Platelet serotonin content correlates inversely with life history of aggression in personality-disordered subjects. *Psychiatry Res* 126:23–32, 2004.

Hollander E, Tracy KA, Swann AC et al. Divalproex in the treatment of impulsive aggression: Efficacy in cluster B personality disorders. *Neuropsychopharmacology* 28:1186–1197, 2003.

Ireland JL, Culpin V. The relationship between sleeping problems and aggression, anger, and impulsivity in a population of juvenile and young offenders. *J Adolesc Health* 38:649–655, 2006.

Judge TA, Scott BA, Ilies R. Hostility, job attitudes, and workplace deviance: Test of a multilevel model. *J Appl Psychol* 91:126–138, 2006.

Kessler RC, Chiu WT, Demler O et al. Prevalence, severity, and comorbidity of 12-month DSM-IV disorders in the National Comorbidity Survey Replication. *Arch Gen Psychiatry* 62:617–627, 2005.

Kessler RC, Coccaro EF, Fava M et al. The prevalence and correlates of DSM-IV intermittent explosive disorder in the National Comorbidity Survey Replication. *Arch Gen Psychiatry* 63:669–678, 2006.

Laurent HK, Kim HK, Capaldi DM. Interaction and relationship development in stable young couples: Effects of positive engagement, psychological aggression, and withdrawal. *J Adolesc* 31:815–835, 2007.

Lawrence E, Bradbury TN. Trajectories of change in physical aggression and marital satisfaction. *J Fam Psychol* 21:236–247, 2007.

Linnoila M, Virkkunen M, Scheinin M et al. Low cerebrospinal fluid 5-hydroxyindoleacetic acid concentration differentiates impulsive from nonimpulsive violent behavior. *Life Sci* 33:2609–2614, 1983.

Mattes JA. Comparative effectiveness of carbamazepine and propranolol for rage outbursts. *J Neuropsychiatry Clin Neurosci* 2:159–164, 1990.

McCloskey MS, Berman ME, Broman-Folks J et al. Preliminary reliability and validity of the Intermittent Explosive Disorder Diagnostic Questionnaire (IED-DQ). *Assessment* (submitted).

McCloskey MS, Berman ME, Noblett KL et al. Intermittent explosive disorder-integrated research diagnostic criteria: Convergent and discriminant validity. *J Psychiatr Res* 40:231–242, 2006.

McCloskey MS, Kleabir K, Chen EY et al. Unhealthy aggression: The association between intermittent explosive disorder and negative health outcomes. *Health Psychol* (submitted).

McCloskey MS, Lee R, Berman ME et al. The relationship between impulsive verbal aggression and intermittent explosive disorder. *Aggress Behav* 34:51–60, 2008a.

McCloskey MS, Noblett KL, Deffenbacher JL et al. Cognitive-behavioral therapy for intermittent explosive disorder: A pilot randomized clinical trial. *J Consult Clin Psychol* 76:876–886, 2008b.

McCloskey MS, Phan KL, Angstadt M et al. Amygdala hyperactivation to angry faces in intermittent explosive disorder. *Neuropsychopharmacology* (submitted).

McElroy SL, Soutullo CA, Beckman DA et al. DSM-IV intermittent explosive disorder: A report of 27 cases. *J Clin Psychiatry* 59:203–210; quiz 211, 1998.

Miller TQ, Markides KS, Chiriboga DA et al. A test of the psychosocial vulnerability and health behavior models of hostility: Results from an 11-year follow-up study of Mexican Americans. *Psychosom Med* 57:572–581, 1995.

New AS, Hazlett EA, Buchsbaum MS et al. Blunted prefrontal cortical 18fluorodeoxyglucose positron emission tomography response to meta-chlorophenylpiperazine in impulsive aggression. *Arch Gen Psychiatry* 59:621–629, 2002.

New AS, Trestman RF, Mitropoulou V et al. Low prolactin response to fenfluramine in impulsive aggression. *J Psychiatr Res* 38:223–230, 2004.

Ortega AN, Canino G, Alegria M. Lifetime and 12-month intermittent explosive disorder in Latinos. *Am J Orthopsychiatry* 78:133–139, 2008.

Ratey JJ, Sorgi P, O'Driscoll GA et al. Nadolol to treat aggression and psychiatric symptomatology in chronic psychiatric inpatients: A double-blind, placebo-controlled study. *J Clin Psychiatry* 53:41–46, 1992.

Salzman C, Wolfson AN, Schatzberg A et al. Effect of fluoxetine on anger in symptomatic volunteers with borderline personality disorder. *J Clin Psychopharmacol* 15:23–29, 1995.

Sheard MH, Marini JL, Bridges CI et al. The effect of lithium on impulsive aggressive behavior in man. *Am J Psychiatry* 133:1409–1413, 1976.

Siever LJ, Buchsbaum MS, New AS et al. d, l-fenfluramine response in impulsive personality disorder assessed with [18F]fluorodeoxyglucose positron emission tomography. *Neuropsychopharmacology* 20:413–423, 1999.

Soloff PH, George RS, Nathan PM et al. Paradoxical effects of amitriptyline on borderline patients. *Am J Psychiatry* 143:1603–1605, 1986.

Swann AC. Treatment of aggression in patients with bipolar disorder. *J Clin Psychiatry* 60(suppl 15): 25–28, 1999.

Tafrate RC. Evaluation of strategies for adult anger disorders, in *Anger Disorders: Definition, Diagnosis & Treatment*. Edited by Kassinove H. Washington, DC: Taylor & Francis, 1995, pp. 109–130.

Vahtera J, Kivimäki M, Koskenvuo M et al. Hostility and registered sickness absences: A prospective study of municipal employees. *Psychol Med* 27:693–701, 1997.

Virkkunen M, Rawlings R, Tokola R et al. CSF biochemistries, glucose metabolism, and diurnal activity rhythms in alcoholic, violent offenders, fire setters, and healthy volunteers. *Arch Gen Psychiatry* 51:20–27, 1994.

Volavka J, Citrome L. Aggression, alcohol and other substances of abuse, in *Neurobiology and Clinical Views on Aggression and Impulsivity*. Edited by Maes M, Coccaro E. London: Wiley, 1998, pp. 29–45.

Wells S, Graham K, West P. Alcohol-related aggression in the general population. *J Stud Alcohol* 61:626–632, 2000.

World Health Organization. *The ICD-10 Classification of Mental and Behavioural Disorders: Clinical Descriptions and Diagnostic Guidelines*. Geneva: World Health Organization, 1992.

Yudofsky S, Silver J, Schneider S. Pharmacologic treatment of aggression. *Psychiatr Ann* 17:397–406, 1987.

21

Violence against Women: Preventing a Social Scourge

Joan C. Chrisler, PhD, and Sheila Ferguson, MD

Introduction

Although the rates of violent crime in the United States have been decreasing in recent years (Bureau of Justice Statistics 2006), the overall national violent crime rate and the homicide rate in several of our large cities are among the highest in the world (Barclay et al. 2003). The United States has been classified as a rape-prone culture (Rozee 1993) that celebrates aggression and eroticizes domination. Violence is so frequent a theme in our films, television shows, video games, comic books, pornography, and popular songs that social psychologists worry that Americans are becoming desensitized to violent aggression. Add to this toxic mix the easy availability of guns and gender role stereotypes that encourage anger and impulsivity in men and anxiety and passivity in women, and the result is conditions conducive to an epidemic of violence against women.

Violence represents an abuse of power in the course of the domination, intimidation, and victimization of one person by another often, but not always, in the context of a relationship (Chrisler and Ferguson 2006). Violence against women and girls can be perpetrated by intimate partners (e.g., domestic or courtship violence, stalking, rape), by family members (e.g., child abuse, elder abuse, incest, injuries incidental to a violent attack on a family member), and by co-workers, casual acquaintances, or strangers (e.g., sexual harassment, stalking, rape, injuries in the course of a crime such as robbery).

Of course, not all violent crimes are perpetrated on women by men. Homicide is a leading cause of death among young men (National Center for Health Statistics 2004), intimate partner violence occurs in lesbians' and gay men's relationships (Island and Letellier 1991; Renzetti 1992), and instances of violence against men by women are now being studied seriously (Anderson 2005; Brush 2005; McHugh 2005). However, because most men are bigger and stronger than most women (and thus able to inflict more serious injuries), because there appear to be many more instances of violence by men than women overall, and there are more data on women's injuries by men, our focus is on the public health effects of violence against women that is usually inflicted by men.

A major concern in studying violence against women is the difficulty of accurately estimating the extent of the problem. Although the Bureau of Justice Statistics collects and reports crime statistics from across the United States, many incidents of domestic violence, rape, sexual harassment, and other crimes against women are never reported to the police. Among the reasons the crimes are not reported are fear (e.g., victims are often threatened with additional violence if they report), embarrassment, depression, denial, social isolation, language difficulties, concern that they will not be believed, worry about stigmatization, and confusion about whether what they experienced was actually a crime. For example, some people do not believe that rape is possible between intimate partners because marriage or previous sexual intercourse implies consent to future sexual intercourse.

Researchers who conduct surveys on acquaintance rape often find respondents who answer "yes" regarding whether they have ever been forced to have sexual intercourse and then answer "no" regarding whether they have ever been raped. Surveys on sexual harassment show a similar phenomenon; women often answer "yes" to questions that define particular types of harassing behavior (e.g., "Has anyone ever touched you in a sexual way or made sexually suggestive remarks to you in your workplace?") and then answer "no" to a question about whether they have ever experienced sexual harassment. Such results could be due to denial, ignorance of the definition of "rape" or "sexual harassment," or mistaken beliefs that rape only occurs between strangers or that only quid-pro-quo threats (e.g., "Have sex with me or you're fired") constitute sexual harassment. Therefore, the situation is probably worse than crime statistics suggest.

Physical Health Consequences

The Centers for Disease Control and Prevention (CDC; National Center for Injury Prevention and Control [NCIPC] 2003) has estimated that about 4,451,000 women are physically assaulted each year by their intimate partners. Forty-one percent of those assaults cause observable injuries, and 28.1% of those injured require medical care. The types of injuries range from minor (e.g., scratches, bruises, welts, sore muscles), to serious (e.g., broken bones, broken teeth, bullet wounds, knife wounds, burns), to death. One study (Wilbur et al. 2001) found that approximately 67% of women who visit emergency rooms after an episode of intimate partner violence (IPV) have symptoms of a head injury, 30% of IPV victims have suffered a loss of consciousness at least once, and 68% have been strangled at least once. Between 1976 and 1996, 30% of femicides in the United States were committed by intimate partners and 41% by someone else the woman knew (Greenfield, Rand, and Craven 1998).

Pregnancy is a high-risk time for IPV. A recent British study (Richardson et al. 2002) reported that pregnancy increases the risk of violence by a factor of 2.11. In a study of 358 low-income U.S. women (O'Campo et al. 1994), 65% reported having experienced either verbal or physical abuse from their male partner or another family member at least once during their pregnancies. The pregnant woman's abdomen is a frequent site of injuries, which are often caused by punching or kicking. Studies have shown that physical abuse during pregnancy delays prenatal care by an average of 6.5 weeks (Taggert and Mattson 1996) and can result in increased risk of miscarriage (Jacoby et al. 1999), premature labor (Cokkinides et al. 1999), anemia, poor weight gain, vaginal infections, and low birth weight (Murphy et al. 2001).

The National Institute of Justice (1996) reported a total of 1,204,265 rapes of women and children in the year 1990; 265 of these victims were murdered. The CDC (National Center for Injury Prevention and Control 2003) has estimated that 322,230 women are raped each year by their intimate partners, and about 36% of these rapes cause physical injuries that require medical care. Marchbanks, Lui, and Mercy (1990) examined the medical records of rape victims and reported that 82% had black eyes and orbital swelling; 25% had bites, burns, scalding, or injuries from restraints or bindings; 19% had internal injuries and had experienced loss of consciousness; 8% had broken bones or teeth; and 2% had knife or gunshot wounds. Rape victims frequently experience vaginal injuries and bruises or other external traumas, usually on the mouth, throat, breasts, and thighs (Banks, Ackerman, and Corbett 1995). Pregnancy, sexually transmitted diseases, and dyspareunia are also common results of rape.

Female victims of rape and IPV frequently report dysmenorrhea, migraines, infections, chronic pain, gastrointestinal disorders, hypertension, musculoskeletal problems (Letourneau, Holmes, and Chasedunn-Roark 1999), low energy, sleep problems, headaches, muscle tension or soreness, fatigue, weight change, back pain, nightmares, dizziness, poor appetite, acid stomach, indigestion, weakness, pounding or racing heart, trembling limbs (Eby et al. 1995), depression (Bonomi et al. 2006), panic attacks (Romito and Grassi 2007), and drug abuse (Burke et al. 2005). These symptoms may be due to residual effects of injuries sustained during the violence, posttraumatic stress disorder, stress-induced changes in immune functioning, or an intensified focus on physical sensations as a result of postviolence concerns about bodily integrity (Koss 1994).

Although some of these symptoms could be appropriately treated by psychotherapy, mental health services are underutilized for several reasons. Medical personnel may not refer patients to psychotherapists, and patients may prefer not to label themselves as victims or as being in need of psychotherapy, may not have health insurance that covers psychotherapy, or may feel more comfortable talking to their family physician than to a psychotherapist or social worker.

The CDC (National Center for Injury Prevention and Control 2003) has estimated that as many as 500,000 women are stalked each year by a current or former intimate partner. This estimate does not include women stalked by strangers or casual acquaintances. Some stalkers are overtly threatening, and some eventually physically assault or even murder their victims, but others do not (Davis and Frieze 2002). Stalking has only recently been recognized as a separate crime category, and finding data about it is difficult. Finding overall estimates of sexual harassment is also difficult because many victims do not report it. The incidence of workplace harassment seems to be highest in male-dominated occupations. For example, the results of one study (Yoder 2001) of women in the military indicate that 76% of participants had been harassed in the previous year. Sexual harassment is rarely accompanied by physical injury.

Mental Health Consequences

The traumatic nature of rape and physical assault, as well as the fear, anxiety, victim blame, and loss of control that accompany rape and IPV, mean that many victims suffer psychologically as a result. The CDC (National Center for Injury Prevention and Control 2003) has estimated that 26% of IPV victims, 33% of rape victims, and 43% of stalking victims seek psychological, psychiatric, or other mental health services. Among the problems commonly diagnosed in women who have been victims of violence are anxiety disorders, depression, posttraumatic stress disorder (PTSD), and antisocial behavior (Bonomi et al. 2006; Fanslow and Robinson 2004; White et al. 2001).

Women also complain of low self-esteem, body image issues, self-perceived poor health, fear of intimacy, and an inability to trust men (Fanslow and Robinson 2004). Higher than average rates of drug and alcohol abuse and eating disorders are often seen in victims (West 2002), and suicidal thoughts are more common among victims than among the general population (Fanslow and Robinson 2004). Victims of sexual harassment often report embarrassment, fear, anxiety, self-blame, depression, and loss of self-confidence (Paludi and Barickman 1998). Although the psychological effects of violence diminish with time, they can be quite severe and greatly distressing to victims.

Economic Consequences

The physical and psychological sequelae of violence against women levy serious economic costs on society. The National Institute of Justice (1996) considered lost productivity (at work and at home), medical care, mental health care, diminished quality of life, ambulance/fire/police services, social/victim services, and property loss/damage, and calculated that costs *per victimization episode* for rape alone totaled more than $3 million for the year 1990; the total annual cost of rape has been estimated at a staggering $127 billion. In view of inflation, those figures would be higher today.

The CDC (National Center for Injury Prevention and Control 2003) has estimated that one-sixth of IPV victims, one-fifth of rape victims, and 35% of stalking victims lose time from paid work; as many as 2.9 million work days may be lost per year because stalking victims are afraid that their current or former partners will follow them into the workplace and cause them humiliation or worse. Victims of IPV have reported greater absenteeism and tardiness, lower productivity, lower wages, lost promotion opportunities, and lost jobs as a result of their experiences of violence (Reeves and O'Leary-Kelly 2007). The CDC (National Center for Injury Prevention and Control 2003) has also estimated that 10.3% of IPV victims, 13.5% of rape victims, and 17.5% of stalking victims are unable to perform child care or housework for a time. Productivity losses also occur when sexual harassment victims take days off from work, change jobs or college majors, or drop out of college or graduate school in order to avoid the harasser (Paludi and Barickman 1998).

The cost of health care services for victims of violence remains high for some time after the original injuries have healed. For example, Koss (1994) found that rape victims increased their physician visits by 56% from an average of 4.1 visits during the year before the rape to an average of 7.3 visits during the following year. Victims of moderate levels of domestic violence increase their visits by a factor of 2, and increased use of medical services may continue for up to 5 years postvictimization (Rivara et al. 2007). Walby (2004) estimated that the British National Health Services spends £1.2 billion ($1.92 billion) per year on direct services to victims of domestic violence. A recent large random-sample telephone survey (Bonomi et al. 2007) found that women who had ever experienced physical or sexual abuse were more likely than those who had not to judge their health status as fair or poor. They also reported more symptoms and had lower scores on the SF-36 Health Survey.

Consequences for the Next Generation

In addition to the damage done to children who are physically or sexually abused themselves, witnessing violence directed against their mothers has physical health, mental health, and behavioral consequences for children. For example, boys who have witnessed their fathers abusing their mothers are at increased risk of committing sexual assault and other violent crimes themselves. Girls who witness their mothers' abuse are at increased risk of teenage prostitution. Both girls and boys are at increased risk of suicide (Jaffe, Wolfe, and Wilson 1990). Children frequently try to protect their mothers from violent attacks, often getting hurt themselves in the process. A large percentage (9%) of adolescent boys and young men who are in jail for homicide were arrested for killing their mothers' batterers (Stahly 2008).

A recent study (Graham-Bermann and Seng 2005) of preschoolers reported that exposure to domestic violence predicted poor physical health and symptoms associated with traumatic stress. A study (Bensley, Van Eenwyk, and Simmons 2003) of adult women found that those who had witnessed or experienced violence as children had poorer general health, more frequent marital distress, and greater risk of physical and emotional abuse by their intimate partners than did those with no such history. Intimate partner violence that occurs before children are born may also have health consequences for them. As noted earlier, pregnancy is a high-risk time for domestic violence, and attacks concentrated on the woman's abdomen can produce miscarriage (Jacoby et al. 1999). Children with low birth weight and exposure to maternal stress often suffer health consequences, as do those whose mothers delay prenatal care (Taggart and Mattson 1996) or cope with the aftermath of the violence with increased use of alcohol, tobacco, and other drugs (Curry, Perrin, and Wall 1998).

Prevention of Violence against Women

The epidemic of violence against women and its societal consequences require a public health response. Most primary prevention work consists of educational efforts to inform the general public about violence against women and girls so that people are able to recognize and label violence (e.g., date rape, sexual harassment), become informed about legal avenues (e.g., restraining orders) and other programs (e.g., battered women's shelters) that women can use to protect themselves, and learn about how to get needed advice and support (e.g., rape crisis hotlines). Other primary prevention efforts have taken the form of lobbying for stiffer sentencing and arrest guidelines for perpetrators; better training of police, medical, and court personnel; and attempts to limit the amount of violence to which children are exposed (e.g., labels on compact discs and video games) (Chrisler and Ferguson 2006). Innovative efforts are needed to reduce the incidence of violence by targeting men and boys (especially those who experienced or witnessed violence themselves as children) for education about alternatives to violence (e.g., assertiveness skills, impulse control, anger management) and to encourage the development of negative attitudes toward violent acts.

Secondary prevention efforts are focused on routine screening (e.g., by internists, pediatricians, obstetricians/gynecologists, psychotherapists) and opportunistic screening (e.g., by emergency medical personnel, social workers) for violence suffered by women and children who are at high risk or present with unusual or suspicious injuries. Screening can be done via questionnaires or face-to-face interviews. Often victims want to be asked about the origin of their injuries, which they are afraid to disclose but might disclose if asked directly (Head and Taft 1995). Medical personnel are often uncomfortable asking patients about violence, even when abuse is suspected, and better training is needed (Richardson et al. 2002). Such training must include not only how to elicit information about assault and abuse but what to do if disclosure of violence is elicited. Disclosure of violence can increase a victim's risk of additional abuse, and steps must be taken to protect her (Chrisler and Ferguson 2006).

Tertiary prevention efforts consist of interventions to prevent additional abuse of the victim as well as referral to appropriate medical care, mental health counseling, and other specialized services that will promote her ability to cope with the aftereffects of the violence and to heal from her physical and psychological traumas. Calls may need to be placed to the police, a rape crisis counselor, or a battered women's shelter. Short-term interventions could include the arrest of the perpetrator; a shelter stay; a protection order; home visits by police or social workers; or advocacy, personal, or vocational counseling. Longer-term interventions could include referral to a psychotherapist, a physical therapist, a victim's services center, a support group, or children's services (Chrisler and Ferguson 2006).

Conclusion

A great deal of work remains to be done to apply what is known to the prevention of violence against women and girls. And much more research is needed to discover more effective prevention efforts. More accurate data on incidents of violence are needed so that researchers can tell whether prevention efforts are successful; perhaps increasing the frequency of screening will provide some of the necessary data. Despite the inadequate data, however, one thing is clear: violence against women is a serious societal problem with consequences not only for the victims but for us all. Efforts to reduce violence must take place at the cultural, institutional, and interpersonal levels, and we must all do our part.

References

Anderson KL. Theorizing gender in intimate partner violence research. *Sex Roles* 52:853–865, 2005.
Banks ME, Ackerman RJ, Corbett CA. Feminist neuropsychology: Issues for physically challenged women, in *Variations on a Theme: Diversity and the Psychology of Women.* Edited by Chrisler JC, Hemstreet AH. Albany: State University of New York Press, 1995, pp. 29–49.

Barclay G, Tavares C, Kenny S et al. International comparisons of criminal justice statistics 2001 [2003]. Available at www.homeoffice.gov.uk/rds/pdfs2/hosb1203.pdf. Accessed May 28, 2008.

Bensley L, Van Eenwyk J, Simmons KW. Childhood family violence history and women's risk for intimate partner violence and poor health. *Am J Prev Med* 25:38–44, 2003.

Bonomi AE, Anderson M, Rivara FP et al. Health outcomes in women with physical and sexual intimate partner violence exposure. *J Women's Health* 16:987–997, 2007.

Bonomi AE, Thompson RS, Anderson M et al. Intimate partner violence and women's physical, mental, and social functioning. *Am J Prev Med* 30:458–466, 2006.

Brush LD. Philosophical and political issues in research on women's violence and aggression. *Sex Roles* 52:867–873, 2005.

Bureau of Justice Statistics. Since 1994, violent crime rates have declined, reaching the lowest level ever in 2005 [2006 report]. Available at www.ojp.usdoj.gov/bjs/glance/viort.htm. Accessed May 28, 2008.

Burke JG, Thieman LK, Gielen AC et al. Intimate partner violence, substance abuse, and HIV among low-income women: Taking a closer look. *Violence Against Women* 11:1140–1161, 2005.

Chrisler JC, Ferguson S. Violence against women as a public health issue. *Ann NY Acad Sci* 1087:235–249, 2006.

Cokkinides VE, Coker AL, Sanderson M et al. Physical violence during pregnancy: Maternal complications and birth outcomes. *Obstet Gynecol* 93:661–666, 1999.

Curry, MA, Perrin N, Wall E. Effects of abuse on maternal complications and birth weight in adult and adolescent women. *Obstet Gynecol* 92:530–534, 1998.

Davis K, Frieze IH. Stalking: What do we know and where do we go? in *Stalking: Perspectives on Victims and Perpetrators.* Edited by Davis K, Frieze IH. New York: Springer, 2002, pp. 353–375.

Eby KK, Campbell JC, Sullivan CM et al. Health effects of experiences of sexual violence for women with abusive partners. *Health Care Women Int* 16:563–576, 1995.

Fanslow JL, Robinson E. Violence against women in New Zealand: Prevalence and health consequences. *J NZ Med Assoc* 117:1173–1206, 2004.

Graham-Bermann SA, Seng J. Violence exposure and traumatic stress symptoms as additional predictors of health problems in high-risk children. *J Pediatr* 146:349–354, 2005.

Greenfield L, Rand M, Craven D. Violence by intimates: Analysis of crimes by current or former spouses, boyfriends, and girlfriends. Washington, DC: U.S. Department of Justice, 1998.

Head C, Taft A. Improving general practitioner management of women experiencing domestic violence: A study of the beliefs and experiences of women victims/survivors and of GPs. Canberra: Australian Department of Health, Housing, and Community Services, 1995.

Island D, Letellier P. *Men Who Beat the Men Who Love Them: Battered Gay Men and Domestic Violence.* Binghamton, NY: Haworth Press, 1991.

Jacoby M, Gorenflo D, Black E et al. Rapid repeat pregnancy and experiences of interpersonal violence among low-income adolescents. *Am J Prev Med* 16:318–321, 1999.

Jaffe PG, Wolfe DA, Wilson SK. *Children of Battered Women: Issues in Child Development and Intervention Planning.* Newbury Park, CA: Sage Publications, 1990.

Koss MP. The negative impact of crime victimization on women's health and medical use, in *Reframing Women's Health: Multidisciplinary Research and Practice.* Edited by Dan AJ. Thousand Oaks, CA: Sage Publications, 1994, pp. 189–200.

Letourneau EJ, Holmes M, Chasedunn-Roark J. Gynecologic health consequences to victims of interpersonal violence. *Women's Health Issues* 9:115–120, 1999.

Marchbanks PA, Lui KJ, Mercy JA. Risk of injury from resisting rape. *Am J Epidemiol* 132:540–549, 1990.

McHugh MC. Understanding gender and intimate partner abuse. *Sex Roles* 52:717–724, 2005.

Murphy CC, Schei B, Myhr TL et al. Abuse: A key factor for low birth weight? *CMAJ* 164:1567–1572, 2001.

National Center for Health Statistics. Deaths, percent of deaths, and death rates for the 15 leading causes of death in 5-year age groups by race and sex: United States, 1999–2004 [2004]. Available at www.cdc.gov/nchs/datawh/statab/unpubd/mortabs/lcwk1_10.htm. Accessed May 28, 2008.

National Center for Injury Prevention and Control. Costs of intimate partner violence against women in the United States [March 2003 report]. Available at www.cdc.gov/ncipc/pub-res/ipv_cost/ipvbook-final-feb18.pdf. Accessed May 28, 2008.

National Institute of Justice. Victim costs and consequences: A new look [1996 report]. Available at www.ncjrs.gov/pdffiles/victcost.pdf. Accessed July 2, 2008.

O'Campo P, Gielen AC, Faden RR et al. Verbal abuse and physical violence among a cohort of low-income pregnant women. *Women's Health Issues* 4:29–37, 1994.

Paludi MA, Barickman RB. *Sexual Harassment, Work, and Education: A Resource Manual for Prevention*, 2nd edition. Albany: State University of New York Press, 1998.

Reeves C, O'Leary-Kelly AM. The effects and costs of intimate partner violence for work and organizations. *J Interpers Violence* 22:327–344, 2007.

Renzetti CM. *Violent Betrayal: Partner Abuse in Lesbian Relationships*. Newbury Park, CA: Sage Publications, 1992.

Richardson J, Coid J, Petruckevitch A et al. Identifying domestic violence: Cross-sectional study in primary care. *BMJ* 324:274–279, 2002.

Rivara FP, Anderson ML, Fishman P et al. Healthcare utilization and costs for women with a history of intimate partner violence. *Am J Prev Med* 32:89–96, 2007.

Romito P, Grassi M. Does violence affect one gender more than the other? The mental health impact of violence among male and female university students. *Soc Sci Med* 65:1222–1234, 2007.

Rozee P. Forbidden or forgiven: Rape in cross-cultural perspective. *Psychol Women Q* 17:499–514, 1993.

Stahly GB. Battered women: Why don't they just leave? in *Lectures on the Psychology of Women*, 4th edition. Edited by Chrisler JC, Golden C, Rozee PD. New York: McGraw-Hill, 2008, pp. 356–375.

Taggart L, Mattson S. Delay in prenatal care as a result of battering in pregnancy: Cross-cultural implications. *Health Care Women Int* 17:25–34, 1996.

Walby, S. The cost of domestic violence [2004]. Available at www.womenandequalityunit.gov.uk. Accessed April 8, 2008.

West CM. Battered black and blue: An overview of violence in the lives of black women. *Women Ther* 25:5–27, 2002.

White JW, Donat PLN, Bondurant B. A developmental examination of violence against girls and women, in *Handbook of the Psychology of Women and Gender*. Edited by Unger RK. New York: Wiley, 2001, pp. 343–357.

Wilbur L, Higley M, Hatfield J et al. Survey results of women who have been strangled while in an abuse relationship. *J Emerg Med* 21:297–302, 2001.

Yoder JD. Military women, in *Encyclopedia of Women and Gender*. Edited by Worell J. San Diego, CA: Academic Press, 2001, pp. 771–782.

22

Intimate Partner Violence: Aggression at Close Quarters

Christy M. McKinney, PhD, MPH, and Raul Caetano, MD, MPH, PhD

Introduction

The purpose of this chapter is to provide an overview of the epidemiology and health-related consequences of intimate partner violence (IPV). We discuss how IPV is defined and measured in epidemiological studies and provide an overview of the national prevalence and incidence of IPV. We describe IPV in selected populations, including pregnant women and adolescents, and across certain demographics, such as sex and race/ethnicity. We also discuss characteristics of IPV victims and perpetrators that are known to increase the risk of IPV. Lastly, we provide an overview of the clinical considerations and prevention of IPV. Because many terms and surveys are abbreviated, we have included a list of IPV-related abbreviations to reference (Table 22.1).

Terms and Definitions

Epidemiological studies have not used a standard definition of IPV, reflecting the complexity of this concept, which encompasses a multitude of social and behavioral constructs. Specifying who is considered an intimate partner and what types of behaviors constitute violence may vary depending on how IPV is conceptualized and measured. Indeed, numerous studies have measured IPV in different populations using a variety of definitions, questions, and time frames (e.g., past 12 months, lifetime). The diverse approaches to assessing IPV have likely contributed to the wide range of IPV prevalence estimates reported across nationwide population-based studies (Breiding, Black, and Ryan 2008; Schafer, Caetano, and Clark 1998; Straus and Gelles 1990; Tjaden and Thoennes 2000b).

In an effort to improve consistency in measuring IPV, the U.S. Centers for Disease Control and Prevention (CDC) has developed guidelines to help researchers adopt a more standardized approach to the terms and measurement of IPV (Saltzman et al. 2002; MP Thompson et al. 2006). This effort will likely contribute to a more consistent definition of IPV. In this section, we provide a summary of the terms proposed by the CDC and their definitions. We also provide information about other commonly used IPV-related terms, describe the Conflict Tactics Scale, the most widely used scale to assess IPV (Straus 1990a), and discuss the implications of collecting IPV-related data from either one or both of the couple.

The CDC's guidelines define the parties involved in IPV and the relationships between them (Saltzman et al. 2002). Intimate partner violence involves a *victim*, the target of violence or abuse, and a *perpetrator*, the individual who inflicts the violence or abuse on the victim. An *intimate partner* may include one or more of the following current or former types of partners: spouse, common-law spouse, boyfriend, girlfriend, dating partner, or date. Intimate partners may be heterosexual or same-sex and may or may not cohabit or

Table 22.1 Abbreviations related to intimate partner violence

Abbreviation	Description
BJS	Bureau of Justice Statistics
BRFSS	Behavioral Risk Factor Surveillance System
CDC	Centers for Disease Control and Prevention
CTS	Conflict Tactics Scale
FMPV	Female-to-male partner violence
IPV	Intimate partner violence
MFPV	Male-to-female partner violence
NCVS	National Crime Victimization Survey
NFVS	National Family Violence Survey
NIJ	National Institute of Justice
NLCS	National Longitudinal Couples Survey
NSFH	National Survey of Families and Households
NVAWS	National Violence Against Women Survey
NVDRS	National Violent Death Reporting System
PRAMS	Pregnancy Risk Assessment Monitoring System
YRBSS	Youth Risk Behavior Surveillance System

be sexually involved. Two people who have had a child together are considered intimate partners, whether or not the couple is still together (Saltzman et al. 2002).

The CDC guidelines also identify four predominant types of IPV: (1) physical violence; (2) sexual violence; (3) psychological or emotional violence or abuse; and (4) threats of physical or sexual violence (Saltzman et al. 2002). *Physical violence* involves the intentional use of physical force with the potential for causing harm and includes behaviors such as pushing, shoving, biting, slapping, hitting, burning, or using a weapon. *Sexual violence* is comprised of three distinct types of behavior: (1) the use of physical force to compel a person to engage in sexual activity against his or her will; (2) an attempted or completed sexual act involving a person who is unable to refuse (i.e., because of the influence of alcohol or because of pressure); and (3) abusive sexual contact that involves intentionally touching genitalia or other private parts against a person's will. *Threats of physical or sexual violence* involve the use of words, gestures, or weapons to communicate an intent to cause physical harm or induce sexual acts without consent. *Psychological or emotional abuse* results from threats of acts or the use of coercive tactics. Examples are behaviors such as humiliating or taking advantage of the victim or smashing objects or destroying property (Saltzman et al. 2002). Though not included in the original CDC guidelines, a fifth type of violence, *stalking*, is also recognized (Centers for Disease Control and Prevention 2000), and one large study has measured it (Tjaden and Thoennes 2000b). However, no proposed uniform definition of this behavior exists.

The CDC defines a *violent IPV episode* as a single violent act or series of acts perceived to be related that occur over a given period of time (Saltzman et al. 2002). An episode may involve one or more types of violence (i.e., physical and sexual violence). The prevalence of IPV typically measures whether *any* violent acts have occurred in the past 12 months or in a person's lifetime. The incidence of IPV measures the number of *new* violent episodes over a specified period of time, which requires each person to report on multiple episodes they experienced.

There are other commonly used terms for which the CDC does not provide uniform definitions. In heterosexual couples, IPV may involve a male perpetrator and female victim (*male-to-female partner violence*, or *MFPV*) or a female perpetrator and male victim (*female-to-male partner violence*, or *FMPV*) and may be reciprocal or nonreciprocal. *Reciprocal violence* is where both partners are perpetrators and victims of violence; in other words, MFPV and FMPV are both present. Reciprocal violence is also referred to as bidirectional or mutual violence. *Nonreciprocal violence* occurs when only one of the couple is a perpetrator and the other is a victim. In heterosexual couples, nonreciprocal violence may be either MFPV or FMPV; nonreciprocal violence is also referred to as unidirectional or nonmutual violence (Caetano, Ramisetty-Mikler, and Field 2005; Whitaker et al. 2007). Often, reciprocity of the violence is unknown and the violence is simply specified according to the sex of the perpetrator and victim. Unless reciprocity is stated, MFPV typically refers to male-to-female partner violence in couples regardless of whether FMPV is also present. Similarly, unless specified, FMPV generally refers to female-to-male partner violence in couples regardless of whether MFPV is present.

In epidemiological data collection, these definitions are operationalized into questions or scales that aim to measure certain types of IPV (i.e., physical assaults). There are numerous assessment scales that operationalize different types of IPV (MP Thompson et al. 2006). Some are developed to measure particular types of IPV such as sexual violence or stalking; others are aimed at a certain subgroup, for example students or abused females (MP Thompson et al. 2006). Perhaps the most widely used scale is the Conflict Tactics Scale (CTS), a broad scale that measures perpetration and victimization of physical violence, sexual violence, and psychological or emotional abuse among both males and females (Straus 1990a). Two version of the CTS have been used most frequently: the CTS Form N (CTS-1) and the more recent CTS Form R (CTS-2) (Straus 1990a, 1996). Both versions measure the 12-month prevalence of various types of IPV. The CTS-1 measured three types of conflict tactics employed by couples: reasoning, verbal aggression, and physical violence (Straus 1979). The CTS-2 expanded the CTS-1 and measures five domains: negotiation, psychological aggression, physical assault, sexual coercion, and injury (Straus et al. 1996). Both the CTS-1 and CTS-2 ask about specific behaviors (i.e., whether their partner pushed or shoved them), and both have demonstrated moderate to high reliability and validity (Straus 1979; Straus et al. 1996). Several national population-based surveys of IPV are based, at least in part, on questions from the CTS (Schafer, Caetano, and Clark 1998; Straus 1990b; Tjaden and Thoennes 2000b). Perhaps because of its widespread use, the CTS is not without its critics, who assert that it is subject to a variety of limitations such as lack of context and its inability to address power and control dynamics (DeKeseredy 2000; Gordon 2000). Nevertheless, this scale is a widely used standardized tool with broad applicability that many have found useful in measuring IPV.

A key decision related to data collection is whether one or both in the couple are asked questions about IPV. When only one of the couple is interviewed, IPV is substantially underreported (Schafer, Caetano, and Clark 1998; Szinovacz and Egley 1995). A positive report for IPV from either of the couple is often used to estimate prevalence in studies that have IPV-related information from both of the couple (Caetano et al. 2005b; Schafer, Caetano, and Clark 1998; Szinovacz and Egley 1995). Alternatively, when data from only one in the couple are ascertained, researchers may utilize information about both victimization and perpetration, if collected, to generate more complete estimates. For example, the National Family Violence Survey interviewed only one of the couple about victimization and perpetration (Straus 1990b). In estimating MFPV, male respondents' information about perpetration and female respondents' information about victimization were used to generate MFPV 1-year prevalence estimates. In cases where only information on victimization is obtained, this approach cannot be used.

Estimates of IPV

Because of the public health importance of IPV, several large-scale nationwide population-based surveys were specifically designed to estimate IPV in the United States. These surveys include the National Family Violence Survey, National Survey of Families and Households,

National Longitudinal Couples Survey, National Violence against Women Survey, and the Behavioral Risk Factor Surveillance System. Other national surveys have obtained information about special types of IPV or specific populations. For example, the National Crime Victimization Survey obtained information about crime-related IPV, while the Pregnancy Risk Assessment Monitoring System measured IPV among new mothers immediately prior to and during pregnancy. In the following section, we provide prevalence and incidence data to the extent available for national surveys that measure IPV overall and among certain subgroups. To put each survey and its estimates into context, we provide information on how an intimate partner was defined, the types of violence measured, the scope of questions used to ascertain IPV, the population studied, the time period of interest, and whether victimization and/or perpetration was measured. Summary estimates of IPV by gender are presented in Table 22.2.

Nationwide General Surveys of IPV

The National Family Violence Survey (NFVS), conducted in 1975, was the first national survey of IPV in the United States (Straus 1990b). The CTS-1 was used to assess IPV (Straus 1979), and the survey included an in-person interviewer-administered questionnaire of randomly selected men and women in married and cohabiting couples. Only one in the couple was interviewed, in either English or Spanish. The respondent was asked questions about conflict tactics employed in disputes with their intimate partner. Questions related to physical violence included how often the respondent acted in the following manner toward their spouse: threw something at; pushed, grabbed, or shoved; threatened to hit or throw something at; or hit or tried to hit (Straus 1979). Data on both perpetration and victimization were used in the calculation of estimates of physical violence. For example, a male participant's affirmative (or negative) response concerning FMPV would be included in the estimate of FMPV, even though the male participant's female intimate partner was not interviewed for the survey. The one-year prevalence of physical violence was 16.0%; MFPV was 12.1% and FMPV was 11.6%. Severe physical violence was reported among 6.1% of respondents; 3.8% and 4.6% of respondents reported severe MFPV and FMPV, respectively (Straus and Gelles 1986).

The NFVS was conducted again in 1985. This time, an abbreviated telephone survey conducted in English was implemented among 6,002 national randomly selected U.S. households in which respondents reported being married, cohabiting, recently divorced or separated, or a single parent. A similar version of the CTS-1 was used to survey one respondent in the household, and reports of both perpetration and victimization of physical violence were used in calculating the estimates. The prevalence of physical violence was similar to the 1975 survey estimates. The 1-year prevalence of physical violence was 16.1%; MFPV was 11.6%, while FMPV was 12.4%. Severe physical violence was reported by 6.3% of respondents; 3.4% and 4.8% of respondents reported severe MFPV and FMPV, respectively (Straus and Gelles 1986).

As part of the 1987–1988 National Survey of Families and Households (NSFH), an estimated 58.3% ($n = 7,589$) of the 13,017 U.S. households overall in this national sample were married or cohabiting couples. These couples responded to questions about perpetration and victimization of physical violence and injury (Sweet, Bumpass, and Call 1988). This was the first large-scale survey in which both partners were interviewed. The survey included an in-person interview and a self-administered questionnaire. Respondents were asked whether they had dealt with a serious argument by hitting or throwing things at each other. Respondents were also asked whether arguments in the past year had ever become physical; for those who responded affirmatively, four additional questions were asked. Two questions were aimed at assessing the sex of the perpetrator and victim, and two questions evaluated whether the respondent had injured the partner or had been injured as a result of the physical violence (Sweet, Bumpass, and Call 1988). A positive report from either

Table 22.2 Estimates of intimate partner violence across broad national surveys

Survey Information	Female Victim (MFPV)	Male Victim (FMPV)
National Family Violence Survey, 1975		
1-year prevalence of physical violence	12.1%	11.6%
National Family Violence Resurvey, 1985		
1-year prevalence of physical violence	11.6%	12.4%
National Survey of Families and Households, 1987		
1-year prevalence of any violence in couple	6.2%	6.7%
Lifetime prevalence of IPV-related injury	2.4%	1.3%
National Longitudinal Couples Survey, 1995		
1-year prevalence of IPV[a]	13.6%	18.2%
National Violence Against Women Survey, 1995–1996		
Lifetime prevalence		
Physical assaults	22.1%	7.4%
Rape	7.7%	0.3%
Stalking	4.8%	0.6%
1-year prevalence		
Physical assaults	1.3%	0.9%
Rape	0.2%	–
Stalking	0.5%	0.2%
1-year incidence per 1,000[b]		
Physical assaults	44.2	31.5
Rape	3.2	–
Stalking	5.0	1.8
Behavioral Risk Factor Surveillance System, 2005		
Lifetime prevalence		
Any IPV[c]	26.4%	15.9%
Physical violence	20.2%	10.7%
Unwanted sex	10.2%	1.5%
1-year prevalence		
Physical violence and/or unwanted sex	1.4%	0.7%
IPV-related injury	0.8%	0.2%
National Crime Victimization Survey, 1998		
1-year incidence of crime-related IPV per 1,000[b]	7.7	1.5
1-year incidence of IPV-related homicide per 1,000[b]	1.2	0.5
Pregnancy Risk Assessment Monitoring System, 2000–2003		
1-year prevalence of physical violence	4.7%	–
During pregnancy prevalence of physical violence	3.7%	–
Youth Behavioral Risk Factor Surveillance System, 2005		
1-year prevalence of dating violence	9.3%	9.0%
Lifetime prevalence of unwanted sex	10.8%	4.2%

[a] IPV includes physical violence, forced sex, and threats of violence with a knife or gun.
[b] For women, the incidence is per 1,000 women; for men, the incidence is per 1,000 men.
[c] IPV includes threatened, attempted, or completed physical violence or unwanted sex.

partner indicated physical violence in the relationship: the 1-year prevalence of MFPV and FMPV were 6.2% and 6.7%, respectively. The one-year prevalence of any physical violence in the couple was 10.4% (Szinovacz and Egley 1995). Estimates derived from a positive report from either partner were substantially higher than those when only one respondent was considered. This suggests that the prevalence of MFPV and FMPV are underestimated in surveys when only one partner is questioned (Szinovacz and Egley 1995). In a 1994 follow-up survey, surviving members of the original sample and their current spouse or partner were interviewed in person. Intimate partner violence was measured in the same manner in 1994 across race/ethnicity and is discussed in detail later (Jasinski 2004).

The 1995 National Longitudinal Couples Survey (NLCS) conducted in-person interviews among a randomly selected sample of married and cohabiting couples throughout the

48 contiguous United States (Schafer, Caetano, and Clark 1997). The survey measured both victimization and perpetration of IPV over the 12 months preceding the survey using an adaptation of the CTS-2 and interviewing both partners in the couple (Straus 1990a). Only physical violence was assessed, and each respondent was asked whether (s)he or their partner had engaged in the following behaviors in the past year: thrown something; pushed, grabbed, or shoved; slapped; kicked, bit, or hit; hit or tried to hit with something; beat up; choked; burned or scalded; forced sex; threatened with a knife or gun; used a knife or gun (Straus 1990a). Each respondent separately reported their behavior toward their partner and their partner's behavior toward them. A positive report from either partner was used in determining the prevalence of IPV. An estimated 21.5% of couples reported a 1-year prevalence of IPV; 13.6% of couples reported MFPV and 18.2% reported FMPV (Lipsky and Caetano 2009; Schafer, Caetano, and Clark 1997). In 2000, an in-person follow-up survey with the couples interviewed in 1995 was conducted; this time, the survey covered all types of violence, including physical, psychological, and sexual (Caetano et al. 2005a). The findings are described in detail later.

The 1995–1996 National Violence Against Women Survey (NVAWS) is a CDC and National Institute of Justice (NIJ) cosponsored nationwide telephone survey among men and women living in residential households (Tjaden and Thoennes 2000a). The survey assessed victimization from physical assaults, rape, and stalking by any type of perpetrator. Whether the perpetrator was an intimate partner was also ascertained for all types of violence reported. Current or former spouses, cohabiting partners, boyfriend or girlfriend and dates were classified as intimate partners (Tjaden and Thoennes 2000a). Only one person in the couple was interviewed. Prevalence (1-year and lifetime) and incidence data were estimated. Questions related to physical assault were taken from a modified version of the CTS-1 (Straus 1990a). Respondents were asked whether any adult had engaged in the following behaviors toward them in the past year: thrown something that could hurt; pushed, grabbed, or shoved; pulled hair; slapped or hit; kicked or bit; choked or attempted to drown; hit with an object; beat up; threatened with a gun; or used a gun, knife, or other weapon. Rape-related questions were based on the National Women's Study, a 1992 survey of rape among women (National Victim Center 1992). Questions included whether a man or boy ever attempted or made the respondent have vaginal, oral, or anal sex by using force or the threat of force; respondents were also asked whether a male or female ever put his (her) fingers or other objects into their vagina or anus against the respondent's will (National Victim Center 1992). To measure stalking, respondents were asked whether any adult had engaged in the following behaviors toward them: spied or followed; sent unsolicited letters; made unsolicited phone calls; stood outside the workplace or home; showed up at places they had no business being; left unwanted items; or vandalized property or destroyed something loved (Tjaden and Thoennes 2000a).

An estimated 22.1% of women and 7.4% of men reported a lifetime prevalence of physical assaults; the lifetime prevalence of rape was 7.7% and 0.3% for women and men, respectively. The lifetime prevalence of stalking was 4.8% for women and 0.6% for men. The 12-month prevalence of physical assaults by an intimate partner was much lower than reported by previous national surveys (Schafer, Caetano, and Clark 1998; Straus and Gelles 1990; Szinovacz and Egley 1995) at 1.3% for women and 0.9% for men. The 12-month prevalence of rape or stalking for women or men were all less than 1.0% (Tjaden and Thoennes 2000a). The 1-year incidence rates of violent incidents involving intimate partners per 1,000 women were 3.2, 44.2, and 5.0 for rape, physical assault, and stalking, respectively. The 1-year incidence rates per 1,000 men were 31.5 and 1.8 for physical assault and stalking; small numbers precluded estimation of the incidence of rape events in men (Tjaden and Thoennes 2000a). Women and men with a history of same-sex cohabitation had a higher lifetime prevalence of physical assault (35.4% and 21.5%, respectively) than did women and men with opposite-sex cohabitation (20.4% and 7.1%, respectively). Women who reported a history of same-sex cohabitation were more likely to have been victimized by a male partner than a female partner in their lifetime. Similarly, men with a history of same-sex cohabitation were also more likely to have been victimized by a male partner than a female partner in their lifetime (Tjaden and Thoennes 2000a).

The Behavioral Risk Factor Surveillance System (BRFSS), a CDC-sponsored ongoing telephone survey of adults in the United States, has an optional module of questions related to victimization by an intimate partner; in 2005, 16 states and over 70,000 respondents responded to questions in the first BRFSS-administered IPV module (Breiding, Black, and Ryan 2008). An intimate partner was defined as a current or former spouse, girlfriend, or boyfriend; only one of the couple was interviewed (Centers for Disease Control and Prevention 2005). The questions asked about specific behaviors and were based on the CDC uniform definitions (Saltzman et al. 2002). Respondents were asked whether an intimate partner had ever threatened, attempted, or actually hit, slapped, pushed, kicked, or hurt the respondent in any way. The respondent was also asked whether they had ever experienced unwanted sex. Respondents who answered affirmatively to any of these questions were asked two follow-up questions related to whether physical or sexual violence had occurred in the last 12-month period and whether the respondents had a related injury in the last 12 months (Breiding, Black, and Ryan 2008). Overall, 26.4% of women and 15.9% of men reported a lifetime prevalence of IPV that included threatened and/or actual physical violence and unwanted sex; an estimated 10.2% of women and 1.5% of men reported unwanted sex. In the past 12 months, 1.4% of women and 0.7% of men reported having experienced physical violence and/or unwanted sex (Breiding, Black, and Ryan 2008).

The 1-year prevalence estimates of IPV were much lower in the NVAWS and BRFSS surveys than in those of the NFSV, NSFH, and NCLS. One major difference between these surveys is that the NVAWS and BRFSS interviewed only one person in the couple about victimization by IPV. This may partially explain the higher prevalence observed in the NSFH and NCLS surveys, which used responses from both couple members to estimate 1-year IPV prevalence. The higher 1-year prevalence in the NFSV may result from using information collected on both victimization and perpetration to estimate FMPV and MFPV. Though the NVAWS, NCLS, and NFSV all used a modified version of the CTS to measure physical violence, the surveys were framed differently. In contrast to the NVAWS, both the NFSV and the NCLS surveys included a preamble to IPV-related questions acknowledging that couples deal with conflict in many different ways (Tjaden and Thoennes 2000a). Though some have suggested that this preamble could be considered leading (Tjaden and Thoennes 2000a), this introduction may have made respondents feel more comfortable about disclosing violent behavior. Additionally, both the NVAWS and BRFSS asked first about ever experiencing IPV-related behavior; only the subset who reported ever experiencing IPV were asked about the previous 12-month period. This pattern of questioning may have facilitated underreporting and contributed to the lower 1-year IPV prevalence estimates in the NVAWS and BRFSS. An alternative explanation is that respondents to the NLCS and NFVS disclosed IPV-related experiences beyond the previous 12-month time frame for which the questions were asked. Though the dissimilarities across surveys may explain at least some of the differences in the 1-year IPV prevalence estimates, the extent to which these methodological differences account for the wide variation in the 1-year IPV prevalence estimates is unclear.

National Estimates of IPV in Special Populations

The National Crime and Victimization Survey (NCVS) is an ongoing nationwide household survey conducted by the U.S. Bureau of Justice Statistics (BJS) on all forms of criminal victimization, including crime-related victimization by an intimate partner. This in-person survey collects information on crime incidents that the victim reports (Rennison and Planty 2003). Because many victims do not consider certain IPV behaviors criminal, this survey appreciably underestimates the overall incidence of IPV and is best considered as information about crime-related IPV, a less common and often more serious form of IPV (Tjaden and Thoennes 2000a). Criminal IPV includes IPV-related rape or sexual assault, robbery, simple or aggravated assault, and other serious violent crimes (Rennison and Planty 2003). Intimate partners included current or former spouses, boyfriends, and girlfriends. In 1998, the annual rate of crime-related IPV was 4.7 per 1,000 persons, with 7.7 per 1,000 among women and 1.5 per 1,000 among men. The annual rate of simple assault in 1998, the majority of IPV-related crimes, was 3.0 per 1,000 persons, with 5.0 per 1,000 among women and 1.0 per 1,000 among men (Rennison and Welchans 2000).

The National Violent Death Reporting System (NVDRS), established in 2003, estimates the incidence rate of violent deaths, including those perpetrated by an intimate partner in the United States (Centers for Disease Control and Prevention 2006a). This system obtains information from death certificates, coroner or medical examiner reports, and law enforcement and crime laboratory data. This reporting system collected information from 12 states in 2004. The age-adjusted homicide rate was 5.4 per 100,000 in 2004; 20% of these deaths (1.1 per 100,000) were classified as intimate partner homicide (Centers for Disease Control and Prevention 2006a). In 2003, 77% of all intimate partner homicide victims were women (Breiding, Black, and Ryan 2008). The NCVS, another source of information about intimate partner homicides, estimated the incidence rate of intimate partner murder to be 0.8 per 100,000 in 1998 and higher among women (1.2 per 100,000) than among men (0.5 per 100,000) (Rennison and Welchans 2000).

The Pregnancy Risk Assessment Monitoring System (PRAMS) is a CDC-sponsored nationwide population-based survey of new mothers and is administered in 26 states. New mothers completed a mailed self-administered questionnaire 2 to 6 months after the birth of their child (Silverman et al. 2006). Respondents were asked whether in the 12 months before or during pregnancy their husband or partner pushed, hit, slapped, kicked, choked, or hurt them in any way. The prevalence of victimization was computed using PRAMS data from the years 2000–2003. Overall, 4.7% of new mothers reported having experienced this type of physical violence by an intimate partner in the 12 months before pregnancy; 3.7% reported physical violence during pregnancy (Silverman et al. 2006).

The Youth Risk Behavioral Surveillance System (YRBSS) is a CDC-sponsored national ongoing survey of high school students (grades 9–12) that includes measures on dating violence and forced sexual intercourse (Centers for Disease Control and Prevention 2004). Students were asked whether in the past 12 months they had been hit, slapped, or physically hurt on purpose by their boyfriend or girlfriend (Centers for Disease Control and Prevention 2006b). An estimated 9.2% of all students reported dating violence (9.3% of female and 9.0% of male students). Students were also asked if they had ever been forced to have sexual intercourse when they did not want to; 7.5% reported a lifetime prevalence of forced sexual intercourse (10.8% among female students and 4.2% among males) (Centers for Disease Control and Prevention 2006b).

Estimates of IPV in Select Subgroups

Several of the surveys discussed have published *racial/ethnic specific prevalence* of IPV (Table 22.3). The 1975 NFVS reported a lower 1-year prevalence of MFPV and FMPV among white couples compared with Hispanic couples (Cazenave and Straus 1990). The 1995 NLCS reported the lowest prevalence of MFPV and FMPV among white couples, an intermediate prevalence of MFPV and FMPV among Hispanic couples, and the highest prevalence of MFPV and FMPV among black couples (Caetano et al. 2000; Lipsky and Caetano 2009). The NVAWS observed similar lifetime prevalence of IPV victimization among white and Hispanic women and men. Black, Native American, and mixed-race women and men all had a higher lifetime prevalence of physical assault compared with their white counterparts. Asian/Pacific Island women had a lower lifetime prevalence of physical assault than white women (Tjaden and Thoennes 2000a). Similar trends were observed across race/ethnicity

Table 22.3 Estimates of intimate partner violence across race/ethnicity in national surveys

Survey Information	White		Black		Hispanic		Native American		Asian/Pacific Islander		Mixed	
	Female	Male	Female	Male	Female	Male	Female	Male	Female	Male	Female	Male
National Family Violence Survey, 1975[a]												
1-year prevalence of physical violence	10.8	11.5			17.3	16.8						
National Longitudinal Couples Survey, 1995[a]												
1-year prevalence of IPV[b]	11.5	15.5	22.9	30.4	17.0	21.2						
National Violence Against Women Survey, 1995–1996[c]												
Lifetime prevalence of physical assault	21.3	7.2	26.3	10.8	21.2	6.5	30.7	11.4	12.8		27.1	8.6
Lifetime prevalence of rape	7.7	0.2	7.4	0.9	7.9		15.9		3.8		8.1	
Behavioral Risk Factor Surveillance System, 2005[a,d]												
Lifetime prevalence of IPV[e]	26.8	15.5	29.2	23.3	20.5	15.5	39.0	18.6	9.7	8.1	43.1	26.0
1-year prevalence of IPV[f]	1.2	0.5	2.2		1.8						1.5	
PRAMS, 2000–2003[c]												
1-year prevalence of physical violence	4.1		7.7		4.7		10.1		3.2			
During pregnancy prevalence of physical violence	3.1		6.9		3.9		7.3		2.3			
YRBSS, 2005[a]												
1-year prevalence of dating violence	8.5	8.0	12.0	11.8	9.0	10.9						
Lifetime prevalence of unwanted sexual intercourse	10.8	3.1	11.5	7.1	9.4	6.4						

[a] White, black, Native American, Asian/Pacific Islander, mixed are non-Hispanic.
[b] IPV includes physical violence, forced sex, and threats of violence with a knife or gun.
[c] White, black, Native American, Asian/Pacific Islander, mixed includes Hispanics.
[d] Estimate for Asian/Pacific Islander is for Asians only and does not include Pacific Islanders.
[e] IPV includes threatened, attempted, or completed physical violence or unwanted sex.
[f] IPV includes actual physical violence and unwanted sex.

for the lifetime prevalence of IPV in the BRFSS survey (Breiding, Black, and Ryan 2008). The PRAMS survey reported that the 1-year prevalence of physical violence in the year prior to pregnancy was higher among Native American and black women compared with white and Hispanic mothers (Silverman et al. 2006). The YRBSS reported a slightly higher 1-year prevalence of dating violence among black male and female students than among Hispanic male and female or white male and female students (Centers for Disease Control and Prevention 2006b).

A few surveys have measured *IPV-related injury*. The NVAWS reported more women (41.5%) than men (19.9%) who were victims of physical assault by an intimate partner were injured (Tjaden and Thoennes 2000a). Among these, 28.1% of women and 21.5% of men received medical care; the majority (59.1% of women and 63.2% of men) were treated in a hospital and seen in the emergency room. An estimated 36.2% of female rape victims were injured, and 31.0% of those injured received medical care; over half received medical care in a hospital emergency room. The most common types of physical injuries among both victims of rape and physical assault were scratches, bruises, or welts, comprising more than 70% of all IPV-related injuries (Tjaden and Thoennes 2000a). The NCVS reported that 50% of women and 32% of men reporting crime-related IPV victimization had injuries (Rennison and Welchans 2000); 37% of injured women were treated. The BRFSS reported that the 1-year prevalence of an IPV-related injury was 0.8% among women and 0.2% among men (Breiding, Black, and Ryan 2008).

Recurrence of IPV

Two surveys, the NSHF and the NLCS, resurveyed the same couples several years later and estimated the recurrence of IPV across race/ethnicity. The NSHF, originally conducted in 1987–1988, followed up with married and cohabiting couples in 1994. In NSHF, the proportion of newly violent couples (couples who reported no MFPV in the year prior to 1987–1988 but reported MFPV in the year prior to 1994) varied across race/ethnicity (Jasinski 2001). A greater proportion of Hispanic (9.7%) compared with black (5.8%) or white (3.8%) men were newly violent toward their partner ($p < 0.05$). Estimates of recurrence were similar across Hispanic (4.1%), black (3.9%), and white (2.8%) male race/ethnicity ($p > 0.05$). In analyses that adjusted for employment status, income, age, and cohabitation, blacks appeared to be at increased risk of being newly violent compared with whites ($p = 0.05$); no other statistically stable differences across male race/ethnicity were observed among newly violent or recurrent violent couples (Jasinski 2001). In 2000, the NLCS resurveyed married and cohabiting couples who took part in the original 1995 couples survey (Caetano et al. 2005a). In the 2000 resurvey, the overall prevalences of MFPV (10%) and FMPV (12%) were lower than those reported in 1995. Recurrent IPV was much higher than that reported in the NSHF: recurrent FMPV and MFPV were 44% and 39%, respectively. Similar proportions of couples reported new FMPV (6.0%) or MFPV (5.7%). In an analysis adjusted for employment status, age, cohabitation, patterns of alcohol intake, and history of family violence, black and Hispanic couples were at increased risk of recurrent or new IPV relative to white couples (Caetano et al. 2005a).

Risk Factors for IPV

The strongest and most consistently identified risk factors for IPV are alcohol-related factors and exposure to violence in childhood. Many have observed strong positive associations between alcohol-related problems or alcohol abuse and IPV (Coker et al. 2000b; Cunradi et al. 2002a; Ernst et al. 1997). Several studies have also reported that illicit drug use is related to an increased risk of IPV (Coker et al. 2000b; Cunradi et al. 2002a; Hotaling and Sugarman 1986; McCauley et al. 1995), as are childhood physical abuse and/or witnessing interparental violence (Hotaling and Sugarman 1986; McKinney et al. 2009; RS Thompson et al. 2006; Tjaden and Thoennes 2000a).

Certain demographic factors have also been associated with IPV across several studies. Younger respondents (male and female) were generally at increased risk of IPV (Mechem et al. 1999; RS Thompson et al. 2006; Vest et al. 2002), as were those in lower income brackets compared with those in higher income groups (Breiding, Black, and Ryan 2008; Cunradi et al. 2002b; McCauley et al. 1995; Sorenson, Upchurch, and Shen 1996; RS Thompson et al. 2006; Tjaden and Thoennes 2000a; Vest et al. 2002). Respondents who were uninsured, on Medicare, or received medical assistance were at increased risk of IPV in some (Coker et al. 2000b; McCauley et al. 1995; Mechem et al. 1999) but not all studies (Ernst et al. 1997). Single or separated/divorced respondents have also reported a higher prevalence of IPV than their married counterparts (Coker et al. 2000b; McCauley et al. 1995; Mechem et al. 1999). Cohabiting couples also appeared to be at increased risk of IPV (Fox and Benson 2006; Tjaden and Thoennes 2000a). The evidence is mixed regarding whether unemployment is associated with an increased risk of IPV (Coker et al. 2000b; Hotaling and Sugarman 1986; McCauley et al. 1995; RS Thompson et al. 2006).

Findings concerning race/ethnicity have been inconsistent (Caetano et al. 2000; Ernst et al. 1997; Mechem et al. 1999; RS Thompson et al. 2006; Tjaden and Thoennes 2000a). Some find that blacks and Hispanics are at increased risk of IPV compared with whites, while others report a decreased risk or no association with IPV. Researchers have observed that, in some cases, when factors such as income and education are accounted for, black or Hispanic race/ethnicity no longer confers an increased risk of male-to-female IPV (Caetano et al. 2000; Cazenave and Straus 1990; Rennison and Planty 2003; Straus and Smith 1990). In the few studies that report on other race/ethnicity groups, Native Americans tend to have an increased risk of IPV, whereas Asians and Pacific Islanders tend to have a decreased risk of IPV compared with whites (Breiding, Black, and Ryan 2008; Silverman et al. 2006; Tjaden and Thoennes 2000a).

One limitation of the data is that most studies of risk factors for IPV are cross-sectional, and it is often unclear whether correlates such as alcohol-related or drug-related problems preceded or followed the onset of IPV. Moreover, most studies have examined risk factors for male-to-female IPV, and less is known about factors related to the risk of FMPV. Nevertheless, these risk factors may help clinicians identify individuals, especially women, who may be likely to experience IPV.

Clinical Considerations and Prevention of IPV

Identification, Education, and Treatment

An estimated 4.8 million women and 2.9 million men are victimized by an intimate partner each year in the United States. Of these, an estimated 1.8 million women and 580,000 men are injured and 550,000 women and 125,000 men receive medical care. Many victims of violence present in outpatient and other primary care clinics; however, the greatest proportion receive medical care in hospital emergency rooms (Tjaden and Thoennes 2000a). By one estimate, 37% of women cared for in hospital emergency rooms for violence-related injuries were victims of IPV (Rand 1997). Both female and male victims of violence are at increased risk of a wide range of mental and physical health problems, including chronic pain, frequent headaches, sexually transmitted infections, substance abuse, depressive symptoms, and mental illness (Bonomi et al. 2006; Carbone-López, Kruttschnitt, and Macmillan 2006; Coker et al. 2000a, 2002; Tjaden and Thoennes 2000a). Clinicians may wish to consider routinely assessing patients with risk factors for IPV or evidence of these mental or physical health conditions.

To date, there has been very limited education and training of primary care providers, emergency medicine physicians, and other relevant health care professionals in diagnosing and treating IPV. In 2001, the Institute of Medicine recognized the high prevalence of IPV, the frequent utilization of health services by IPV victims, and the lack of knowledge concerning IPV among health care providers and published a detailed report on the need to educate and train health professionals about family violence (Institute of Medicine 2002). More recently, the Family Violence Prevention Fund partnered with the National Health Care Standards Campaign on Domestic Violence to create a national advisory committee comprised of a coalition of health care providers and public health and policy professionals. The national advisory committee developed the updated *National Consensus Guidelines on Identifying and Responding to Domestic Violence Victimization in Health Care Settings* (The Family Violence Prevention Fund 2004). These guidelines provide information on the routine assessment of IPV and indicate the kinds of providers who should be trained, where identification and response to IPV victims should occur, what providers should ask, who should be routinely screened, and how to assess a victim's current safety, maintain confidentiality, and document appropriately. These diagnostic and treatment guidelines are free and available online through the Family Violence Prevention Fund Web site at http://endabuse.org/programs/healthcare/files/Consensus.pdf.

In clinical practice, the first step in identifying victims of IPV is screening. In 2004, the U.S. Preventive Services Task Force evaluated the screening of women for IPV. Screening tools such as the Women's Experience with Battering (WEB) scale and the Partner Abuse Inventory, an 11-item questionnaire based on the CTS, show fair to good internal consistency (Smith, Earp, and DeVellis 1995). However, there have been no studies that examine whether these screening tools are effective in reducing IPV or whether screening puts victims at increased risk of IPV (Nelson et al. 2004). Nevertheless, several professional medical organizations, such as the American Medical Association, American Academy of Family Physicians, and the American College of Obstetricians and Gynecologists, do recommend screening and treating identified victims of IPV (American College of Obstetricians and Gynecologists 2002).

Once identified, many victims of IPV do not immediately leave their intimate partner (Coker 2006). However, providing victims with the resources to consider their options and make informed decisions may help them make decisions about their future. Clinicians can provide several resources to patients in need of IPV victimization information and services. The National Domestic Violence hotline (800)799-SAFE (7233) is a 24-hour resource available in English and Spanish as well as 140 other languages through interpreter services. The National Domestic Hotline gives women information about domestic violence and also provides services such as crisis intervention, safety planning, and referrals to local area providers such as shelters. Their Web site is http://www.ndvh.org. The National Sexual Assault Hotline (800)656-HOPE (4673) provides 24-hour free confidential counseling to victims of sexual violence and is maintained by the Rape, Abuse and Incest National Network (Web site www.rainn.org). This National Sexual Assault Hotline provides crisis and intervention support and information about medical evidence and other medical issues, explains the criminal justice system, answers questions about recovery, and connects victims with services in their area. The Family Violence Prevention Fund (http://www.endabuse.org) also provides direct services such as information about how to create a personal and/or work safety plan and has a wide range of fact sheets and other IPV-related information.

Prevention

Efforts to develop effective and appropriate prevention programs have been limited. The CDC has sponsored several projects aimed at identifying effective strategies for primary and secondary IPV prevention. The CDC is also tracking the development of cost-effective prevention programs (Centers for Disease Control and Prevention 2007). A number of studies aimed at primary prevention of IPV have been conducted in adolescents, and though a few programs are promising, there is no gold standard as yet (Whitaker et al. 2006). Similarly, interventions to prevent abuse or reabuse are limited. As mentioned earlier, studies of the effectiveness of screening to improve outcomes for IPV victims have not been completed (Nelson et al. 2004; Wathen and MacMillan 2003). Additional research into primary and secondary IPV prevention is urgently needed to reduce its tragic burden and adverse consequences.

Conclusion

A substantial proportion of women and men are victims and/or perpetrators of IPV at some point in their lives. We have provided an overview of the estimates of IPV across broad national surveys and in specific subgroups. We also described several of the most frequently identified risk factors that may help providers identify female and male victims and perpetrators of IPV. Health care professionals, especially primary care providers and emergency room physicians, are often in a unique position to identify and connect victims of IPV with resources that can facilitate treatment and address safety. Recent guidelines provide comprehensive information regarding how to diagnose and treat victims while ensuring their safety. Further research on effective primary and secondary prevention programs is needed in order to develop strategies and programs that will prevent IPV.

References

American College of Obstetricians and Gynecologists (ACOG). *Guidelines for Women's Health Care*, 2nd edition. Washington, DC: American College of Obstetricians and Gynecologists, 2002.

Bonomi AE, Thompson RS, Anderson M et al. Intimate partner violence and women's physical, mental, and social functioning. *Am J Prev Med* 30:458–466, 2006.

Breiding MJ, Black MC, Ryan GW. Prevalence and risk factors of intimate partner violence in eighteen U.S. states/territories, 2005. *Am J Prev Med* 34:112–118, 2008.

Caetano R, Cunradi CB, Clark CL et al. Intimate partner violence and drinking patterns among white, black, and Hispanic couples in the U.S. *J Subst Abuse* 11:123–138, 2000.

Caetano R, Field CA, Ramisetty-Mikler S et al. The five-year course of intimate partner violence among White, Black and Hispanic couples in the U.S. *J Interpers Violence* 20:1039–1057, 2005a.

Caetano R, McGrath C, Ramisetty-Mikler S et al. Drinking, alcohol problems and the five-year recurrence and incidence of male to female and female to male partner violence. *Alcohol Clin Exp Res* 29:98–106, 2005b.

Caetano R, Ramisetty-Mikler S, Field CA. Unidirectional and bidirectional intimate partner violence among White, Black, and Hispanic couples in the United States. *Violence Vict* 20:393–406, 2005.

Carbone-López K, Kruttschnitt C, Macmillan R. Patterns of intimate partner violence and their associations with physical health, psychological distress, and substance use. *Public Health Rep* 121:382–392, 2006.

Cazenave NA, Straus MA. Race, class, network embeddedness, and family violence: A search for potent support systems, in *Physical Violence in American Families: Risk Factors and Adaptations to Violence in 8,145 Families.* Edited by Straus MA, Gelles RJ. New Brunswick, NJ: Transaction Publishers, 1990, pp. 321–339.

Centers for Disease Control and Prevention. Building data systems for monitoring and responding to violence against women. *MMWR Recomm Rep* 49:1–18, 2000.

Centers for Disease Control and Prevention. Methodology of the Youth Risk Behavior Surveillance System. *MMWR Recomm Rep* 53:1–13, 2004.

Centers for Disease Control and Prevention. *Behavioral Risk Factor Surveillance System questionnaire.* Atlanta, GA: Centers for Disease Control and Prevention, 2005.

Centers for Disease Control and Prevention. Homicides and suicides – National Violent Death Reporting System, United States, 2003–2004. *MMWR Morb Mortal Wkly Rep* 55:721–724, 2006a.

Centers for Disease Control and Prevention. Youth Risk Behavior Surveillance – United States, 2005. *MMWR CDC Surveill Summ* 55:1–108, 2006b.

Centers for Disease Control and Prevention. Preventing Violence against Women: Program Activities Guide. Atlanta, GA: Centers for Disease Control and Prevention, 2007.

Coker AL. Preventing intimate partner violence: How we will rise to this challenge. *Am J Prev Med* 30:528–529, 2006.

Coker AL, Davis KE, Arias I et al. Physical and mental health effects of intimate partner violence for men and women. *Am J Prev Med* 23:260–268, 2002.

Coker AL, Smith PH, Bethea L et al. Physical health consequences of physical and psychological intimate partner violence. *Arch Fam Med* 9:451–457, 2000a.

Coker AL, Smith PH, McKeown RE et al. Frequency and correlates of intimate partner violence by type: Physical, sexual, and psychological battering. *Am J Public Health* 90:553–559, 2000b.

Cunradi CB, Caetano R, Schafer J. Alcohol-related problems, drug use, and male intimate partner violence severity among US couples. *Alcohol Clin Exp Res* 26:493–500, 2002a.

Cunradi CB, Caetano R, Schafer J. Socioeconomic predictors of intimate partner violence among White, Black, and Hispanic couples in the United States. *J Fam Violence* 17:377–389, 2002b.

DeKeseredy WS. Current controversies on defining nonlethal violence against women in intimate heterosexual relationships: Empirical implications. *Violence Against Women* 6:728–746, 2000.

Ernst AA, Nick TG, Weiss SJ et al. Domestic violence in an inner-city ED. *Ann Emerg Med* 30:190–197, 1997.

The Family Violence Prevention Fund. *National Consensus Guidelines on Identifying and Responding to Domestic Violence Victimization in Health Care Settings.* San Francisco, CA: The Family Violence Prevention Fund, 2004.

Fox GL, Benson ML. Household and neighborhood contexts of intimate partner violence. *Public Health Rep* 121:419–427, 2006.

Gordon M. Definitional issues in violence against women: Surveillance and research from a violence research perspective. *Violence Against Women* 6:747–783, 2000.

Hotaling GT, Sugarman DB. An analysis of risk markers in husband to wife violence: The current state of knowledge. *Violence Vict* 1:101–124, 1986.

Institute of Medicine. Executive summary, in *Confronting Chronic Neglect: The Education and Training of Health Professionals on Family Violence.* Edited by Cohn F, Salmon ME, Stobo JD. Washington, DC: National Academy Press, 2002, pp. 1–11.

Jasinski JL. Physical violence among Anglo, African American, and Hispanic couples: Ethnic differences in persistence and cessation. *Violence Vict* 16:479–490, 2001.

Jasinski JL. Physical violence among white, African American, and Hispanic couples: Ethnic differences in initiation, persistence, and cessation, in *Violence Against Women and Family Violence: Developments in Research, Practice, and Policy.* Edited by Fisher BS. Washington, DC: U.S. Department of Justice, 2004, pp. I-3-1–I-3-11.

Lipsky S, Caetano R. Definitions, surveillance systems and the prevalence and incidence of intimate partner violence in the United States, in *Preventing Partner Violence: Research and Evidence-Based Intervention Strategies.* Edited by Whitaker DJ, Lutzker JR. Washington, DC: American Psychological Association, 2009, pp. 17–40.

McCauley J, Kern DE, Kolodner K et al. The "battering syndrome": Prevalence and clinical characteristics of domestic violence in primary care internal medicine practices. *Ann Intern Med* 123:737–746, 1995.

McKinney CM, Caetano R, Ramisetty-Mikler S et al. Childhood family violence and perpetration and victimization of intimate partner violence: Findings from a national population-based study of couples. *Ann Epidemiol* 19(1): 25–32, 2009.

Mechem CC, Shofer FS, Reinhard SS et al. History of domestic violence among male patients presenting to an urban emergency department. *Acad Emerg Med* 6:786–791, 1999.

National Victim Center. *Rape in America: A Report to the Nation.* Arlington, VA: National Victim Center & Crime Victims Research and Treatment Center, 1992.

Nelson HD, Nygren P, McInerney Y et al. Screening women and elderly adults for family and intimate partner violence: A review of the evidence for the US Preventive Services Task Force. *Ann Intern Med* 140:387–396, 2004.

Rand MR. *Violence-Related Injuries Treated in Hospital Emergency Departments.* Washington, DC: U.S. Department of Justice, 1997.

Rennison C, Planty M. Nonlethal intimate partner violence: Examining race, gender, and income patterns. *Violence Vict* 18:433–443, 2003.

Rennison CM, Welchans S. *Intimate Partner Violence.* Washington, DC: U.S. Department of Justice, 2000.

Saltzman LE, Fanslow JL, McMahon PM et al. *Intimate partner violence surveillance: Uniform definitions and recommended data elements, Version 1.0.* Atlanta, GA: Centers for Disease Control and Prevention, 2002.

Schafer J, Caetano R, Clark CL. *Intimate Partner Violence in the US: Results of the National Couples Study*. Berkeley: Alcohol Research Group, 1997.

Schafer J, Caetano R, Clark CL. Rates of intimate partner violence in the United States. *Am J Public Health* 88:1702–1704, 1998.

Silverman JG, Decker MR, Reed E et al. Intimate partner violence around the time of pregnancy: Association with breastfeeding behavior. *J Womens Health* 15:934–940, 2006.

Smith PH, Earp JA, DeVellis R. Measuring battering: Development of the Women's Experience with Battering (WEB) scale. *Womens Health* 1:273–288, 1995.

Sorenson SB, Upchurch DM, Shen H. Violence and injury in marital arguments: Risk patterns and gender differences. *Am J Public Health* 86:35–40, 1996.

Straus MA. Measuring intrafamily conflict and violence: The Conflict Tactics (CT) scales. *J Marriage Fam* 7:75–88, 1979.

Straus MA. Measuring intrafamily conflict and violence: The Conflict Tactics (CT) scales, in *Physical Violence in American Families: Risk Factors and Adaptations to Violence in 8,145 Families*. Edited by Straus MA, Gelles RJ. New Brunswick, NJ: Transaction Publishers, 1990a, pp. 29–47.

Straus MA. The National Family Violence Surveys, in *Physical Violence in American Families: Risk Factors and Adaptations to Violence in 8,145 Families*. Edited by Straus MA, Gelles RJ. New Brunswick, NJ: Transaction Publishers, 1990b, pp. 3–16.

Straus MA, Gelles R. How violent are American families? Estimates from the National Family Violence Resurvey and other studies, in *Physical Violence in American Families: Risk Factors and Adaptations to Violence in 8,145 Families*. Edited by Straus M, Gelles R. New Brunswick, NJ: Transaction Publishers, 1990, pp. 95–112.

Straus MA, Gelles RJ. Societal change and change in family violence from 1975 to 1985 as revealed by two national surveys. *J Marriage Fam* 48:465–479, 1986.

Straus MA, Hamby SL, Boney-McCoy S et al. The revised Conflict Tactics Scales (CTS2): Development and preliminary psychometric data. *J Fam Issues* 17:283–316, 1996.

Straus MA, Smith C. Violence in Hispanic families in the United States: Incidence rates and structural interpretations, in *Physical Violence in American Families: Risk Factors and Adaptations to Violence in 8,145 Families*. Edited by Straus MA, Gelles RJ. New Brunswick, NJ: Transactions Publishers, 1990, pp. 341–367.

Sweet J, Bumpass L, Call V. *The Design and Content of the National Survey of Families and Households*. Working Paper, University of Wisconsin, Madison, 1988.

Szinovacz ME, Egley LC. Comparing one-partner and couple data on sensitive marital behaviors: The case of marital violence. *J Marriage Fam* 57:995–1010, 1995.

Thompson MP, Basile KC, Hertz MF et al. *Measuring Intimate Partner Violence Victimization and Perpetration: A Compendium of Assessment Tools*. Atlanta, GA: Centers for Disease Control and Prevention, 2006a.

Thompson RS, Bonomi AE, Anderson M et al. Intimate partner violence: Prevalence, types, and chronicity in adult women. *Am J Prev Med* 30:447–457, 2006b.

Tjaden P, Thoennes N. *Extent, Nature, and Consequences of Intimate Partner Violence: Findings from the National Violence Against Women Survey*. Washington, DC: U.S. Department of Justice, 2000a.

Tjaden P, Thoennes N. *Full Report of the Prevalence, Incidence, and Consequences of Violence against Women: Findings from the National Violence Against Women Survey*. Washington, DC: U.S. Department of Justice, 2000b.

Vest JR, Catlin TK, Chen JJ et al. Multistate analysis of factors associated with intimate partner violence. *Am J Prev Med* 22:156–164, 2002.

Wathen CN, MacMillan HL. Interventions for violence against women: Scientific review. *JAMA* 289:589–600, 2003.

Whitaker DJ, Haileyesus T, Swahn M et al. Differences in frequency of violence and reported injury between relationships with reciprocal and nonreciprocal intimate partner violence. *Am J Public Health* 97:941–947, 2007.

Whitaker DJ, Morrison S, Lindquist C et al. A critical review of interventions for the primary prevention of perpetration of partner violence. *Aggress Violent Behav* 11:151–166, 2006.

23

Pyromania: Clinical Aspects

Candice Germain, MD, and Michel Lejoyeux, MD, PhD

History of Psychiatric Attention to the Disorder

Pyromania is defined as an impulsive behavior leading to fire setting without an identifiable motive other than taking pleasure in viewing the fire and its effects. The essential features are deliberate and purposeful (rather than accidental) fire setting on more than one occasion. The term pyromania was introduced in 1833 by Marc, a French psychiatrist, who described it as a form of "instinctive and impulsive monomania." At that time, monomania meant an abnormal behavior, "a crime against nature, so monstrous and without reason, as to be explicable only through insanity, yet perpetrated by subjects apparently in full possession of their sanity" (Marc 1833). In 1845, Esquirol classified pyromania as a reasoning monomania caused by an instinctive desire to burn (Esquirol 1845). The word pyromania was transported from the French to the English medical vocabulary in the early nineteenth century.

Ray (1844) was the first American psychiatrist to address the question of pathologic arson. In his text on medical jurisprudence of insanity, he described pyromania as a "distinct form of insanity, annulling responsibility for the acts to which it leads." In the 1850s and 1860s, debates separated the authors who supported the idea that pyromania was a mental disorder and those who rejected this idea. President Garfield's assassination in 1881 put into disfavor the use of the insanity plea to defend against criminal charges, and through the remainder of the nineteenth century, most American authorities rejected the concept of pyromania.

After Marc, Griesinger, a German psychiatrist, stated, "Away with the term pyromania, and let there be a careful investigation in every case into the individual psychological peculiarities which lie at the bottom and give rise to this impulse.... To include cases of fire setting under the title of 'pyromania' is the necessary but evil result of a superficial classification" (Griesinger 1867). One hundred forty years later, however, the pyromania diagnosis, is still present, now in the fourth edition of *Diagnostic and Statistical Manual of Mental Disorders* (DSM-IV) (American Psychiatric Association 1994).

In nineteenth-century Europe, the typical arsonist was thought to be a female domestic in her teens, uprooted from her home and family and suffering from nostalgia. In the early twentieth century, Stekel (1924) and Freud (1932) postulated sexual roots of fire setting and advanced a psychoanalytic formulation centered on disordered psychosexual development, specifically fixation at or regression to the phallic-urethral stage of psychosexual development.

Until 1950, the case history approach to the study of fire setting, with all its weaknesses, was dominant. In 1951, Lewis and Yarnell, in their important monograph on pathologic fire setting, described several groups of arsonists, having reviewed the case histories of 1,626 arsonists collected largely from the National Board of Fire Underwriters (Lewis and Yarnell 1951). In 688 cases (42%), no objective reason explained the fire setting. From these cases, Lewis and Yarnell derived a still modern conception of pyromania: "Unexplained cases of fire-setting may correspond to pyromaniacs, acting under irrational impulses, with possible internal tension, agitation, or derealisation." Their paper has been cited by almost all later scholars working on this topic. Although research has continued, our understanding of pyromania remains poor.

While DSM-I (American Psychiatric Association 1952) classified pyromania as an obsessive-compulsive reaction, the majority of American medical literature in the 1960s rejected the concept of pyromania as a specific mental disorder. In 1968, DSM-II (American Psychiatric Association 1968) did not mention the term at all. In the 1970s, pyromania reemerged as a distinct impulse control disorder (Mavromatis and Lion 1977) and returned in DSM-III (American Psychiatric Association 1980) under the category of "disorders of impulse control not elsewhere classified."

Definitions and Differential Diagnosis

Many pathological behaviors in addition to pyromania are forms of deliberate fire setting. Most of these behaviors are criminal rather than psychiatric.

"Fire setting" is the broadest term because it does not require the act to be intentional.

"Arson" refers to the act of deliberately setting fire to property of any kind. Authors writing in the field of criminology and law presume that most cases of arson are motivated by financial benefit to the individual. Most of these criminal acts are frauds committed in order to get money from insurance companies. Arson is a major source of property damage, injury, and death, and its incidence appears to have increased in both the United States and Europe (see Chapter 24, this volume). Some studies suggest that the frequency of criminal fire setting increases in times of economic recession, whereas in times of high inflation, the frequency is low (Lejoyeux, McLoughlin, and Ades 2006). Other criminal reasons for arson include the attempt to prepare or to conceal another crime or to threaten or blackmail people.

"Pathologic arson or fire setting" designates the act as secondary to a medical, neurological, or psychiatric disorder.

According to the DSM-IV-TR (text revision) diagnostic criteria, fire setting by pyromaniacs is not done for criminal reasons, for profit or sabotage, for monetary gain, as an expression of sociopolitical ideology (an act of terrorism or protest) or anger, or for revenge. Pyromania must be distinguished from fire-setting behavior better explained by schizophrenia, bipolar disorder, substance abuse, personality disorders, dementia, and mental retardation. The DSM-IV-TR also excludes self-immolation and "communicative arson." (Some individuals with mental disorders use fire to communicate a desire or need; see Geller 1992a.) Pyromania, in the sense of arson without a separate motive, is a rare phenomenon that seldom explains repeated fire-setting behavior. The validity of pyromania as a psychiatric diagnosis continues to be questioned in that some do not believe that this mental disorder really exists.

A Broad Classification of Arson

Geller (1992b) has presented a clinically focused classification of arson (Table 23.1). He emphasized the complexity of establishing such a classification because methodological difficulties interfere: (a) samples are often derived from very specialized populations (hospital, prison, etc.), and (b) while typologies artificially segregate fire setters into two groups, the so-called motivated group and the so-called motiveless group, pathological fire setters assigned to the latter category may have motives. Among schizophrenic patients, for example, a significant percentage of fire setting can be accounted for by reasons other than delusional ideation or hallucinations. Some patients can be sophisticated enough to set fires for reasons independent of hallucinations but then blame the arson on "the voices"!

Diagnosis

In the DSM-IV-TR, pyromania (Code 312.33) is classified as an impulse control disorder (ICD) not elsewhere classified. The DSM-IV-TR diagnostic criteria (Table 23.2) exclude fire

Table 23.1 Classification of arson

Arson Unassociated with Psychobiologic Disorders	Arson Associated with Mental Disorders
Arson for profit	Disorders of thought or perception
Insurance fraud	Delusions
Welfare fraud	Hallucinations
Bankruptcy scam	Disorders of mood
Property improvements	Depression
Building strippers	Mania
Burglary	Disorders of judgment
Business modifications	Developmental disorders
Employment	Dementia
Crime concealment	Psychoactive substance-induced disorders
Revenge	Disorders of impulse control
Vanity of recognition	Intermittent explosive disorder
Hero syndrome	Pyromania
Fire buff	Communicative arson
Vagrant	
Vandalism	
Political	
Riot	
Terrorism	
Protest	
Arson Associated with Medical or Neurologic Disorders	Juvenile Fire
Chromosomal disorders	Fire setting
Klinefelter's syndrome	Fire play
XYY syndrome	
Central nervous system disorders	
Epilepsy	
Head trauma	
Brain tumor	
Infectious diseases	
Acquired Immune Deficiency Syndrome (AIDS)	
Endocrine and metabolic disorders	
Late luteal phase dysphoric disorder	
Hypoglycemia	

Table 23.2 Pyromania (Code 312.33) DSM-IV-TR criteria

A. Deliberate and purposeful fire setting on more than one occasion.
B. Tension or affective arousal before the act.
C. Fascination with, interest in, curiosity about, or attraction to fire and its situational contexts (i.e., utensils, utilization, and consequences).
D. Pleasure, gratification, or relief when setting fires or when witnessing or participating in their aftermath.
E. The fire setting is not done for monetary gain, sociopolitical ideology, criminal purpose, out of anger or revenge, or in response to delusional ideas, hallucinations, or judgment disorder (i.e., dementia, mental retardation, or substance intoxication).
F. The fire setting is not better explained by a conduct disorder, a manic episode, or an antisocial personality.

setting better explained by any other diagnosis. Pyromania is characterized by a failure to resist impulsive, repetitive, deliberate fire-setting urges that are unrelated to external reward (money, revenge, or political act).

In the *International Classification of Diseases*, tenth edition (ICD-10) (World Health Organization 2002), pyromania is listed in the category "habit and impulsive disorders"

(Code F63). The definition closely resembles the DSM-IV-TR definition (Table 23.2), but substitutes the phrase "persistent preoccupation with subjects related to fire and burning" for the "fascination" and "interest" mentioned in DSM-IV-TR.

Apart from the DSM-IV-TR and ICD-10 definitions, the term "pyromania" has sometimes been used to denote all acts of fire setting motivated by the pleasure in watching the fire (Vreeland and Lewin 1980). Some authors have used this term for individuals who seem to attain sexual satisfaction from fire setting (Prins 1980). Others have used the term as a diagnostic label for individuals who are motivated by an irresistible impulse to set fires (Mavromatis and Lion 1977). Pyromania could also be considered a compulsive behavior, but no published study justifies this label. To our knowledge, a relationship between pyromania and the obsessive-compulsive spectrum has not been demonstrated.

The notion of behavioral addiction could also be applied to pyromania. The recent work of Grant and Kim (2007), described later in this chapter, confirms that pyromania shares many phenomenological characteristics with other impulse control disorders and addictive disorders:

Urge or craving state prior to engaging in the behavior
Pleasure derived from the behavior
Repetitive engagement in the behavior despite negative consequences
Diminished control over the behavior
Increased frequency and intensity of the behavior over time (tolerance)

Clinical Picture of Pyromania and Fire Setting

The essential feature of pyromania is the presence of multiple deliberate fire settings for the purpose of pleasure or gratification. Another important clinical feature is the individual's fascination with fire. Patients present an urge to engage in fire setting, along with a loss of control, despite the negative consequences. Some pyromaniacs, however, make meticulous preparations before acting on the urge and experience tension or emotional arousal during this preparation phase.

Pyromaniacs like watching fire. They are often recognized as regular "watchers" at fires in their neighborhoods. They may activate false fire alarms. They often have a passion for the institutions, equipment, and persons who struggle against fire. They may spend time in the local fire station or even work as firefighters. Some collect firemen's tools and fire photos. Pyromaniacs are usually indifferent to the material or human consequences of a fire they have caused. Some may experience a certain pleasure while viewing the resulting destruction.

Grant and Kim (2007) described the features of 21 individuals with a DSM–IV lifetime diagnosis of pyromania. The mean ($\pm$ SD) age at onset of pyromania was 18.1 ($\pm$ 5.8) years. Eighteen subjects (85.7%) reported urges to set fires. Subjects reported setting a fire a mean ($\pm$ SD) of once every 5.9 ($\pm$ 3.8) weeks. Most fire settings did not meet the legal definition of arson: subjects reported setting "controlled" fires in their bathrooms, in dumpsters, in backyards, or in vacant lots. They found pleasure in setting fires, regardless of what they were burning, and were aware of the significant amount of time they spent on this behavior. The majority (66.7%) described planning the fires, buying utensils to set them, and planning what items would burn most intensely; 57.2% reported watching fires, even those they had not set; and 38.1% reported traveling to fires when they heard fire engines. All subjects reported a "rush" when setting or watching a fire, and most reported a sexual feeling. Of these 21 subjects, 76.2% reported that the frequency of fire setting and the intensity of the fires increased over time. This element is reminiscent of the tolerance phenomenon that occurs in substance use disorders. Triggers for setting fires were most often stress or boredom. All subjects reported pleasure or relief when setting fires, but 19 subjects (90.5%) reported feeling severe distress afterward. Some had thoughts of suicide.

More data are needed to elucidate the course of pyromania. Adolescence is a period of increased risk-taking, and controversy exists about how frequently adolescent fire-setting behavior continues into adulthood (Barnett and Spitzer 1994).

The "normal" human interest in fire starts between 2 and 3 years of age (Nurcombe 1964). Kafry's (1980) study of normal schoolboys at the ages of 6, 8, and 10 found that fire interest was almost universal. Among children (Kosky and Silburn 1984), the distinction between normal interest in fire and excessive interest leading to pyromania is not always clear. Simply playing with matches is not, however, a symptom of pyromania. Kolko and Kazdin (1989a, 1989b) found that children who set fires had more curiosity about fire, recent involvement in fire-related activities, early experience with fire, and contact with peers or family members involved with fire than did children who had not set fires. Thus a continuum may exist between excessive interest in fire and pyromania.

Slavkin (2002) summarized the characteristics of juveniles who set fires. Predictors of fire setting include heightened aggression, social skill deficits, level of deviancy (lying, truancy, running away from home), covert antisocial behavior, and family dynamics (family conflicts, lax discipline, violence at home, parental alcohol or drug abuse, physical or sexual abuse, or emotional neglect).

An abnormal interest in fire is especially important in populations of fire officers who become pyromaniacs. Lewis and Yarnell (1951) described a series of 90 volunteer firemen who deliberately set fires. A notable proportion of fire fetishists is found among pyromaniacs, whether or not they are working as fire officers. McGuire, Carlisle, and Young (1965) showed that a "fire experience" may become a "fire fetish." A fire fantasy – whether imagined or a recollection of a real event – occurring just before orgasm is conditioned by the positive feedback of orgasm to become more and more exciting.

Noblett and Nelson (2001) studied females presenting with pyromania or arson. Arsonists more frequently had histories of deliberate self-harm and sexual abuse, but both groups had often suffered psychosocial traumas and difficulties. Noblett and Nelson (2001) state that pyromania may be a displacement of aggressivity. Patients with pyromania could be unable to confront people directly and could channel their aggression into fire-setting behavior as an attempt to influence their environment and improve their self-esteem where other means have failed. Geller (1987) explained fire setting as an attempt at communication by individuals with few social skills.

Barnett and Spitzer (1994) reviewed the motives of individuals setting fires. Revenge, hatred, envy, jealousy, and disappointed love are most often seen in adults. In adolescents, motives such as malignity, anger, rage, the fun of extinguishing fire, arrogance, and the craving for recognition prevail. In quite a few cases, several motives are present, revenge often being one of them (Hill et al. 1982). In many cases, the act of fire setting is carried out under the influence of alcohol (Geller 1987; Hill et al. 1982).

Many cases of nonpsychotic fire setters who had no obvious motive have also been documented. In these cases, the forensic psychiatric expert is considerably handicapped. Psychological research into the personality of such fire setters is, however, suggestive of personality disorders characterized by intolerance of frustration, overinhibition of aggression in ordinary behavior, striving for power, readily feeling insulted, and a tendency to act aggressively (Lejoyeux et al. 2002).

Group Fire Setters

In general, riot fires represent multiple acts of fire setting in slum suburbs of large cities in times of social and racial strain. The phenomenon is most common in the United States. However, recent acts of fire setting in shelters for refugees in Germany and in suburbs of large cities in France are just as much the result of social and racial tensions. Gangs of fire setters are also sometimes involved in acts of fire setting for political reasons. Fire setting by adolescents, as an act of vandalism motivated by boredom, is found in most societies. In most cases, the vandals are driven not so much by the desire to destroy as by the excitement involved in carrying out the act. Delinquents who commit the criminal act with a group of fire setters are mentally healthier than those who commit the crime individually (Molnar, Keitner, and Harwood 1984).

Assessment

No clinical interview is especially designed to assess pyromania. Most assessment scales of impulse control disorders do not include a section on pyromania. Fire setting is included, however, in the MIDI (Minnesota Impulsive Disorders Interview), a semistructured clinical interview with excellent classification accuracy in adults with ICDs (Grant et al. 2005). The MIDI includes questions for each ICD, with additional follow-up questions reflecting DSM-IV criteria. With regard to fire setting, patients are invited to indicate whether they have lit a fire intentionally and are asked about their urge to set a fire. The MIDI excludes fire setting for financial motives and during periods of anger and examines fires lit to escape from a depressive mood. The last question concerns fascination with fire.

Several instruments are available to detect children at risk for fire setting: Lowenstein Fire Raising Diagnostic Test (Lowenstein 1981, 1989), the Children's Fire-setting Interview (Kolko and Kazdin 1989a), and the Fire-setting Risk Interview (Kolko and Kazdin 1989b). No such instruments are available for the adult population.

Prevalence

To our knowledge, there are no prevalence data for pyromania in the general population. The majority of epidemiological studies have focused on fire setting in childhood or adolescence: prevalence has been estimated at between 2.4% (Jacobson 1985) and 3.5% (Kolko and Kadzin 1989b; Kosky and Silbrun 1984). Sixty percent of all fires in large U.S. cities are lit by individuals under 18 years of age (Raines and Foy 1994). Among juveniles, fire setting is more prevalent in males than in females (Soltys 1992).

Pyromania is rare in recent studies of psychiatric populations, in contrast to results from earlier periods. This contrast may result in part from the fact that, before the publication of DSM-III, the term pyromania was often misapplied in the psychiatric literature and referred to all pathologic fire setters. This still may be the case in the nonpsychiatric literature on arsonists, in which the prevalence of pyromania is reported as considerably higher than in the psychiatric literature.

The prevalence of pyromania among adult arsonists is not well established. In a prospective study between 1983 and 1993 of 153 adult arsonists in Yorkshire, the next most common motive after revenge (31%) was excitement (11%), which could correspond to pyromania (Rix 1994). In a retrospective study of 282 arsonists, the rate of pyromania was high: pyromania was found in 23% of arsonists who had committed other nonviolent crimes and in 12% of arsonists with a history of violent crimes (Repo et al. 1997). In a recent Finnish study describing a forensic psychiatric population of 90 arson recidivists, only three subjects (3.3%) fulfilled the diagnostic criteria for pyromania (Lindberg et al. 2005).

The current prevalence of pyromania in 204 adult psychiatric inpatients was 3.4% ($n = 7$) and the lifetime prevalence 5.9% ($n = 12$) (Grant et al. 2005). A French study involving 107 depressed patients found that 3 (2.8%) met the DSM-IV-TR criteria for pyromania (Lejoyeux et al. 2002). Another study of 79 alcoholic inpatients found no case of pyromania (Lejoyeux et al. 1999).

In one study in a child psychiatric outpatient population, the diagnosis of pyromania applied in only 2 of 32 fire setters (6.3%) (Heath et al. 1985). A recent study looking for ICDs in 102 adolescent psychiatric inpatients found a 6.9% current prevalence rate for pyromania, with a statistically significantly higher rate in girls (Grant, Williams, and Potenza 2007).

Grant and Kim (2007) constructed a detailed demographic picture of 21 individuals meeting DSM-IV lifetime criteria for pyromania. Fourteen were adults, of whom 3 (21.4%) were female, and 7 were adolescents, all of whom were female. The subjects' ages ranged from 15 to 49 years (mean ± SD = 26.1 ± 11.8). The majority of the subjects were white (85.7%) and single or divorced (71% of the adults and all adolescents). Adults had good educational attainment (57.1% were high school graduates), and most (71.4%) were employed. Five (23.8%) alleged histories of sexual abuse, and 7 (33.3%) reported histories of physical abuse.

Comorbidities of Arson and Pyromania

Establishing rates of psychiatric comorbidities among individuals with pyromania is difficult because most data are reported for broader groups such as fire setters or arsonists. These heterogeneous data are summarized here, while attempting to keep clear the groups described.

Only one study has examined psychiatric comorbidity in a sample of individuals ($n = 21$) with a history of pyromania (Grant and Kim 2007). Thirteen subjects (61.9%) had a current comorbid mood disorder, 10 (47.6%) met criteria for another ICD, and 7 (33.3%) had a diagnosis of a substance use disorder. Some subjects felt that their mood symptoms and substance abuse were responses to their distress over setting fires. Of the 21 subjects, 95% had at least one lifetime comorbid psychiatric disorder, particularly major depression (48%), bipolar disorder (14%), another impulse control disorder (67%), or a substance use disorder (33%). Interestingly, all subjects who no longer met criteria for pyromania reported that symptoms of another ICD or substance use disorder had started since they stopped setting fires (Grant and Kim 2007).

The true rate of mental illness in fire setters is hard to establish, in part because many fire setters are not apprehended. Hence, rates from about 10% to 20% (U.S. Department of Justice 1982) to over 60% (Taylor and Gunn 1984) have been reported. The disorders most frequently present are personality disorders, psychotic disorders, and mental retardation (Barnett and Spitzer 1994 [fire setters]; Lindberg et al. 2005 [arsonists]; Rix 1994 [arsonists]).

In a study of 106 cases of fire setting referred for psychiatric examination (Gunzel 1987), 56% of these fire setters suffered from mental retardation, a personality disorder, dementia, or alcoholism; 7.6% had a psychotic disorder; more than 30% had no apparent separate motive; and the act was rationally motivated in only 3%.

In a Finnish study (Joukamaa and Touvinen 1983), fire setters for whom a psychiatric expert opinion had been obtained received a diagnosis of psychosis or borderline personality disorder more frequently than other delinquents. Alcoholism and mood disorders are also frequent diagnoses among arsonists (Koson and Dvoskin 1982).

In a study of mental health records and/or prison files of 283 arsonists, Ritchie and Huff (1999) found that 36% had a diagnosis of schizophrenia or bipolar disorder and 64% were abusing alcohol or drugs at the time of fire setting; only 3 cases carried a pyromania diagnosis. Other authors have noted a close link between fire setting, aggression, and antisocial behavior in juvenile fire setters (Stickle and Blechman 2002).

The reported prevalence of personality disorders in arsonists and fire setters varies between 25% and 66% (Bourget and Bradford 1989; Bradford 1982; Bradford and Dimock 1986; Hill et al. 1982; O'Sullivan and Kelleher 1987; Rice and Harris 1990). A study by Virkkunen et al. (1989) in which subjects were selected for the impulsive character of their fire setting reported a prevalence of 90%. When specific diagnoses are provided, the most common personality disorders are antisocial and borderline (Bradford and Dimock 1986; Virkkunen et al. 1989). Forehand et al. (1991) suggest that juvenile fire setting represents an advanced stage of antisocial behavior and is not a unique syndrome. In their study, juvenile fire setters and non–fire setters who had a comparable number of conduct disorder symptoms did not differ on the child behavior checklist subscales of adolescent psychopathology.

Arson has also been reported to be associated with schizophrenia and other psychotic disorders (Geller 1987; Koson and Dvoskin 1982; Lewis and Yarnell 1951; O'Sullivan and Kelleher 1987; Virkkunen 1974). Many studies of schizophrenic fire setters show that they may set fires under the influence of their psychotic symptoms. However, all studies of psychotic fire setters note that, in the majority of cases, nonpsychotic motives such as revenge or hatred prevail.

In some cases, arson is secondary to major depressive disorder (Lewis and Yarnell 1951; O'Sullivan and Kelleher 1987) or to mania in bipolar disorder (Geller 1987; Koson and Dvoskin 1982; Lewis and Yarnell 1951). Arson has been frequently associated with mental retardation (Bradford 1982; Bradford and Dimock 1986; Geller 1987; Harris and Rice 1984; Hill et al. 1982; Koson and Dvoskin 1982; Lewis and Yarnell 1951; O'Sullivan and Kelleher 1987) and dementia (Harris and Rice 1984; Lewis and Yarnell 1951; Yesavage et al. 1983).

Lastly, arsonists may be under the influence of psychoactive substances, especially alcohol (Bourget and Bradford 1989; Bradford 1982; Bradford and Dimock 1986; Hill et al. 1983; Koson and Dvoskin 1982; Lewis and Yarnell 1951; Yesavage et al. 1983).

A French study (Yesavage et al. 1983) compared a group of fire setters who had been found not guilty for psychiatric reasons with mentally healthy fire setters. Motives such as revenge and "fun with fire" were much more frequent in the psychiatric group compared with the nonpsychiatric group. In the latter group, the act was frequently denied or motives were unknown to the delinquents. In both groups, however, broken homes, with divorced parents, especially absence of the father, were frequently found.

Studies of fire-setting psychiatric inpatients show that most suffer from schizophrenia (Geller 1987; Geller and Bertsch 1985) or borderline personality disorder (Boling and Brotman 1975; Rosenstock et al. 1980), whereas mental retardation, mood disorders, and other personality disorders are less frequent (Geller 1987; Geller and Bertsch 1985). One must keep in mind that these diagnoses were not made using current diagnostic criteria.

Medical and neurologic disorders associated with cases of arson include:

Chromosomal disorders such as Klinefelter's syndrome and XYY syndrome (Cowen and Mullen 1979; Eberle 1989; Kaler, White, and Kruesi 1989; Miller and Sulkes 1988; Nielsen 1970)

Epilepsy (Byrne and Walsh 1989; Carpenter and King 1989; Singer et al. 1978; Stone 1986)

Head trauma (Hurley and Monaham 1969)

Brain tumors (Tonkonogy and Geller 1992)

Cerebellar arachnoid cyst (Heidrich et al. 1996)

Huntington's chorea (Yoshimasu 1965)

Moebius syndrome (congenital palsy of the sixth and seventh cranial nerves, often associated with other nerve palsies and other abnormalities) (Woolf 1977)

Infectious disorders, especially AIDS (Cohen et al. 1990)

Endocrine and metabolic disorders include:

Late luteal phase dysphoric disorder (Dalton 1980)

Reactive hypoglycemia measured by the glucose tolerance test (Virkkunen 1982, 1984)

Biological Approaches to Pyromania

A low 5-HIAA concentration in the cerebrospinal fluid (CSF) is associated with disorders of impulse control (Linnoilam et al. 1983). In one study, impulsive fire setters had lower CSF concentrations of 5-HIAA and 3-methoxy-4-hydroxyphenylglycol (MHPG) than a control group matched for age, sex, and height (Virkkunen et al. 1989). In this study, the recidivists who set fires during the follow-up period had lower CSF 5-HIAA and MHPG concentrations than did the nonrecidivists. As noted above, acts of fire setting have been reported in patients with various organic brain disorders.

The observed switch from one impulsive behavior to another, as well as the high rates of co-occurring impulsive and addictive disorders in pyromania, have raised the question of whether a similar neuropathophysiology underlies various pathological behaviors that are strongly characterized by reward seeking (Grant and Kim 2007).

Pyromania may reflect a mixture of impulsive and planned thrill-seeking to alleviate dysphoric states and may not be an independent disorder with a unique neurobiology. As with other impulse control disorders, neuroimaging, genetic studies, and clinical trials will be needed to identify its pathophysiology (Lejoyeux, McLoughlin, and Ades 2006).

Psychodynamic Models

The psychoanalytic approach aims to explore the unconscious motivation behind fire setting and the symbolism of fire. One of the first descriptions of fire setting refers to Samson, the biblical hero (Barker 1994). "Samson set the torches alight and set the jackal loose in the standing corn of Philistines. And he burnt up standing corn and stocks as well, and vineyards, and olive groves." A symbol of comfort and warmth, but also of hell, destruction, valor, and power, fire still pervades cultural imagery.

Wilhelm Stekel (1924), discussing 95 cases of fire setting, asserted that "awakening and ungratified sexuality impel the individual to seek a symbolic solution to his conflict between instinct and reality." Writing before psychoanalytic theory was created, Marc (1833) also noted a sexual dimension to pyromania: "Incendiary acts are chiefly manifested in young persons, in consequence of the abnormal development of the sexual function, corresponding with the period of life between twelve and twenty."

Freud postulated that, in fantasy, fire is extinguished with the stream of urine. Hence, psychoanalysts suggest that fire setters are fixated at the urethral or phallic-urethral phase of psychosexual development (Freud 1932; Grinstein 1952; Schumacher 1991). Freud (1932) turned to classical mythology to support his formulation, citing the story of Prometheus, the Titan who brought mankind the fire he had stolen from the gods, hidden in a fennel stalk, a hollow rod. Freud saw the fennel stalk as a penis symbol and, invoking the mechanism of reversal, he suggested that it was not fire that man harbors in his penis but the means of extinguishing fire: the water of his stream of urine.

In related material, it has been claimed that adult fire setters suffered from enuresis as children (Gold 1962; Greenberg 1966). However, the theoretical relationship between fire setting and urethral fixation has been controversial. Fire setting has also been interpreted to be a result of oral fixation (Kaufman, Heims, and Reiser 1961).

A study of fire-setting children aged 6 to 12 years, using the Rorschach technique, detected two types of personalities: one interpreted as a borderline personality, where fire represents the outward projection of internal tension, and the second as a neurotic personality, where fire setting is related to sexual conflict (Rothstein 1963).

Impulsivity and Sensation Seeking

We compared the levels of impulsivity and sensation seeking in depressed patients presenting with ($n = 31$) and without ($n = 76$) impulse control disorders (ICDs) (Lejoyeux et al. 2002).

The Zuckerman Sensation Seeking Scale (Zuckerman, Eysenck, and Eysenck 1978) did not reveal statistically significant differences between the two groups in the overall score or in subscale scores (thrill and adventure seeking, disinhibition, boredom susceptibility, and experience seeking). Sensation seeking did not differ between subtypes of impulse control disorders. Mean total impulsivity scores, assessed with the Barratt scale (Barratt and Patton 1983), were not significantly different in the ICD+ (53.5) and the ICD– (47.8) group. But, the ICD+ and ICD– groups differed significantly in Barratt Scale mean motor impulsivity scores (18.1 versus 14.3, $p = 0.01$). Barratt Scale motor impulsiveness is defined as acting without thinking, while cognitive impulsiveness is characterized by quick cognitive decisions and nonplanned impulsiveness by a lack of anticipation. Barratt Scale motor, cognitive, and nonplanned impulsivities were not increased in patients with pyromania ($n = 3$) compared with the other ICD patients.

Impulse control disorders in general and pyromania in particular were not associated with antisocial or borderline personality disorders. These two disorders correspond to a behavior style that is impulsive and unable to tolerate frustration. In depressed patients, these personality types do not seem to bring about unusual impulsive behavior. Surprisingly, patients with ICDs were more often married. Other authors have suggested that ICDs induce marital disruption and affective loneliness (McElroy et al. 1992). Our three pyromania patients were married.

Treatments

Treatment options for ICDs include both pharmacotherapy and psychotherapy. However, systematic research regarding pharmacotherapy for pyromania and fire setting is still lacking, and no treatment is well established as effective. Nonpharmacological interventions for fire setters, including forms of cognitive-behavioral therapy (Kolko 2001) counseling and day treatment programs (Slavkin 2002), have shown some efficacy.

The most important consideration determining the treatment plan is the presence or absence of comorbid psychiatric conditions such as affective, psychotic, and addictive disorders. Assessing the relationship of fire setting to comorbid disorders is not only of theoretical interest but also provides guidance for pharmacological treatments and behavioral interventions.

The majority of treatment studies regarding pathological fire setting deal with children and adolescents. A number of case studies report on behavioral therapy methods. In older literature, encouraging results were reported with the use of aversive stimuli (Carstens 1982; Royer, Flynn, and Osadea 1971), a combination of aversive stimuli and positive reinforcement (Holland 1969), alternative behavior substitution (Stawar 1976), procedures for stimulus satiation (Welsh 1971; Wolff 1984), and complex schedules of reinforcement (Kolko 1983). In addition, cases in which psychodynamic psychotherapy was used have also been reported (Awad and Harrison 1976; Siegel 1957). Because marked disturbance in family relationships has been found in many cases of recurrent fire-setting behavior by children, family therapy methods have been used (Birchill 1984; Minuchin 1974). Finally, multimodal interventions have been described using behavioral intervention, education and relaxation training (Koles and Jenson 1985; MacGrath et al. 1979), family treatment and art therapy (Schaeffer and Millman 1978), and individual psychotherapy, family therapy, and education (Dalton, Haslett, and Daul 1986).

In the United States, the prevention of fire setting in children has been promoted using videos and movies in various education programs. In community-based programs developed by the Federal Emergency Management Agency (FEMA) and by the National Firehawk Foundation, child and adolescent fire setters have been treated, in part with their families, to reduce the relapse rate (Kolko 1988). FEMA offers program manuals and technical training materials, which the Firehawk program augments.

Webb et al. (1990) highlight interdisciplinary collaboration between fire departments and mental health services as a key factor in identifying and treating juvenile fire setters and their families.

Remarkably little work has been done on the treatment of adult fire setters. This lack of study reflects the moral dilemma in conducting controlled trials on a highly dangerous behavior and the practical dilemma of evaluating treatments for a low-frequency event. Medication treatments are indicated only for an underlying or associated disorder (e.g., depression, schizophrenia, mania). Chromosome analysis should be considered in male fire setters who have any of the clinical features of Klinefelter's syndrome. Recognizing these individuals is important because testosterone therapy may be helpful in controlling their fire-setting behavior (Miller and Sulkes 1988).

Rice and Chaplin (1979) have outlined a social skills program for adult arsonists. Based largely on assertiveness training, and using behavioral rehearsal, modeling, coaching, instruction, and feedback, this intervention is rooted in the social skills deficit model of adult pathologic fire setting.

Conclusion

Most pyromania subjects who are arrested are judged to be criminals and are condemned to jail sentences rather than managed via psychiatric care. The psychopathological context of their act remains unknown and untreated. Pyromania is associated with significant morbidity and mortality, as well as material and psychological damage. Some evidence suggests that if pyromania is more systematically assessed and diagnosed, it can be treated effectively with behavioral therapy.

The recognition of pyromania has major implications for risk management. The diagnosis of comorbid mental disorders and pathological impulsivity when an individual is arrested for fire setting will allow useful treatment to be provided, perhaps helping to prevent additional episodes. Forming an expert psychiatric prognosis regarding future pathological impulsive behavior is difficult, however, given both the lack of data regarding recidivism and the danger that these patients pose.

Additional research and clinical efforts are needed to better understand, prevent, identify, and treat pyromania in both adult and youth populations.

References

American Psychiatric Association. *Diagnostic and Statistical Manual of Mental Disorders*. Washington, DC: American Psychiatric Association, 1952.

American Psychiatric Association. *Diagnostic and Statistical Manual of Mental Disorders*, 2nd edition. Washington, DC: American Psychiatric Association, 1968.

American Psychiatric Association. *Diagnostic and Statistical Manual of Mental Disorders*, 3rd edition. Washington, DC: American Psychiatric Association, 1980.

American Psychiatric Association. *Diagnostic and Statistical Manual of Mental Disorders*, 4th edition, text revision. Washington, DC: American Psychiatric Association, 2000.

Awad GA, Harrison SI. A female firesetter: A case report. *J Nerv Ment Dis* 163:432–437, 1976.

Barker AF. *Arson: A Review of the Psychiatric Literature*. Institute of Psychiatry, Maudsley Monographs no. 35. Oxford: Oxford University Press, 1994.

Barnett W, Spitzer M. Pathological fire-setting, 1951–1991: A review. *Med Sci Law* 34:4–20, 1994.

Barratt ES, Patton JH. Impulsivity: Cognitive, behavioral and psychophysiological correlates, in *Biological Bases of Sensation Seeking, Impulsivity and Anxiety*. Edited by Zuckerman M. Hillsdale, NJ: Erlbaum, 1983.

Birchill LE. Portland's firesetters program involves both child and family. *Am Fire J* 23:15–16, 1984.

Boling L, Brotman C. A fire-setting epidemic in a state mental health center. *Am J Psychiatry* 132:946–950, 1975.

Bourget D, Bradford JMW. Female arsonists: A clinical study. *Bull Am Acad Psychiatry Law* 17:293–300, 1989.

Bradford JMW. Arson: A clinical study. *Can J Psychiatry* 27:188–193, 1982.

Bradford JMW, Dimock J. A comparative study of adolescents and adults who willfully set fires. *Psychiatr J Univ Ott* 11:228–234, 1986.

Byrne A, Walsh JB. The epileptic arsonist. *Br J Psychiatry* 155:268, 1989.

Carpenter PK, King AL. Epilepsy and arson. *Br J Psychiatry* 154:554–556, 1989.

Carstens C. Application of a work penalty threat in the treatment of a case of juvenile firesetting. *J Behav Ther Exp Psychiatry* 13:159–161, 1982.

Cohen MAA, Aladjem AD, Bremin D et al. Firesetting by patients with the Acquired Immuno Deficiency Syndrome (AIDS). *Ann Intern Med* 112:386–387, 1990.

Cowen P, Mullen PE. An XYY man. *Br J Psychiatry* 135:79–81, 1979.

Dalton K. Cyclical criminal acts in premenstrual syndrome. *Lancet* 2:1070–1071, 1980.

Dalton R, Haslett N, Daul G. Alternative therapy with a recalcitrant fire-setter. *J Am Acad Child Psychiatry* 25:713–717, 1986.

Eberle AJ. Klinefelter syndrome and fire-setting behavior. *Pediatrics* 83:649, 1989.

Esquirol JED. *Mental Maladies: A Treatise on Insanity*. Philadelphia: Lea & Blanchard, 1845.

Forehand R, Wierson M, Frame CL et al. Juvenile firesetting: A unique syndrome or an advanced level of antisocial behavior. *Behav Res Ther* 29:125–128, 1991.

Freud S. The acquisition of power over fire. *Int J Psychoanal* 13:405–410, 1932.

Geller JL. Firesetting in the adult psychiatric population. *Hosp Community Psychiatry* 38:501–506, 1987.

Geller JL. Arson in review: From profit to pathology. *Psychiatr Clin North Am* 15:623–645, 1992a.

Geller JL. Pathological firesetting in adults. *Int J Law Psychiatry* 15:283–302, 1992b.

Geller JL, Bertsch G. Fire-setting behavior in the histories of a state hospital population. *Am J Psychiatry* 142:464–468, 1985.

Gold JH. Psychiatric profile of the firesetter. *J Forensic Sci* 7:203–228, 1962.

Grant JE, Kim SW. Clinical characteristics and psychiatric comorbidity of pyromania. *J Clin Psychiatry* 68:1717–1722, 2007.

Grant JE, Levine L, Kim D et al. Impulse control disorders in adult psychiatric inpatients. *Am J Psychiatry* 162:2184–2188, 2005.

Grant JE, Williams KA, Potenza MN. Impulse control disorders in adolescent psychiatric inpatients: Co-occurring disorders and sex differences. *J Clin Psychiatry* 68:1584–1592, 2007.

Greenberg A. Pyromania in a woman. *Psychoanalysis* 35:256–262, 1966.

Griesinger W. *Mental Pathology and Therapeutics*. London: The New Sydenham Society, 1867.

Grinstein A. Stages in the development of control over fire. *Int J Psychoanal Bull Int Psychoanal Assoc* 33:416–420, 1952.

Gunzel H. Brandstiftung bei psychosen und unter alkoholischer beeinflussung. *Krim Forensische Wiss* 66:175–180, 1987.

Harris GT, Rice ME. Mentally disordered firesetters: Psychodynamic versus empirical approaches. *Int J Law Psychiatry* 7:19–34, 1984.

Heath GA, Hardesty VA, Goldfine PE et al. Diagnosis and childhood firesetting. *J Clin Psychol* 41:571–575, 1985.

Heidrich H, Schmidtke A, Lesch KP et al. Cerebellar arachnoid cyst in a firesetter: The weight of organic lesions in arson. *J Psychiatry Neurosci* 21:202–206, 1996.

Hill RW, Langevin R, Paitich D et al. Is arson an aggressive act or a property offense? A controlled study of psychiatric referrals. *Can J Psychiatry* 27:648–654, 1982.

Holland CJ. Elimination by parents of fire-setting behavior in a 7 year-old boy. *Behav Res Ther* 7:135–137, 1969.

Hurley W, Monaham TM. Arson: The criminal and the crime. *Br J Criminol* 9:4–21, 1969.

Jacobson RR. The subclassification of child firesetters. *J Child Psychol Psychiatry* 26:769–775, 1985.

Joukamaa M, Touvinen M. Criminality and psychological disturbance of Finns remanded for psychiatric examination. *J Forensic Sci Soc* 23:170, 1983.

Kafry D. Playing with matches: Children and fire, in *Fires and Human Behavior*. Edited by Canter D. New York: Wiley, 1980.

Kaler SG, White BJ, Kruesi MJP. Firesetting and Klinefelter's syndrome. *Pediatrics* 84:749, 1989.

Kaufman I, Heims LW, Reiser DE. A re-evaluation of the psychodynamics of firesetting. *Am J Orthopsychiatry* 31:123–136, 1961.

Koles MR, Jenson WR. Comprehensive treatment of chronic firesettings in a severely disordered boy. *J Behav Ther Exp Psychiatry* 16:81–85, 1985.

Kolko DJ. Multicomponent parental treatment of firesetting in a six year old boy. *J Behav Ther Exp Psychiatry* 14:349–353, 1983.

Kolko DJ. Community interventions for juvenile firesetters: A survey of two national programs. *Hosp Community Psychiatry* 39:973–979, 1988.

Kolko DJ. Efficacy of cognitive-behavioral treatment and fire safety education for children who set fires: Initial and follow up outcomes. *J Child Psychol Psychiatry* 42:359–369, 2001.

Kolko DJ, Kazdin AE. Assessment of dimensions of childhood firesetting among patients and non-patients: The Firesetting Risk Interview. *J Abnorm Child Psychol* 17:157–176, 1989a.

Kolko DJ, Kazdin AE. The Children's Firesetting Interview with psychiatrically referred and nonreferred children. *J Abnorm Child Psychol* 17:609–624, 1989b.

Kosky RJ, Silburn S. Children who light fires: A comparison between fire-setters and non fire-setters referred to a child psychiatric outpatient service. *Aust NZ J Psychiatry* 18:251–255, 1984.

Koson DF, Dvoskin J. Arson: A diagnostic study. *Bull Am Acad Psychiatry Law* 10:39–49, 1982.

Lejoyeux M, Arbaretaz M, McLoughlin M et al. Impulse-control disorders and depression. *J Nerv Ment Dis* 190:310–314, 2002.

Lejoyeux M, Feuche N, Loi S et al. Study of impulse-control disorders among alcohol-dependent patients. *J Clin Psychiatry* 60:302–305, 1999.

Lejoyeux M, McLoughlin M, Ades J. Pyromania, in *Clinical Manual of Impulse-Control Disorders.* Edited by Hollander E, Stein DJ. Washington, DC: APPI, pp. 229–250, 2006.

Lewis NDC, Yarnell H. *Pathological Firesetting (Pyromania).* Nervous and Mental Disease Monographs no. 82. New York: Coolidge Foundation, 1951.

Lindberg N, Holi MM, Tani P et al. Looking for pyromania: Characteristics of a consecutive sample of Finnish male criminals with histories of recidivist fire-setting between 1973 and 1983. *BMC Psychiatry* 5:47, 2005.

Linnoilam M, Virkkunen M, Seneinin M et al. Low cerebral spinal fluid 5-hydroindolacetic acid concentration differentiates impulsive from nonimpulsive violent behavior. *Life Sci* 33:2609–2614, 1983.

Lowenstein LF. The diagnosis of child arsonists. *Acta Paedopsychiatrica* 47:151–154, 1981.

Lowenstein LF. The etiology, diagnosis and treatment of the fire-setting behavior of children. *Child Psychiatry Hum Dev* 19:186–194, 1989.

MacGrath P, Marshall PG, Prior K. A comprehensive treatment program for a firesetting child. *J Behav Ther Exp Psychiatry* 10:69–72, 1979.

Marc M. Considérations médico-légales sur la monomanie et particulièrement sur la monomanie incendiaire. *Ann Hyg Publ Med Leg* 10:367–484, 1833.

Mavromatis M, Lion JR. A primer on pyromania. *Dis Neur Syst* 38:954–955, 1977.

McElroy SL, Hudson JL, Pope HG et al. The DSM-III-R impulse control disorders not elsewhere classified: Clinical characteristics and relationships to other psychiatric disorders. *Am J Psychiatry* 149:318–327, 1992.

McGuire RJ, Carlisle JM, Young BG. Sexual deviations as conditioned behavior: A hypothesis. *Behav Res Ther* 2:185–190, 1965.

Miller M, Sulkes S. Fire-setting behavior in individuals with Klinefelter syndrome. *Pediatrics* 82:115–117, 1988.

Minuchin S. *Families and Family Therapy.* Cambridge, MA: Harvard University Press, 1974.

Molnar G, Keitner L, Harwood BT. A comparison of partner and solo arsonists. *J Forensic Sci* 29:574–583, 1984.

Nielsen J. Criminality among patients with Klinefelter's syndrome and the XYY syndrome. *Br J Psychiatry* 117:365–369, 1970.

Noblett S, Nelson B. A psychosocial approach to arson – a case controlled study of female offenders. *Med Sci Law* 41:325–330, 2001.

Nurcombe B. Children who set fires. *Med J Aust* 1:579–584, 1964.

O'Sullivan GH, Kelleher MJ. A study of fire-setters in the south-west of Ireland. *Br J Psychiatry* 151:818–823, 1987.

Prins H. *Offenders, Deviants, or Patients?* London: Tavistock, 1980.

Raines JC, Foy CW. Extinguishing the fires within: Treating juvenile firesetters. *Fam Soc* 75:595–604, 1994.

Ray I. *A Treatise of Medical Jurisprudence of Insanity,* 2nd edition. Boston: Tickner, 1844.

Repo E, Virkkunen M, Rawlings R et al. Criminal and psychiatric histories of Finnish arsonists. *Acta Psychiatr Scand* 95:318–323, 1997.

Rice ME, Chaplin TC. Social skill training for hospitalized male arsonists. *J Behav Ther Exp Psychiatry* 10:105–108, 1979.

Rice ME, Harris GT. Firesetters admitted to a maximum security psychiatric institution: Characteristics of offenders and offenses. *Penetanguishene Ment Health Centre Res Rep* 7:1–27, 1990.

Ritchie EC, Huff TG. Psychiatric aspects of arsonists. *J Forensic Sci* 44:733–740, 1999.

Rix KJ. A psychiatric study of adult arsonists. *Med Sci Law* 34:21–34, 1994.

Rosenstock HA, Holland A, Jones PH. Fire-setting on an adolescent in-patient unit: An analysis. *J Clin Psychol* 41:20–22, 1980.

Rothstein R. Explorations of ego structures of firesetting children. *Arch Gen Psychiatry* 9:246–253, 1963.

Royer FL, Flynn WF, Osadca BS. Case history: Aversion therapy for fire-setting by a deteriorated schizophrenic. *Behav Ther* 2:229–232, 1971.

Schaefer CE, Millman HL. *Therapies for Children.* San Francisco: Jossey-Bass, 1978.

Schumacher W. Das brandstiftersyndrom in psychodynamischer sicht, in *Medizinrecht Psychopathologie Recht-medizin: diesseits und jenseits der Grenzen von Recht und Medizin.* Festschrift für Günter Schewe. Edited by Schutz H, Schewe G, Kaatsch HJ et al. Berlin: Springer, 1991, pp. 290–300.

Siegel L. Case study of a thirteen year old firesetter: A catalyst in the growing pains of a residential treatment unit. *Am J Orthopsychiatry* 27:396–410, 1957.

Singer L, Dautais G, Freyman Jr et al. Passages à l'acte meurtriers et incendiaires avec amnésie lacunaire chez deux malades épileptiques. *Ann Med Psychol (Paris)* 136:609–617, 1978.

Slavkin ML. Child and adolescent psychiatry: What every clinician needs to know about juvenile firesetters. *Psychiatr Serv* 53:1237–1238, 2002.

Soltys SM. Pyromania and fire setting behaviors. *Psychiatr Ann* 22:79–83, 1992.

Stawar TL, Fable MOD. Operantly structured fantasies as an adjunct in the modification of firesetting behavior. *J Behav Ther Exp Psychiatry* 7:285–287, 1976.

Stekel WC. *Peculiarities of Behavior.* New York: Boni & Liveright, 1924.

Stickle TR, Blechman EA. Aggression and fire: Antisocial behavior in fire setting and nonfire setting juvenile offenders. *J Psychopathol Behav Assess* 24:177–193, 2002.

Stone AA. Vernon adopts Tarasoff: A real barn-burner. *Am J Psychiatry* 143:352–355, 1986.

Taylor PJ, Gunn J. Violence and psychosis. *BMJ* 228:1945–1949, 1984.

Tonkonogy JM, Geller JL. Hypothalamic lesions and intermittent explosive disorder. *J Neuropsychiatry Clin Neurosci* 4:45–50, 1992.

U.S. Department of Justice, Federal Bureau of Investigations. *Uniform Crime Report for the United States.* Washington, DC: U.S. Department of Justice, Federal Bureau of Investigation, 1982.

Virkkunen M. On arson commited by schizophrenics. *Acta Psychiatrica Scand* 50:152–160, 1974.

Virkkunen M. Reactive hypoglycaemic tendency among violent offenders: A further study by means of the glucose tolerance test. *Neuropsychobiology* 8:35–40, 1982.

Virkkunen M. Reactive hypoglycaemic tendency among arsonists. *Acta Psychiatrica Scand* 69:445–452, 1984.

Virkkunen M, De Jong J, Bartko J et al. Relationship of psychobiological variables to recidivism in violent offenders and impulsive fire setters. *Arch Gen Psychiatry* 46:600–603, 1989.

Vreeland RG, Lewin BM. Psychological aspects of firesetting, in *Fires and Human Behaviour.* Edited by Canter D. New York: Wiley, 1980, pp. 31–46.

Webb NB, Sakheim GA, Town-Miranda L et al. Collaborative treatment of juvenile firesetters: Assessment and outreach. *Am J Orthopsychiatry* 60:305–310, 1990.

Welsh RS. The use of stimulus satiation in the elimination of juvenile fire-setting behavior, in *Behavior Therapy with Children.* Edited by Graziano AM. Chicago: Aldine, 1971, pp. 283–289.

Woolf PG. Arson and Moebius syndrome: Case study of stigmatization. *Med Sci Law* 17:68–70, 1977.

Wolff R. Satiation in the treatment of inappropriate firesetting. *J Behav Ther Exp Psychiatry* 15:337–40, 1984.

World Health Organization. *International Classification of Diseases,* 10th edition. Geneva: World Health Organization, 2002.

Yesavage JA, Benezech M, Ceccaldi P et al. Arson in mentally ill and criminal populations. *J Clin Psychiatry* 44:128–130, 1983.

Yoshimasu S. Two cases of arson in the prodromal stage of Huntington's chorea. *Acta Criminol Med Leg Jpn* 31:25–31, 1965.

Zuckerman M, Eysenck SBG, Eysenck HJ. Sensation seeking in England and America: Cross-cultural, age and sex comparisons. *J Consult Clin Psychol* 46:139–149, 1978.

24

Arson: Choking off the Flames

Paul Schwartzman, MS, DAPA, LMHC

Introduction

The massive Santiago Canyon Fire of 2007 consumed 28,445 acres east of Irvine, California. The fire destroyed 14 homes and 24 outbuildings, with an additional 8 homes and 3 outbuildings seriously damaged. Sixteen firefighters were injured fighting the blaze, and about 3,000 people were evacuated. The fire caused an estimated $10 million in damage. Individuals interviewed in the evacuation shelters expressed extreme anxiety regarding their pets, homes, and belongings. They had no idea what they would find when they were allowed to return to their neighborhoods.

The Federal Bureau of Investigation, Bureau of Alcohol, Tobacco and Firearms, the Orange County Fire Authority, and the California Department of Forestry worked together to determine the origin and cause of this fire. Investigators found two points of origin where they believe the fire was set, and they officially declared this an arson fire (CBS News 2007; Wikipedia 2008).

In another incident, in the city of Passaic, New Jersey, a 1985 fire destroyed 10 city blocks, gutted 18 factories, and destroyed or seriously damaged 23 homes. The factories housed 60 different manufacturers and companies and contained paints, chemicals, solvents, and other materials that provided an incredible fuel source as well as creating toxic emissions. One of the buildings warehoused the costumes for most of the New York City Opera's productions; these were entirely destroyed and were estimated to be worth several million dollars. In all, 2.2 million square feet of factory space valued at $400 million was destroyed. In addition, the 60 companies had employed more than 2,000 people who were now without jobs. The Red Cross reported that 150 families, more than 400 people, were displaced and needed emergency shelter. All of these families needed to leave their homes with only the clothing on their backs.

This was a very difficult fire to combat and was complicated by low water pressure in the area. A 65-year-old firefighter suffered a fatal heart attack while fighting the fire. The fire was determined to have been set by two boys, 12 and 13 years old. They were igniting matches and putting them into a large trash container in an alley next to one of the factories. The boys were charged with arson, criminal mischief, and reckless endangerment causing wide damage (*New York Times* 1985).

These two case examples clearly illustrate the devastation and the social, emotional, and financial consequences of arson. This chapter presents information, statistics, and perspective on the magnitude of arson in the United States and some of the systems and methods that have evolved to address this destructive force.

Magnitude of the Problem

In 2005, there were about 1,602,000 reported fires, amounting to a fire department response to a fire somewhere in the United States every 20 seconds. The majority of these fires were

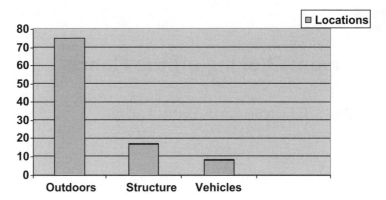

Figure 24.1   FBI/NFPA/USFA location reports (percentage).

the result of cooking, careless smoking, heating equipment, chimney fires, and lightning strikes. Twenty percent of these fires, or an estimated 323,900, were intentional fires and arson (Hall 2007).

In 2005, the most recent year for which data are available, intentional fires and arson resulted in 490 civilian fire deaths, 1,500 civilian injuries, and $1.1 billion in direct property damage. Intentional fires and arson further led to three on-duty firefighter fatalities and 7,600 on-duty firefighter injuries (Hall 2007). The National Fire Incident Reporting System, which collects information on firefighter deaths and injuries, suggests that arson fires are the most dangerous for firefighters.

While these numbers are unsettling, the good news is that intentional fires and arson have been on a steady decline for the past 20 years. In 1980, there were 859,800 intentional fires, nearly 1,000 civilian deaths, and 24 on-duty firefighter deaths (Hall 2007). Some publications report that intentional fires and arson are likely to increase in bad economic times such as those being experienced in the United States currently. However, trend analysis of economic recession periods over the past several decades illustrates that no such trends have occurred (Hall 2008).

Intentional Fire and Arson Locations

The majority (75%, or 242,000) of intentional fires occur outside and in unoccupied structures such as fields and woods, garages, and dumpsters. About 17% (55,000) occur in structures that the fire service characterizes as single- and multiple-family residences, schools, and factories. When intentional fires occur in public assembly structures, the point of origin is most often (23%) in bathrooms, locker rooms, or coat rooms. The second most prevalent location is exterior wall surfaces (6%) (Hall 2007). The remaining 8% (26,000) of intentional fires are set to vehicles (see Figure 24.1).

Community size impacts the location of fires to some extent. A larger percentage of intentional structure fires occur in larger communities in cities with populations larger than 100,000 persons (Hall 2007).

Defining Intentional Fires and Arson

An *intentional fire* is generally defined as a fire that is deliberately ignited, typically using an incendiary device such as a match, lighter, candle, or explosive device. The fact that a fire is intentional within this definition does not mean that it necessarily has ill intent.

This chapter will use a narrower definition of intentional fire, in which the determining factor is the ill intent. An individual may ignite a trash pile to dispose of the trash. In this

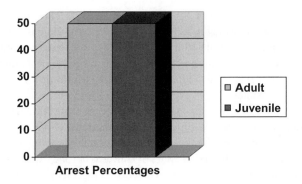

Figure 24.2   FBI UCR report.

example, the intent is to burn trash, and even if the fire causes damage beyond its intent, it would be considered a reckless or careless fire or an unintentional fire. The hypothetical fire was started with a socially appropriate purpose and was intended to be controlled. This chapter will use the term *intentional* fire to mean a fire that is started in order to cause harm.

When does intentional fire become arson? Arson is a legal term. The Federal Bureau of Investigation (FBI) Uniform Crime Reporting Program defines arson as "any willing or malicious burning or attempt to burn, with or without intent to defraud, a dwelling house, public building, motor vehicle or aircraft, personal property of another, etc." This chapter refers to both intentional fires and arson because intentionally set fires do not always match the legal definition of arson. This distinction is influenced by several nuances in local jurisdiction law that vary from state to state. The threshold for arson is typically reached when the intent of the fire can be demonstrated to be hostile, there is harm to property or persons, and there is evidence to demonstrate that the fire was caused by incendiary means.

It can be argued that the problem of intentionally set fires is greater than is documented. If an individual intentionally burns paper towels in a school lavatory sink and the smoke alarm is tripped, this individual would probably not be charged with arson in many areas of the United States because there was no physical damage to the porcelain sink. The most likely charge would be vandalism, and the intentional fire statistic would be lost.

Intentional Fires and Arson Arrests

It is a myth that arson is hard to solve because all evidence is destroyed. Often incendiary fires do leave evidence or characteristics of intentionally set fires that can be uncovered when investigated by a trained investigator. Too often, these fires are not sufficiently investigated or evidence at the scene is not properly preserved.

In spite of these complexities, one of every six arson offenses (18% in 2005) was cleared by arrest, and approximately 7% of these arrests led to convictions. This percentage is consistent with other serious crimes in which typically there are no witnesses and investigations, as mentioned, are not diligent (U.S. Department of Justice 2007).

The FBI Uniform Crime Reporting Program further documents that half of all those arrested for arson in the United States are juveniles under the age of 18. Arson arrests account for a much larger proportion of arrests for youths under the age of 10 than any other crime that the FBI tracks (3% of all arson arrests were youths under age 10 in 2005). In 2005, 83% of all arson arrests from youth to adult were males (see Figure 24.2).

Intentional Fires and Arson and Community Responses

Because juveniles are so highly represented in this population, there has been a trend over the past 25 years to develop Juvenile Firesetter Intervention Programs (JFIP) in communities across the United States (Schwartzman et al. 2000). These programs typically are organized and managed by the fire service, but in some communities they are administered by a local burn center or mental health agency. The programs train personnel within the fire service to respond by conducting an initial screening to determine a motivation for fire involvement when there are actual fire incidents involving youths or concerns when there is fire misuse or unusual interest.

If the youth's involvement is deemed to be motivated primarily by curiosity or experimentation, a comprehensive educational intervention is provided. Recidivism rates following the intervention are quite low for this population (Schwartzman et al. 2000). If the fire misuse appears to be motivated by issues or concerns beyond experimentation, then a coordinated community response is initiated that brings together relevant community agencies, including mental health, social service, and juvenile justice systems, to intervene with individual, family, or other dynamics associated with the fire-setting behavior.

As a result of this program concept, a body of research has been emerging that allows us to better understand fire-setting behavior among youths (Schwartzman et al. 2000). Juveniles who start intentional fires are a heterogeneous group and present with a myriad of different motivations for their fire setting. A common motivation is a crisis, and the fire setting is a "cry for help" to bring attention to untenable family situations, often involving chronic neglect and physical or sexual abuse.

Fire setting may also be part of a constellation of aggressive behaviors in conduct-disordered youths. In individuals with this diagnosis, there is not necessarily any specific attachment to fire. It happens to be an available tool. If a lighter is handy, something is ignited, but if a rock is more convenient, it will be thrown through a window. Fire setting may be an indication of poor impulse control and may be reinforced by associated sensory responses. Regardless, the community-based response to juvenile fire setting has provided an opportunity to conduct comprehensive assessments and acquire more complete information about fire-setting behavior. This enhanced understanding further leads to better developed, targeted treatment plans (Schwartzman et al. 2000).

Unfortunately, the adult population is rarely managed with this approach. Adults who present with fire-setting behavior are most often steered directly to the criminal justice system, with minimal or no contact with the mental health system. Intentional fire setters who clearly present with psychotic symptoms, however, may be diverted to a forensic psychiatric facility. Much of the research concerning adult fire setters comes from case studies among hospitalized populations. Additional information has been generated from FBI profilers examining serial arsonists and murderers (U.S. Department of Justice 2007) (see Figure 24.3). It is often stated that serial murderers have fire-setting behavior in their repertoire. The result is a highly skewed perspective on this behavior, with a popular perception among the general population and professionals that fire setting is practiced by individuals with severe, chronic illness or that it is arson for profit, which in actuality rarely occurs. In either portrayal of fire setting, treatment is not considered a viable option.

The lack of treatment programs for adult fire setters is exacerbated by the fact that mental health professionals receive virtually no systematic training regarding fire-setting behaviors. If training is provided, it is usually in the context of understanding the diagnosis of pyromania specified in the current edition of the *Diagnostic and Statistical Manual of Mental Disorders* (American Psychiatric Association 2000; Schwartzman et al. 2000).

As mentioned, much of what is understood about adult intentional fire setters has been generated by FBI and forensic reviews of intentional and arson fires. Criminal investigations suggest that the leading motive for intentional fires is revenge, which may involve domestic violence followed by vandalism. This motive accounts for more than half of the fires investigated.

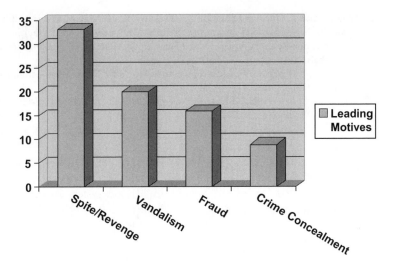

Figure 24.3   FBI UCR motives mentioned (percentage).

Implications for Treatment

Fire setters are not a homogenous group, and their motivations for choosing fire are often complex. Systematic and comprehensive assessments of this behavior are imperative if treatment interventions are to be effective.

Mental health professionals have a critical role in responding to this dangerous and frightening behavior. The majority of mental health professionals possess the skills and techniques to intervene with fire setters. However, there are important differences between working with this population and working with individuals who do not present with fire-setting behaviors.

One important difference is that the mental health treatment providers need to interface with the criminal justice system and other community support systems. Working to develop a collaborative relationship will greatly enhance the mental health system's response to intentional fires and arson.

Historically, treatments have ignored the fire-setting behavior and have emphasized the dynamics surrounding the fire setting, such as family conflict and depression. The fire-setting behavior needs to be specifically examined in terms of its context. Comprehensive assessments should include a thorough psychosocial examination of the individual and family, the history of fire use and exposure, whether there are current stressors or crises that might trigger this behavior, careful documentation of the cognitive and emotional processes before, during, and after the fire, and, finally, understanding the internal and external reinforcements for the behavior. This detailed assessment will help to determine whether or not the fire-setting behavior is related to impulse control disorders and is therefore likely to respond to the treatment modalities described in Chapter 23 of this volume, on pyromania.

References

American Psychiatric Association. *Diagnostic and Statistical Manual of Mental Disorders*, 4th edition, text revision. Washington, DC: American Psychiatric Association, 2000.

CBS News. Arson behind the Santiago Fire. October 25, 2007.

Hall JR Jr. *Intentional Fires and Arson.* Quincy, MA: National Fire Protection Association, 2007.

Hall JR Jr. Arson and economic conditions: Is there a link? *Nal Fire Protect J Online Rep*, February 2008.

New York Times. Two Boys Accused of Starting Huge Passaic Fire. September 5, 1985.

Schwartzman P, Fineman K, Slavkin M, et al. *Juvenile Firesetter Mental Health Intervention: A Comprehensive Discussion of Treatment, Service Delivery and Training of Providers.* Juvenile Firesetter Intervention Research Project Phase I Final Report. Albany, NY: National Association of State Fire Marshals, 2000.

United States Department of Justice. *Crime in the United States.* Washington, DC: Criminal Justice Information Services, 2007.

Wikipedia. http://en.wikipedia.org/wiki/October_2007_California_wildfire#Other_fires. Accessed December 20, 2008.

Appendix I: Treatment Guidelines

Compulsive Buying Disorder: Guide to Treatment Planning

- Assess motivations for treatment
- Rule out hypomania or mania as the source of compulsive buying
- Assess motivations for compulsive buying and help the patient confront them
- Assess the emotional, financial, familial, and occupational consequences of compulsive buying
- Assess and treat comorbid:
  - Mood disorders
  - Anxiety disorders
  - Impulse control disorders
  - Substance abuse disorders
- Consider a trial of cognitive-behavioral therapy
  - Self-monitoring
  - Exposure and response prevention
  - Correction of cognitive distortions
  - Behavioral leisure time alternatives to shopping
  - Discourage shopping alone
  - Encourage leaving checks and credit cards at home
- Consider recommending and helping the patient review self-help materials
- Consider referral to Debtors Anonymous
- Consider psychodynamic attention to motivations for buying
- Consider couple or family therapy when collusion or consequences indicate
- Consider next a 6-week trial of an SSRI
- Consider next a 6-week trial of naltrexone and/or an SSRI

Kleptomania: Guide to Treatment Planning

- Assess motivations for treatment
- Rule out hypomania or mania and neurological disorders (rare) as the cause of the stealing
- Assess the triggers, frequency, urge intensity, and the patient's degree of control over stealing urges
- Assess the emotional, familial, occupational, and legal consequences of kleptomania and intervene
- Assess and treat comorbid disorders, evaluating especially for:
  - Mood disorders
  - Anxiety disorders
  - Eating disorders
  - Impulse control disorders
  - Substance abuse disorders

- Consider trials of cognitive-behavioral therapy methods
  - Covert sensitization
  - Aversion therapy
  - Systematic desensitization
  - Imaginal sensitization
  - No shopping alone
- Consider prescribing and helping the patient review self-help materials
- Consider a 6-week trial of an SSRI at the highest comfortably tolerated dose
- Consider next a 6-week trial of naltrexone and/or an SSRI
- Consider next trials of mood stabilizers (lithium, valproate, topiramate)

Pathological Gambling: Guide to Treatment Planning

- Assess motivations for treatment
- Assess motivations for pathological gambling, and help the patient eliminate them
- Assess related interpersonal, occupational, financial, and legal problems
- Rule out bipolar disorders and medications inducing gambling behaviors
- Assess suicide risk and intervene
- Identify and treat comorbid disorders
  - Mood disorders
  - Anxiety disorders
  - Substance abuse disorders
  - Antisocial personality disorder
- Assess irrational beliefs about gambling
- Require or strongly encourage attendance at Gamblers Anonymous meetings
- Initiate couple or family therapy as needed (including Gam-Anon)
- Initiate multicomponent cognitive-behavioral therapy (trying various combinations)
- Refer to social agencies for help with vocational, social, and legal problems
- Add relapse-prevention techniques to successful treatment
- Consider an 8-week trial of naltrexone at 50 mg/day
- Consider next an 8-week trial of n-acetyl cysteine titrated to 1,800 mg/day
- Consider recommending self-help materials

Trichotillomania: Guide to Treatment Planning

- Assess motivation for treatment
- Assess all sites of pulling, and measure baseline rates
- Inquire about trichophagia; if present, order serum iron and complete blood count
- Assess effects of trichotillomania on functioning
- Assess and treat comorbid anxiety, mood, substance abuse, and impulse control disorders
- Institute modified habit-reversal treatment (HRT)
- Guide the patient to educational and support groups
- Consider next pharmacotherapy, first with:
  - Clomipramine at 50–250 mg/day, 6-week trial
  - An SSRI, 6-week trial
- Consider adding:
  - Acceptance and Commitment Therapy to HRT
  - Hypnosis to HRT, or hypnosis alone
  - An SSRI to HRT
- Consider additional 4-week to 8-week pharmacotherapy trials with:
  - n-acety lcysteine at 1200–2400 mg/day, 8-week trial
  - Lithium carbonate at 900–1,500 mg/day
  - Naltrexone at 50–250 mg/day

- ○ Adding a low dose of an atypical antipsychotic to an SSRI (4 weeks)
  - ○ Topiramate at 25–250 mg/day
- Institute monthly "booster/relapse-prevention sessions" after successful psychotherapy

Skin Picking: Guide to Treatment Planning

- Rule out disorders inducing skin picking:
  - ○ Dermatological disorders (e.g., psoriasis, prurigo nodularis)
  - ○ Medical disorders (e.g., lymphoma, diabetes mellitus)
  - ○ Medications (e.g., anticholinergic drugs, stimulants)
- Evaluate for underlying body dysmorphic disorder and treat if present
- Evaluate for other self-injurious behaviors (e.g., cutting), and treat
- Assess:
  - ○ Motivations for seeking treatment
  - ○ Motivations for skin picking
  - ○ Subjective experiences before, during, and after picking
  - ○ Impacts of skin picking on self-perception, social relationships, and work
- Consider using a rating scale to quantify skin-picking severity
- Treat comorbid mood, anxiety, substance abuse, and impulse control disorders
- Help the patient cope with or resolve social stressors
- Initiate a 6-week trial of an SSRI at a high dose and monitor for side effects
- If necessary, consider next either:
  - ○ A trial of habit-reversal therapy alone or as augmentation
  - ○ A 4-week augmentation trial with a low dose of an atypical antipsychotic
- Consider next a trial of naltrexone at up to 250 mg/day (monitor liver function if dose exceeds 50 mg/day)
- Consider next an 8-week trial of lamotrigine

Nail Biting: Guide to Treatment Planning

- Assess motivations for treatment
- Assess apparent triggers or exacerbating factors
- Assess the medical and dental complications of nail biting (e.g., paronychia), and consider referral to specialists
- Help the patient cope with or resolve stressors exacerbating nail biting
- Treat comorbid anxiety disorders
- Institute self-monitoring (e.g., a log of episodes, repeated measures of nail length)
- Consider next modified habit-reversal treatment
  - ○ Institute or continue self-monitoring
  - ○ Design and implement a competing response
  - ○ Institute relaxation exercises
  - ○ Enhance motivation for stopping nail biting by written motivation review
- Consider next sequential 6-week trials of SSRIs
- Consider next a trial of naltrexone at 50 mg/day and/or an SSRI

Problematic Internet Use: Guide to Treatment Planning

- Assess reasons for seeking treatment
- Assess for:
  - ○ Preoccupation with the Internet
  - ○ Adverse relationship, job, educational, or career consequences
  - ○ Use of the Internet to escape problems or to relieve dysphoric mood
  - ○ Tolerance or withdrawal symptoms of Internet use
  - ○ Lack of control over Internet use

- Rule out mania, hypomania, social anxiety, and other Axis I disorders as cause of excessive use
- Assess for comorbid conditions and treat if present, such as:
  - Mood disorders
  - Anxiety disorders
  - Attention deficit hyperactivity disorder
  - Substance abuse disorders
- Consider cognitive-behavioral therapy:
  - Keeping a daily Internet log (time spent, triggers, moods)
  - Correcting cognitive distortions
  - Teaching time-management skills
  - Teaching coping strategies
- Consider family-based interventions for children and adolescents
- Consider next a 10-week trial of an SSRI
- Consider use of a support group

Nonparaphilic Sexual Disorders: Guide to Treatment Planning

- Establish recurrent failure to control nondeviant, sexually arousing fantasies, urges or behaviors, with clinically significant distress or impaired functioning
- Rule out hypomania/mania, schizophrenia, delusional disorder (erotomania), and brain lesions, seizure disorder, degenerative neurological disorders
- Assess motivation for treatment
- Obtain a full description of the behaviors and their contexts:
  - Compulsive masturbation
  - Protracted promiscuity or excessive prostitution
  - Pornography, telephone sex, cybersex dependence
  - Severe sexual desire incompatibility with partner
  - Sexual harassment
  - Ego-dystonic sexual fantasizing
- Obtain a full sexual history
- Assess for associated familial, intimate partner, financial, legal and medical problems (e.g., HIV/AIDS, syphilis, genital injury, use of enhancement drugs)
- Assess and treat comorbid disorders (especially mood disorders, anxiety disorders, substance abuse, and attention deficit disorder [ADD])
- Inform the patient about the therapeutic options and strategies
- Address suicidal risk and potential harm to others and treat
- Reduce access to the "drug of choice" (e.g., for those who use the Internet for sex)
- Consider the need for hospitalization (e.g., for medical difficulty, risk of harm, need to interrupt a cycle of behavior after unsuccessful outpatient treatment)
- Consider psychotherapy (cognitive-behavioral, psychodynamic, interpersonal)
- Consider 4-week to 6-week trials of several SSRIs
- Consider adding a psychostimulant when ADD is present
- Consider a trial of naltrexone 150–250 mg/day
- Institute relapse prevention techniques
- Advise the patient about evaluating and using self-help groups

Intermittent Explosive Disorder: Guide to Treatment Planning

- Assess motivations for treatment
- Assess the type, frequency, triggers, and target(s) of the verbal or physical aggression
- Assess for related interpersonal, occupational, and legal problems

- Rule out bipolar disorders, depression, substance abuse, and PTSD as the cause of the aggressive behavior
- Identify and treat comorbid disorders
  ○ Mood disorders
  ○ Anxiety disorders
  ○ Substance abuse disorders
  ○ Antisocial personality disorder
  ○ Borderline personality disorder
- Start fluoxetine (or another SSRI), and titrate to highest comfortably tolerated dose as needed
- For patients with a comorbid Cluster B personality disorder, consider divalproex, titrated to plasma level of 80–120 ng/ml
- Use multicomponent cognitive-behavioral therapy incorporating cognitive restructuring, relaxation training, and coping skills training
- Consider combining pharmacotherapy and cognitive-behavioral therapy
- Initiate couple or family therapy as needed
- Refer to social agencies for help with vocational, social, and legal problems
- Add relapse-prevention techniques to successful treatment

Pyromania: Guide to Treatment Planning

- Assess motivations for treatment
- Assess potential or actual criminal behavior related to fire setting
- Rule out (or treat) Axis I disorders motivating fire setting, such as:
  ○ Schizophrenia
  ○ Mania
  ○ Developmental delay
  ○ Dementia
- Assess for conduct disorder, antisocial personality disorder, and borderline personality disorder associated with fire setting
- Assess for medical and neurological disorders associated with arson, such as:
  ○ Chromosomal disorders
  ○ Epilepsy
  ○ Head trauma
  ○ Brain tumors
- Assess contributing factors:
  ○ Social skill deficits
  ○ Family dysfunction, including:
    ■ Violence at home
    ■ Parental alcohol or drug abuse
    ■ Physical or sexual abuse
    ■ Emotional neglect
- Assess motives for setting fires
- Consider behavioral and other psychotherapies (aversive stimuli, positive reinforcement, alternative behavior substitution, social skills training)
- Consider family therapy for children and adolescents

Appendix II: List of Scales and Assessment Instruments

Minnesota Impulsive Disorders Questionnaire
Compulsive Buying Scale
Kleptomania Assessment Scale
South Oaks Gambling Screen
Massachusetts General Hospital Hair Pulling Scale
The Massachusetts General Hospital (MGH) Skin Picking Scale
Internet Addiction Test
Intermittent Explosive Disorder – Diagnostic Questionnaire

Minnesota Impulse Disorders Interview

General Information

1. (Check) _____ male   _____ female
2. (Check) _____ white   _____ black   _____ Hispanic
   _____ Asian   _____ Native American
   _____ other
3. How old are you? _____ (years)
4. What do you do for a living? _____
5. What is your sexual orientation / gender identity?
   _____ heterosexual _____ bisexual _____ gay _____ transgender
6. What is your marital status?
   _____ single
   _____ married
   _____ separated
   _____ divorced
   _____ widowed
7a. Do you have children?   Y   N
   7b. (if yes) How many children do you have? _____
   7c. (if yes) How old are they? _____
8a. How many years of school have you completed? _____
   8b. (if more than high school) What is the highest degree that you have
   obtained? _____
9. What is your approximate yearly household income? _____

Buying Disorder Screen

1. Do you or others think that you have a problem with buying things too often or with
   spending too much money?   Y   N
   1b. (if yes) Why? _____

2a. Do you ever experience an irresistible urge or uncontrollable need to buy things or mounting tension that can only be relieved by buying?   Y   N

    2b. (if yes) Do these urges or thoughts about buying seem to be forced into your thinking or intrusive?   Y   N

    2c. (if yes) Do you attempt to resist these urges or thoughts?   Y   N

3a. Is bying followed by release of tension or a sense of gratification even if only for the moment?   Y   N

4a. Has problem buying led to social, marital, family, financial, or work problems or caused you to experience significant distress?   Y   N

    4b. (if yes) In which of these areas has there been a problem?

        social _____

        marital _____

        family _____

        financial _____

        work _____

        personal distress _____

        other (specify) _____

    4c. (if yes) How has buying affected these areas?

    _____

    _____

(if yes to questions 1 and 4, go to complete buying disorder interview; if no to question 1 or 4, end module)

Kleptomania Screen

1a. Have you ever stolen anything?   Y   N   (if no, skip to the next module)

    1b. (if yes) When did this occur? _____

    1c. (if yes) What did you steal? _____

    1d. (if yes) Do you currently steal?   Y   N

    (if yes) Please describe your current pattern of stealing:

    _____

    1e. (subject demonstrates a recurrent pattern of theft not limited to a few isolated events)   Y   N   (if no, end module)

    1f. Some people steal for their own personal use or for the value things might bring in selling or trading them. Others steal for no reason obvious to others or even themselves, with stealing seeming senseless or impulsive. Why do you steal?

    _____

    _____

    1g. What percentage of your stealing is for your own use, for sale or trade, and for no apparent reason?

    steals for monetary value   _____%

    steals for personal use   _____%

    steals objects not necessary   _____%

    for personal use or for monetary value   _____%

2a. Do you experience an irresistible urge or uncontrollable need to steal things or mounting tension that can only be relieved by stealing?   Y   N

    2b. (if yes) Do these urges or thoughts about stealing seem to be forced into your thinking or intrusive?   Y   N

    2c. (if yes) Do you attempt to resist these urges or thoughts?   Y   N

3a. Is stealing followed by release of tension or a sense of gratification even if only for the moment?   Y   N

4a. Has stealing led to social, marital, family, financial, or work problems or caused you personal distress?   Y   N

    4b. (if yes) In which of these areas has there been a problem?

        social _____

        marital _____

        family _____

        financial _____

        work _____

        personal distress _____

        other (specify) _____

    4c. (if yes) How has stealing affected these areas?

    _____

    _____

Trichotillomania Screen

1. Have you ever pulled out scalp, eyelash, eyebrow, pubic, or any other body hair other than for cosmetic reasons? (e.g., eyebrow plucking, pubic hair plucking for swimsuits, gray hair removal, facial hair removal)   Y   N   (if no, skip to the next module)

2. From the following list, please indicate which hair sites you have ever pulled from. (check only those not pulled exclusively for cosmetic reasons; check even if subject indicates that no visible loss has been evident)

    scalp _____

    lashes _____

    brows _____

    pubic _____

    beard _____

    mustache _____

    legs _____

    arms _____

    axillary _____

    chest _____

    abdomen _____

3. Has hair pulling ever resulted in visible hair loss such as hair thinning, bald patches, or, in the case of eyelashes, gaps along the eyelid?   Y   N   (if no, end module)

4a. Do you ever experience a mounting or building tension or urge to pull hair prior to pulling hair from any site?   Y   N

    4b. (if yes) Is this different from a more general tension or anxiety that might be attributable to stressors at the time?   Y   N

5. Do you experience tension relief after pulling out hair even if only momentarily?   Y   N

6. Do you experience a sense of pleasure or gratification after pulling out hair even if only momentarily?   Y   N

Intermittent Explosive Disorder

The following included questions about assaultiveness. Because the law requires me to report to the authorities threat of physical harm to others and child abuse, I strongly recommend that you not supply any more detail to questions other than that asked of you and that you answer all yes/no questions with a yes or no response only. By following these guidelines, none of your answers will be reportable. You may choose not to answer any or all of these questions.

1a. Have you ever lost control and assaulted someone or destroyed property?   Y   N
  1b. (if yes) Has this happened on several occasions?   Y   N
  1c. (if yes) Did you cause serious injury or destruction of property during these episodes?   Y   N
  1d. Did you or others feel that these episodes were grossly out of proportion to the situation?   Y   N
  1e. Are these episodes unlike you?   Y   N
  1f. Are these episodes always associated with using alcohol or other psychoactive drugs?   Y   N
  1g. At what age did you first experience this loss of control?
2. Are you often on the edge of losing control?   Y   N

Pyromania Module

1a. Have you deliberately or purposefully set a fire on more than one occasion?   Y   N
  (if no, skip to the next module)
  (if yes) Have more than one of these fires:
  1b. not been set for monetary gain?   Y   N
  1c. not been to conceal criminal activity?   Y   N
  1d. not been out of anger or vengeance?   Y   N
  1e. not been to improve your living circumstances?   Y   N
  (Note: Hallucinations, delusions not addressed in this module)
2. Have you experienced any kind of urge or mounting tension prior to setting a fire?   Y   N
3. Have certain mood changes made you feel like you had to set a fire?   Y   N
4. Are you fascinated with, interested in, curious about, or attracted to fire, situations in which fires occur, things used to set fires, or the consequences of fires?   Y   N
5. Do you experience pleasure, gratification, or relief when setting fires, watching fires, or being involved with the aftermath of fires?   Y   N

Gambling Screen

1. Do you gamble?   Y   N   (if no, skip to the next module)
2. Do you or others think that you have ever had a problem with gambling?   Y   N
3. Have you ever felt guilty about the way you gamble or what happens when you gamble?   Y   N
4. Have you often been preoccupied with gambling or obtaining money to gamble?   Y   N
5. Have you frequently gambled larger amounts of money or over longer periods of time than you intended to?   Y   N
6. Have you found that you need to increase the size or frequency of bets to obtain the same excitement?   Y   N
7. Have you felt restless or irritable when you were unable to gamble?   Y   N
8. Have you ever tried to stop gambling and had difficulty?   Y   N
9. Have you ever decreased your involvement with, or quit some important social, work, or recreational activity in order to gamble?   Y   N
10. Have you ever continued to gamble despite having significant money, social, family, or occupational problems caused or exacerbated by gambling?   Y   N

11. Have you returned to gambling despite repeatedly losing money gambling in an attempt to win back losses?   Y   N
12. Have you frequently gambled when you were expected to meet social or occupational obligations?   Y   N

Compulsive Sexual Behavior Screen

The following section includes questions about sexual behavior. The law requires us to report to the authorities acts of physical harm to others and child abuse. We strongly recommend that you do not supply answers to the questions below if your answers indicate that your sexual activities involve threatening others or sexual relationships with minors that you would not want reported. If you choose to answer only the yes/no questions none of your answers will be reportable. You may choose not to answer any or all of these questions.

1. Do you or others that you know think that you have a problem with being overly preoccupied with some aspect of your sexuality or being overly sexually active?   Y   N
2a. Do you have repetitive sexual fantasies that you feel are out of your control or cause you distress?   Y   N
   2b. (if yes) Can you give me examples? (if yes) Please describe this: _____
_____
   2c. (if yes) Does the fantasy above frequently intrude into your mind?   Y   N
   2d. (if yes) Do you try to resist thinking about this (above) fantasy?   Y   N
   2e. (if yes) When you are having the fantasy, does it cause you to feel good or bad about yourself?   _____ Good   _____ Bad
   2f. Do you feel ashamed about having had the fantasy after the fact?   Y   N
3a. Do you have repetitive sexual urges that you feel are out of your control or cause you distress?   Y   N
   3b. (if yes) Can you give me examples? (if yes) Please describe this: _____
_____
   3c. (if yes) Do the urges above frequently intrude into your mind?   Y   N
   3d. (if yes) Do you try to resist thinking about the urges above?   Y   N
   3e. (if yes) When you are having the urges, do they cause you to feel good or bad about yourself?   _____ Good   _____ Bad
   3f. (if yes) Do you feel ashamed about having had these urges after the fact?   Y   N
4a. Do you engage in repetitive sexual behavior that you feel is out of control or a cause of distress?   Y   N
   4b. (if yes) Can you give me examples? (if yes) Please describe this: _____
_____
   4c. (if yes) Do thoughts of the behaviors above frequently intrude into your mind?   Y   N
   4d. (if yes) Do you try to resist engaging in this behavior?   Y   N
   4e. (if yes) When you are engaged in this behavior, does if cause you to feel good or bad about yourself?   _____ Good   _____ Bad
   4f. Do you feel ashamed about having engaged in the behavior after the fact?   Y   N

Compulsive Bying Scale

1. Please indicate how much you agree or disagree with each of the statements below. Place an X on the line that best indicates how you feel about each statement.

	Strongly agree	Somewhat agree	Neither agree nor disagree	Somewhat disagree	Strongly disagree
a. If I have any money left at the end of the pay period, I just have to spend it.	(1)	(2)	(3)	(4)	(5)

2. Please indicate how often you have done each of the following things by placing an X on the appropriate line.

	Very Often	Often	Some-times	Rarely	Never
a. Felt others would be horrified if they knew of my spending habits.	(1)	(2)	(3)	(4)	(5)
b. Bought things even though I couldn't afford them.	——	——	——	——	——
c. Wrote a cheek when I knew I didn't have enough money in the bank to cover it.	——	——	——	——	——
d. Bought myself something in order to make myself feel better.	——	——	——	——	——
e. Felt anxious or nervous on days I didn't go shopping.	——	——	——	——	——
f. Made only the minimum payments on my credit cards.	——	——	——	——	——

$$\text{Scoring equation} = -9.69 + (Q1a \times .33) + (Q2a \times .34) + (Q2b \times .50)$$
$$+ (Q2c \times .47) + (Q2d \times .33) + (Q2e \times .38) + (Q2f \times .31).$$

If score is ≤ -1.34, subject is classified as a compulsive buyer.

From Ronald J. Faber and Thomas O'Guinn, "A Clinical Screener for Compulsive Buying," *Journal of Consumer Research* 19(3): 459–469, 1992. Published by the University of Chicago Press. © Journal of Consumer Research, Inc., 1992. All rights reserved.

Kleptomania Symptom Assessment Scale (K-SAS)

The following questions are aimed at evaluating kleptomania symptoms. Please **read** the questions **carefully** before you answer.

1) **If you had urges to steal during the past WEEK, on average, how strong were your urges? Please circle the most appropriate number:**

None	Mild	Moderate	Severe	Extreme
0	1	2	3	4

2) **During the past WEEK, how many times did you experience urges to steal? Please circle the most appropriate number.**

0) None
1) Once
2) Two or three times
3) Several to many times
4) Constant or near constant

3) **During the past WEEK, how many hours (add up hours) were you preoccupied with your urges to steal? Please circle the most appropriate number.**

None	1 hr or less	1 to 4 hr	4 to 10 hr	over 10 hr
0	1	2	3	4

4) **During the past WEEK, how much were you able to control your urges? Please circle the most appropriate number.**

Very much	Much	Moderate	Minimal	No control
0	1	2	3	4

5) **During the past WEEK, how often did thoughts about stealing come up? Please circle the most appropriate number.**

0) None
1) Once
2) Two to four times
3) Several to many times
4) Constantly or nearly constantly

6) **During the past WEEK, approximately how many hours (add up hours) did you spend thinking about stealing? Please circle the most appropriate number.**

None	1 hr or less	1 to 4 hr	4 to 10 hr	over 10 hr
0	1	2	3	4

7) **During the past WEEK, how much were you able to control your thoughts of stealing? Please circle the most appropriate number.**

Very much	Much	Moderate	Minimal	None
0	1	2	3	4

8) **During the past WEEK, on average, how much tension or excitement did you have shortly before you committed a theft? If you did not actually steal anything, please estimate how much anticipatory tension or excitement you believe you would have experienced if you had committed a theft. Please circle the most appropriate number.**

None	Minimal	Moderate	Much	Very much
0	1	2	3	4

9) During the past WEEK, on average, how much excitement and pleasure did you feel when you successfully committed a theft? If you did not actually steal, please estimate how much excitement and pleasure you believe you would have experienced if you had committed a theft. Please circle the most appropriate number.

None	Minimal	Moderate	Much	Very much
0	1	2	3	4

10) During the past WEEK, how much emotional distress (mental pain or anguish, shame, guilt, embarrassment) has your stealing caused you? Please circle the most appropriate number.

None	Minimal	Moderate	Much	Very much
0	1	2	3	4

11) During the past WEEK, how much personal trouble (relationship, financial, legal, job, medical or health) has your stealing caused you? Please circle the most appropriate number.

None	Minimal	Moderate	Much	Very much
0	1	2	3	4

South Oaks Gambling Screen

1. Indicate which of the following types of gambling you have done in your lifetime.	Not at all	Less than once a week	Once a week or more
a. played cards for money	❏	❏	❏
b. bet on horses, dogs or other animals (in off-track betting, at the track or with a bookie)	❏	❏	❏
c. bet on sports (parlay cards, with a bookie or at jai alai)	❏	❏	❏
d. played dice games (including craps, over and under or other dice games) for money	❏	❏	❏
e. went to casino (legal or otherwise)	❏	❏	❏
f. played the numbers or bet on lotteries	❏	❏	❏
g. played bingo	❏	❏	❏
h. played the stock and/or commodities market	❏	❏	❏
i. played slot machines, poker machines, or other gambling machines	❏	❏	❏
j. bowled, shot pool, played golf or played some other game of skill for money	❏	❏	❏

2. What is the largest amount of money you have ever gambled with on any one day?

Never have gambled ❏
$1 or less ❏
More than $1 up to $10 ❏
More than $10 up to $100 ❏
More than $100 up to $1,000 ❏
More than $1,000 up to $10,000 ❏
More than $10,000 ❏

3. Do (did) your parents have a gambling problem?

Both my father and mother gamble (or gambled too much) ❏
My father gambles (or gambled) too much ❏
My mother gambles (or gambled) too much ❏
Neither gambles (or gambled) too much ❏

4. When you gamble, how often do you go back another day to win back money you lost?

Never ❏
Some of the time (less than half the time) I lost ❏
Most of the time I lost ❏
Every time I lost ❏

5. Have you ever claimed to be winning money gambling when in fact you lost?

Never (or never gamble) ❏
Yes, less than half the time I lsot ❏
Yes, most of the time ❏

6. Do you feel you have ever had a problem with gambling?

No ❏
Yes, in the past, but not now ❏
Yes ❏

	Yes	No
7. Did you ever gamble more than you intended to?	❏	❏
8. Have people criticized your gambling?	❏	❏
9. Have you ever felt guilty about the way you gamble or what happens when you gamble?	❏	❏
10. Have you ever felt like you would like to stop gambling but didn't think you could?	❏	❏
11. Have you ever hidden betting slips, lottery tickets, gambling money, or other signs of gambling from your spouse, children, or other important people in your life?	❏	❏
12. Have you ever argued with people you live with over how you handle money?	❏	❏
13. *If you answered "yes" to question 12:* Have money arguments ever centered on your gambling?	❏	❏
14. Have you ever borrowed from someone and not paid them back as a result of your gambling?	❏	❏
15. Have you ever lost time from work (or school) due to gambling?	❏	❏

	Yes	No
16. If you borrowed money to gamble or to pay gambling debts, where did you borrow from? (Check "yes" or "no" for each)		
a. from household money	❏	❏
b. from your spouse	❏	❏
c. from other relatives or in-laws	❏	❏
d. from banks–loan companies or credit unions	❏	❏
e. from credit cards	❏	❏
f. from loan sharks (Shylocks)	❏	❏
g. you cashed in stocks, bonds, or other securities	❏	❏
h. you sold personal or family property	❏	❏
i. you borrowed on your checking account (passed bad checks)	❏	❏
j. you have (had) a credit line with a bookie	❏	❏
k. you have (had) a credit line with a casino	❏	❏

Reference: Lesieur HR, Blume SB. The South Oaks Gambling Screens (SOGS): a new instrument for the identification of pathological gamblers. Am J Psychiatry 1987; 144:1184–8.

The Massachusetts General Hospital (MGH) Hair Pulling Scale

Instructions: For each question, choose the one statement in that group that best describes your behaviors and/or feelings over the past week. If you have been having ups and downs, try to estimate an average for the past week. Be sure to read all the statements in each group before making your choice.

For the next three questions, rate only the urges to pull your hair.

1. **Frequency of urges.** On an average day, how often did you feel the urge to pull your hair?
   0 This week I felt no urges to pull my hair.
   1 This week I felt an **occasional** urge to pull my hair.
   2 This week I felt an urge to pull my hair **often.**
   3 This week I felt an urge to pull my hair **very often.**
   4 This week I felt **near constant** urges to pull my hair.

2. **Intensity of urges.** On an average day, how intense or "strong" were the urges to pull your hair?
   0 This week I did not feel any urges to pull my hair.
   1 This week I felt mild urges to pull my hair.
   2 This week Melt **moderate** urges to pull my hair.
   3 This week I felt **severe** urges to pull my hair.
   4 This week I felt **extreme** urges to pull my hair.

3. **Ability to control the urges.** On an average day, how much control do you have over the urges to pull your hair?
   0 This week I could **always** control the urges, or I did not feel any urges to pull my hair.
   1 This week I was able to distract myself from the urges to pull my hair **most of the time.**
   2 This week I was able to distract myself from the urges to pull my hair **some of the time.**
   3 This week I was able to distract myself from the urges to pull my hair **rarely.**
   4 This week I was **never** able to distract myself from the urges to pull my hair.

For the next three questions, rate only the actual hairpulling.

4. **Frequency of hairpulling.** On an average day, how often did you actually pull your hair?
   0 This week I did not pull my hair.
   1 This week I pulled my hair **occasionally.**
   2 This week I pulled my hair **often.**
   3 This week I pulled my hair **very often.**
   4 This week I pulled my hair so often it felt like I was **always** doing it.

Subject Number: Date:

5. **Attempts to resist hairpulling.** On an average day, how often did you make an attempt to stop yourself from actually pulling your hair?
   0 This week I felt no urges to pull my hair.
   1 This week I tried to resist the urge to pull my hair **almost all of the time.**
   2 This week I tried to resist the urge to pull my hair **some of the time.**
   3 This week I tried to resist the urge to pull my hair **rarely.**
   4 This week I **never** tried to resist the urge to pull my hair.

6. **Control over hairpulling.** On an average day, how often were you successful at actually stopping yourself from pulling your hair?

   0 This week I did not pull my hair.

   1 This week I was able to resist pulling my hair **almost all of the time.**

   2 This week I was able to resist pulling my hair **most of the time.**

   3 This week I was able to resist pulling my hair **some of the time.**

   4 This week I was **rarely** able to resist pulling my hair.

For the last question, rate the consequences of your hairpulling.

7. **Associated distress.** Hairpulling can make some people feel moody, "on edge," or sad. During the past week, how uncomfortable did your hairpulling make you feel?

   0 This week I did not feel uncomfortable about my hairpulling.

   1 This week I felt **vaguely uncomfortable** about my hairpulling.

   2 This week I felt **noticeably uncomfortable** about my hairpulling.

   3 This week I felt **significantly uncomfortable** about my hairpulling.

   4 This week I felt **intensely uncomfortable** about my hairpulling.

From "The Massachusetts General Hospital (MGH) Hairpulling Scale: 1. Development and Factor Analysis," by NJ Keuthen et al., *Psychother Psychosom* 64:141–145, 1995. Reprinted with permission of S. Karger AG, Basel.

The Massachusetts General Hospital (MGH) Skin-Picking Scale

Instructions: For each question, choose the one statement in that group that best describes your behavior and/or feelings over the past week. If you have been having ups and downs, try to estimate an average for the past week. Be sure to read all the statements in each group before making your choice.

For the next three questions, rate only the <u>urges</u> to pick your skin.

1. Frequency of urges. On an average day, how often did you feel the urge to pick your skin?
   - 0 This week I felt no urges to pick my skin.
   - 1 This week I felt an occasional urge to pick my skin.
   - 2 This week I felt an urge to pick my skin often.
   - 3 This week I felt an urge to pick my skin very often.
   - 4 This week I felt near constant urges to pick my skin.

2. *Intensity of urges.* On an average day, how intense or "strong" were the urges to pick your skin?
   - 0 This week I did not feel any urges to pick my skin.
   - 1 This week I felt mild urges to pick my skin.
   - 2 This week I felt moderate urges to pick my skin.
   - 3 This week felt severe urges to pick my skin.
   - 4 This week I felt extreme urges to pick my skin.

3. *Ability to control the urges.* On an average day, how much control do you have over the urges to pick your skin?
   - 0 This week I could always control the urges, or I did not feel urges to pick my skin.
   - 1 This week I was able to distract myself from the urges to pick my skin most of the time.
   - 2 This week I was able to distract myself from the urges to pick my skin some of the time.
   - 3 This week I was able to distract myself from the urges to pick my skin rarely.
   - 4 This week I was never able to distract myself from the urges to pick my skin.

For the next three questions, rate only the <u>actual</u> skin picking.

4. *Frequency of skin picking. On an average day, how often did you actually pick your skin?*
   - 0 This week I did not pick my skin.
   - 1 This week I picked my skin occasionally.
   - 2 This week I picked my skin often.
   - 3 This week I picked my skin very often.
   - 4 This week I picked my skin so often it felt like I was always doing it.

5. *Attempts to resist skin picking.* On an average day, how often did you make an attempt to stop yourself from actually picking your skin?
   - 0 This week I felt no urges to pick my skin.
   - 1 This week I tried to resist the urge to pick my skin almost all of the time.
   - 2 This week I tried to resist the urge to pick my skin some of the time.
   - 3 This week I tried to resist the urge to pick my skin rarely.
   - 4 This week I never tried to resist the urge to pick my skin.

6. *Control over skin picking.* On an average day, how often were you successful in actually stopping yourself from picking your skin?
   - 0 This week I did not pick my skin.
   - 1 This week I was able to resist picking my skin almost all of the time.
   - 2 This week I was able to resist picking my skin most of the time.
   - 3 This week I was able to resist picking my skin some of the time.
   - 4 This week I was rarely able to resist picking my skin.

For the last question, rate the <u>consequences</u> of your skin picking.

7. *Associated distress. Skin picking can make some people feel moody, "on edge," or sad. During the past week, how uncomfortable did your skin picking make you feel?*

   0 This week I did not feel uncomfortable about my skin picking.

   1 This week I felt vaguely uncomfortable about my skin picking.

   2 This week I felt noticeably uncomfortable about my skin picking.

   3 This week I felt significantly uncomfortable about my skin picking.

   4 This week I felt intensely uncomfortable about my skin picking.

Reprinted from the *Journal of Psychosomatic Research*, vol. 50, NJ Keuthen et al., "The Skin Picking Scale (SPS): Scale Construction and Psychosomatic Analyses," pp. 337–341, 2001, with permission from Elsevier.

Internet Addiction TEST (IAT)

Based on the following 5-point Likert scale, select the response that best represents the frequency of the behavior described in the following 20-item questionnaire.

0 = Not Applicable
1 = Rarely
2 = Occasionally
3 = Frequently
4 = Often
5 = Always

1. ___ How often do you find that you stay online longer than you intended?
2. ___ How often do you neglect household chores to spend more time online?
3. ___ How often do you prefer the excitement of the Internet to intimacy with your partner?
4. ___ How often do you form new relationships with fellow online users?
5. ___ How often do others in your life complain to you about the amount of time you spend online?
6. ___ How often do your grades or schoolwork suffer because of the amount of time you spend online?
7. ___ How often do you check your email before something else that you need to do?
8. ___ How often does your job performance or productivity suffer because of the Internet?
9. ___ How often do you become defensive or secretive when anyone asks you what you do online?
10. ___ How often do you block out disturbing thoughts about your life with soothing thoughts of the Internet?
11. ___ How often do you find yourself anticipating when you will go online again?
12. ___ How often do you fear that life without the Internet would be boring, empty, and joyless?
13. ___ How often do you snap, yell, or act annoyed if someone bothers you while you are online?
14. ___ How often do you lose sleep due to late-night log-ins?
15. ___ How often do you feel preoccupied with the Internet when offline or fantasize about being online?
16. ___ How often do you find yourself saying "just a few more minutes" when online?
17. ___ How often do you try to cut down the amount of time you spend online and fail?
18. ___ How often do you try to hide how long you've been online?
19. ___ How often do you choose to spend more time online over going out with others?
20. ___ How often do you feel depressed, moody, or nervous when you are offline, which goes away once you are back online?

After all the questions have been answered, add the numbers for each response to obtain a final score. The higher the score, the greater the level of addiction and creation of problems resulting from such Internet use. The severity impairment index is as follows:

NONE 0–30 points

MILD 31–49 points: You are an average online user. You may surf the Web a bit too long at times, but you have control over your use.

MODERATE 50–79 points: You are experiencing occasional or frequent problems because of the Internet. You should consider their full impact on your life.

SEVERE 80–100 points: Your Internet use is causing significant problems in your life. You should evaluate the impact of the Internet on your life and address the problems directly caused by your Internet use.

Reprinted with permission from Dr. Kimberly Young, Director of the Center for Internet Addition Recovery.

Intermittent Explosive Disorder – Diagnostic Questionnaire

Most everyone experiences aggressive thoughts or behaviors at different points in life. Please answer the following questions about your experiences with this as accurately as possible. Your responses will remain completely confidential.

For the following questions we would like you to think about a time since you turned age 13. So, from your 13th birthday to the present . . .

1. What was longest number of consecutive weeks in which you had at least two "arguments" each week? _____ (**# of weeks**)

   IF YOUR ANSWER TO QUESTION 1 IS LESS THAN 4, THEN PLEASE SKIP TO QUESTION 2

   1a. How old were you when you last had two (2) or more arguments each week for at least four weeks in a row? _____ (**age in years**)

2. What is the greatest number of times you broke something and/or hit someone in anger over the course of a year? (Your answer should be a total of the number of times you broke objects *plus* the number of times hitting someone) _____ (**# of times breaking + hitting**)

   IF YOUR ANSWER TO QUESTION 2 IS LESS THAN 3, THEN PLEASE SKIP TO QUESTION 3

   2a. How old were you when you most recently broke things and/or hit someone three or more times over the course of a year _____ (**age in years**)

3. Has the frequency and intensity of your "arguing," "breaking things," and/or "hitting others" <u>ever</u> bothered you? Circle one: **Yes**   *or*   **No**

4. Has the frequency and intensity of your "arguing," "breaking things," and/or "hitting others" ever caused you <u>any</u> problems (e.g., at work or school, or with family, friends, partners or acquaintances)? Circle one: **Yes**   *or*   **No**

5. Was most of the "arguing", "breaking things", and/or "hitting" done as a part of a plan to gain some advantage (e.g., intimidation) or was it usually an unplanned response to becoming angry? Circle one: **Planned**   *or*   **Unplanned**

6. During some of the times you were "arguing," "breaking things," and/or "hitting others," were you taking any medication, drinking alcohol, or experiencing the effects (high or withdrawal) of any drug? Circle one   **Yes**   *or*   **No**

IF YOUR ANSWER TO QUESTION 6 IS "NO", THEN PLEASE SKIP TO QUESTION 7

   6a. Has there been a time in your life when you were getting into 2 or more "arguments" a week for 4 or more weeks <u>when you were not taking any medication, drinking alcohol, or experiencing the effects (high or withdrawal) of any drug?</u> Circle one: **Yes**   *or*   **No**

   6b. Has there been a time in your life when you hit individuals and/or "broke things" in anger a total of or more times in a year <u>when you were not taking any medication, drinking alcohol, or experiencing the effects (high or withdrawal) of any drug?</u> Circle one: **Yes**   *or*   **No**

7. How many times since age 13 have you <u>destroyed something</u> and/or injured someone in anger? _____ (**# of times**)

Reprinted with permission from Michael S. McCloskey.

Index

AA. *See* Alcoholics Anonymous
ABS. *See* Addictive Buying Scale
acquisitive impulses, 3, 89–93. *See also* compulsive
  buying; compulsive buying disorder;
  gambling; gambling, pathological;
  kleptomania
Addictive Buying Scale (ABS), 10
ADHD. *See* Attention deficit hyperactivity disorder
advertising, compulsive buying and, 29
advocacy organizations. *See* national advocacy
  organizations
African Americans, trichotillomania and, 99–100
age
  compulsive buying disorder and, 12
  intermittent explosive disorder, 225
  kleptomania by, 37
  nail biting by, 148
  paraphilia related disorders by, 203
  pathological gambling by, 52–53
  problematic Internet use by, 175
  psychogenic excoriation by, 138–139
  pyromania and, 259
  skin-picking disorder by, 129–130
  trichotillomania by, 101–102, 111–112
    treatment for, 115–116
aggressive disorders. *See* intermittent explosive
  disorder; intimate partner violence
Al-Anon, 209
alcohol abuse
  IED and, 223
  pathological gambling and, 55
  problematic Internet use and, 177
  SPD and, 131
Alcoholics Anonymous (AA), 209
ALI test. *See* American Law Institute test
alopecia, 113–114
alprazolam, for kleptomania, 42
AMA. *See* American Medical Association
American Law Institute (ALI) test, 46
American Medical Association (AMA), 78
amitriptyline, for skin-picking disorder, 133
antidepressants. *See* selective serotonin reuptake
  inhibitors
antipsychotic medications, for SPD, 133
antisocial personality disorder (AsPD), 223–224
  kleptomania and, 35, 37, 39, 47
arson, 269–273. *See also* pyromania
  arrests for, 271
  classification of, 256, 257
  community responses to, 272–273

  for adults, 272
  comorbidities with, 261–262
    medical and neurologic disorders as, 262
    personality disorders as, 261–262
    schizophrenia as, 262
  fatalities as result of, 269–270
  locations for, 270
  pyromania and, 255–256
  Santiago Canyon Fire as, 269
  treatment strategies for, 273
AsPD. *See* antisocial personality disorder
attention deficit hyperactivity disorder (ADHD),
  176–177
  paraphilia related disorders and, 205
atypical antipsychotics, for pathological
  gambling, 68

Barratt Impulsiveness Scale, 39
Behavioral Risk Factor Surveillance System
  (BRFSS), 243, 246
behavioral therapy, for pathological gambling, 63
  cognitive behavioral therapy, 63–64
bibliotherapy, for compulsive buying disorder, 18
biofeedback and relaxation training, for oral
  parafunctions, 161
bipolar disorder
  compulsive buying disorder as result of, 7
  skin-picking disorder and, 129
borderline personality disorder (BPD), 199–200
  intermittent explosive disorder and, 223–224
BPD. *See* borderline personality disorder
BRFSS. *See* Behavioral Risk Factor Surveillance
  System
bruxism, 157
bupropion, for compulsive buying disorder, 17

California v. Cabazon Band of Mission Indians,
  92
casinos. *See* tribal casinos
CBD. *See* compulsive buying disorder
CBS. *See* Compulsive Buying Scale
CBT. *See* cognitive behavioral therapy
Centers for Disease Control and Prevention (CDC),
  intimate partner violence guidelines of,
  240–241
Cherokee Nation v. Georgia, 91
citalopram
  for compulsive buying disorder, 17
  for hypersexuality, 207
  for skin-picking disorder, 133